M. Schein · J.C. Marshall

Source Control

Springer

Berlin
Heidelberg
New York
Hong Kong
London
Milan
Paris
Tokyo

M. Schein   J.C. Marshall (Eds.)

Source Control

A Guide to the Management
of Surgical Infections

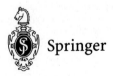 Springer

MOSHE SCHEIN
Professor of Surgery
Weill Medical College
of Cornell University

Department of Surgery
Bronx Lebanon Hospital Center
1650 Selwyn Avenue
4th Floor, Suite 4F
Bronx, NY 10457, USA
(e-mail: mschein1@mindspring.com)

JOHN C. MARSHALL
Professor of Surgery
Eaton North 9-234
Toronto General Hospital
University Health Network
200 Elizabeth Street
Toronto, Ontario M5G 2C4, Canada
(e-mail: john.marshall@uhn.on.ca)

ISBN 3-540-42973-5 Springer-Verlag Berlin Heidelberg New York

Library of Congress Cataloging-in-Publication Data

Source control : A Guide to the management of surgical infections /
M. Schein, J.C. Marshall (eds.).
    p. cm.
  Includes bibliographical references and index.
  ISBN 3540429735 (alk. paper)
  1. Surgical wound infections--Treatment. I. Schein, Moshe. II. Marshall, J. (John),
1949-
RD98.3 .S67 2002
617'.01--dc21

                                                        2002026898

Springer-Verlag Berlin Heidelberg New York
a member of Bertelsmann Springer Science+Business Media GmbH

http://www.springer.de

© Springer-Verlag Berlin Heidelberg 2003
Printed in Italy

Cover design: design and production, Heidelberg
Typesetting: Goldener Schnitt, Sinzheim

SPIN: 10769410   24/3130   5 4 3 2 1 0 – Printed on acid-free paper

Preface

Surgical infections are infections that develop in surgical patients. They may develop before the operation or occur postoperatively. In fact, many surgical infections arise in patients who have not undergone an operation or who do not need one. Using such a broad definition, surgical infections form an integral and significant part of any general, thoracic, and vascular surgery practice. We believe that the best infectious disease specialist for the surgical patient is the educated surgeon.

The concept of *source control* encompasses all of those physical interventions – surgical and otherwise – that are used to treat infection. Although source control is one of the most important aspects of the treatment of serious infection, it is a topic that in the past has received relatively little attention. Our goal, in this book, is to correct this deficiency. This project grew out of an initiative of the Source Control Working Group of the Surgical Infection Society (SIS) and almost all contributors are members of SIS or SIS-Europe. Each of the individual chapters – which cover general aspects of source control, as well as source control for specific conditions and anatomical sites – is followed by a balancing invited commentary by another expert. A certain amount of overlap is inevitable in such a multi-authored book; however, the many opinions expressed here reflect the dimensions of consensus and controversy in the field.

This book is aimed principally at the practicing surgeon and surgical trainee, but will also be useful to the non-surgeon who takes part in the care of infected surgical patients in the intensive care environment, as well as to the infectious disease specialist.

The most potent antibiotics, and the best supportive care, are meaningless if principles of source control are not adhered to with obsessiveness.

Moshe Schein, Bronx, New York   October 2002
John C. Marshall, Toronto, Ontario

Dedication

This book had its genesis in a project initiated by the Surgical Infection Society to develop greater structure for the description and evaluation of the surgical management of infection. We are deeply grateful to the membership of the Surgical Infection Societies of North America and Europe, who not only supported this ambitious project, but also provided their experience and insights as authors. We are immeasurably indebted to our families – the Schein family, my wife Heidi and sons Omri, Yariv, and Dan; and the Marshall clan, my wife and partner Mary Morison and our daughter Kate – for their love and tolerance of yet another intrusion into family life as the project took shape. We owe a huge vote of thanks to Mrs. Stephanie Benko from Springer-Verlag in Heidelberg, for shepherding the undertaking through to completion. And we dedicate our book to those who have experienced the ravages of infection, either themselves or through the tribulations of a loved one, in the hope that it may contribute to improving the care of future victims.

Moshe Schein, New York May 2002
John C. Marshall, Toronto May 2002

Contents

Part III: Special Problems

Contributors

Andersson, Roland E.B., MD, PhD
  Department of Surgery, Ryhov Hospital,
  55185 Jönköping, Sweden

Barbul, Adrian, MD, FACS
  Professor of Surgery, Johns Hopkins School of Medicine,
  Chief, Department of Surgery Sinai Hospital of Baltimore,
  2401 W. Belvedere Avenue, Baltimore, MD 21215, USA

Barie, Philip S., MD, FCCM, FACS
  Professor of Surgery, Weill Medical College of Cornell
  University, Anne and Max M. Cohen Surgical Intensive
  Care Unit, Department of Surgery,
  P-713A, New York Presbyterian Hospital, 525 E. 68th Street,
  New York, NY 10021, USA

Baue, Arthur E., MD
  Professor of Surgery Emeritus, Saint Louis University School
  of Medicine, Vice President for the Medical Center Emeritus,
  Saint Louis University, Box 396, Fishers Island,
  NY 06390, USA

Bauhofer, Artur, PhD
  Institute of Theoretical Surgery,
  Philipps University Marburg,
  Baldingerstraße, 35033 Marburg, Germany

Beilman, Gregory J., MD, FACS
  Department of Surgery, University of Minnesota,
  Box 11, UMHC, 420 Delaware Street S.E., Minneapolis,
  MN 55455, USA

Bohnen, John, MD, FACS
  Division of General Surgery; Med Director, Health Care
  Improvement Unit, St. Michael's Hospital, Director,
  Postgraduate Surgical Education and Associate Professor,
  University of Toronto; St. Michael's Hospital,
  38 Shuter Street, Room 5027, Toronto, ON M5B1A6, Canada

Brolin, Robert E., MD, FACS
  Professor of Surgery, Director, Bariatric Surgery,
  Saint Peter's University Hospital,
  254 Easton Avenue, New Brunswick, NJ 08903, USA

Büchler, Markus W., MD, FACS
  Professor and Chairman, Department of General Surgery,
  University of Heidelberg,
  Im Neuenheimer Feld 10, 69120 Heidelberg, Germany

Burrows, Lori L., PhD
  Director, Centre for Infection and Biomaterials Research,
  Department of Surgery, University of Toronto,
  714A-555 University Avenue, Toronto, ON M5G 1X8, Canada

Carriquiry, Luis A., MD
  Professor and Chairman, Second Surgical Clinic,
  Macial Hospital, School of Medicine,
  University of the Republic
  R. Pastoriza 1451, ap. 502
  Montevideo 11600, Uruguay

Chaudry, Irshad H., MD
  Professor, Departments of Surgery, Microbiology,
  Physiology and Biophysics, Center for Surgical Research,
  The University of Alabama at Birmingham School
  of Medicine, Birmingham,
  AL 35294-0019, USA

Cheadle, William G., MD, FACS
  Professor of Surgery, University of Louisville,
  Department of Surgery,
  2nd Floor Ambulatory Care Building,
  550 S. Jackson Street, Louisville, KY 40292, USA

Christou, Nicolas V., MD, PhD,
  Professor of Surgery, McGill University,
  Head, Division of General Surgery,
  McGill University and McGill University,
  Health Centre, Suite C5.53,
  698 Pine Avenue West, Montral, QC 113A 1A1, Canada

Cioffi, William G., MD
  Professor of Surgery, Brown Medical School,
  593 Eddy Street, APC 110, Providence, RI 02903, USA

Clavien, Pierre-Alain, MD, PhD, FACS
Professor and Chairman, Department of Visceral and
Transplant Surgery, University Hospital Zurich,
Raemistrasse 100, 8091 Zurich, Switzerland

Condon, Robert E., MD, MSc, FACS
Clinical Professor of Surgery, University of Washington,
Seattle; Professor and Chairman of Surgery, Emeritus,
The Medical College of Wisconsin, Milwaukee,
2722 86th Ave NE, Clyde Hill WA 98004-1653 USA

Dahn, Michael S., MD, PhD, FACS
Professor of Surgery, University of Missouri at Kansas City,
University Missouri/Trauma Medical Center,
2301 Holmes Street, Kansas City, MO 64108, USA

Danielson, Daren, MD
Hennepin County Medical Center
Department of Surgery
701 Park Ave, MC#813B
Minneapolis, MN 55415, USA

Deglinomini, John, MD
Department of Surgery,
Saint Vincents Catholic Medical Centers, Manhattan,
New York Medical College, Metropolitan Hospital Center,
New York, NY 10029, USA

Deitch, Edwin A., MD, FACS
Professor and Chair Department of Surgery,
New Jersey Medical School,
185 S. Orange Avenue, MSB-G-506, Newark, NJ 07103-2714, USA

Dellinger, Patchen, MD, FACS
Professor of Surgery, University of Washington Medical
Center, Department of Surgery,
Box 356410, 1959 N.E. Pacific Street, Seattle, WA 98195-6410,
USA

DiPiro, Joseph, PhD
College of Pharmacy, Department of Surgery,
Medical College of Georgia,
Atlanta, GA, 30303, USA

Dunican, Annemarie L., MD
    Rhode Island Hospital
    Department of Surgery
    593 Eddy Street, APC 110
    Providence, RI 02903, USA

Dunn, David L. , MD, PhD, FACS
    Professor and Chairman of Surgery,
    Department of Surgery, University of Minnesota,
    MMC 195, 420 Delaware Street SE, Minneapolis, MN 55455, USA

Eachempati, Soumitra R., MD
    Assistant Professor of Surgery,
    Weill Medical College of Cornell University,
    Department of Surgery,
    P-718A, New York Presbyterian Hospital
    925 E. 68th Street, New York, NY 10021, USA

Escallon, Jaime, MD, FACS, FRCSC
    Associate Professor of Surgery, Javeriana University,
    Department of Surgery, Medical Center,
    Fundación Santa Fe de Bogotá,
    Avenue 9 1170-20, Cons 518, Bogotá, Colombia

Fabian, Timothy C., MD, FACS
    Professor and Chairman, Department of Surgery,
    University of Tennessee, College of Medicine,
    965 Court Avenue G228, Memphis, TN 38163, USA

Faist, Eugen, MD
    University of Munich, Department of Surgery,
    Marchioninistraße 15, 81377 Munich, Germany

Fingerhut, Abe, MD, FACS
    Chief of Surgery, Centre Hospitalier Intercommunal,
    Rue du Champ Gaillard, 78303 Poissy, Paris, France;
    Clinical Professor of Surgery, University of Louisiana State
    Medical Center, New Orleans, LA 78303, USA

Fink, Mitchell P., MD
    Professor and Chair, Department of Critical Care Medicine,
    Watson Chair in Surgery,
    University of Pittsburgh School of Medicine,
    3550 Terrace Street, Room 616 Scaife Hall,
    Pittsburgh, PA 15261, USA

Fishel, Rhonda S., MD
   Assistant Professor of Surgery,
   Johns Hopkins School of Medicine,
   Associate Surgeon and Chief, Department of Surgery,
   Sinai Hospital of Baltimore,
   2401 W. Belvedere Avenue, Baltimore, MD 21215, USA

Flint, Lewis, MD, FACS
   Professor of Surgery, USF College of Medicine,
   Medical Director, Regional Trauma Center,
   Tampa General Hospital,
   P.O. Box 1289, Suite G417, Tampa, FL 33601, USA

Förster, E., MD
   Department of Surgery,
   Nordwest-Krankenhaus Sanderbusch, 26452 Sande,
   Germany

Fry, Donald E., MD, FACS
   Professor and Chairman, Department of Surgery,
   University of New Mexico School of Medicine,
   915 Camino de Salud NE, Albuquerque, NM 87131, USA

Frykberg, Eric R., MD, FACS
   Professor of Surgery, Chief, Division General Surgery,
   University of Florida Health Science Center,
   653-2 West 8th Street, Jacksonville, FL 32209-6511, USA

Függer, Reinhold, MD, PhD
   Department of Surgery, Elisabethinen Hospital,
   Fadingerstraße 1, 4010 Linz, Austria

Gang, Gyu I., MD
   Department of Surgery,
   The University of Cincinnati College of Medicine,
   231 Albert Sabin Way, Cincinnati, OH 45267-0558, USA

Götzinger, Peter, MD
   Department of Surgery, University of Vienna,
   Währinger Gürtel 18-20, 1090 Vienna, Austria

Gloor, Beat, MD
   Department of Viczeral and Transplantation Surgery,
   University of Bern, Inselspital,
   Freiburgstrasse, 3010 Bern, Switzerland

Goor, Harry Van, MD
Associate Professor of Surgery,
University Medical Center Nijmegen,
P.O. Box 9101, 6500 HB Nijmegen, The Netherlands

Gorecki, Piotr, MD
Assistant Professor of Surgery,
State Univerity of New York at Stony Brook,
Chief, Division of Laparoscopic Surgery,
New York Methodist Hospital,
506 6th Street, Brooklyn, NY 11215, USA

Górecki, Wojciech J., MD, PhD
Assistant Professor, Department of Pediatric Surgery,
Jagiellonian University Krakow,
265 Wielicka st, 30-663, Krakow, Poland

Goris, R.J.A., MD, PhD
Professor of Surgery, Department of Surgery,
University Hospital Nijmegen,
Postbus 9101, 6500 HB Nijmegen, The Netherlands

Hau, Toni, MD, FACS
Professor and Chief, Department of Surgery,
Nordwest-Krankenhaus Sanderbusch, 26452 Sande, Germany

Henley, Bradford, MD, MBA
Harborview Medical Center,
Department of Orthopaedics
325 Ninth Avenue Box 359798, Seattle, WA 98104, USA

Hirshberg, Asher, MD
Associate Professor of Surgery,
Baylor College of Medicine,
One Baylor Plaza, Houston, TX 77030, USA

Horn, Jan K., MD
Professor of Clinical Surgery, Department of Surgery,
San Francisco General Hospital,
University of California, San Francisco, CA 94110, USA

Jimenez, Maria F., MD
Associate Professor of Surgery, Javeriana University,
Department of Surgery Medical Center,
Fundación Santa Fe de Bogotá,
Avenue 9 1170-20, Cons 518, Bogotá, Colombia

Kadry, Zakiyah, MD
Department of Visceral and Transplant Surgery,
University Hospital Zurich,
Raemistrasse 100, 8091 Zurich, Switzerland

Kao, Lillian S., MD
Assistant Professor of Surgery, University of Washington,
Division of General Surgery and Trauma, Harborview
Medical Center, Department of Surgery,
Box 359796, Seattle, WA 98104, USA

Kell, Malcolm R., MD
Cork University Hospital, Wilton, Cork, Ireland

Khaneja, Satish C., MD, FACS
Chief of Thoracic Surgery, Department of Surgery,
Bronx Lebanon Hospital Center,
1650 Selwyn Ave, Bronx, NY 10457, USA

Krukowski, Zygmunt H., PhD, FRCS, FRCP
Consultant Surgeon, Aberdeen Royal Infirmary,
Professor of Surgery, University of Aberdeen,
Aberdeen AB25 2ZN, Scotland, UK

Kudsk, Kenneth A., MD
Professor of Surgery, Vice Chairman of Surgical Research,
University of Wisconsin, Madison School of Medicine,
Department of Surgery, H 4/736 C.S.C., 600 Highland Ave.,
Madison, WI 53792-7375, USA

Lazaron, Victor, MD
Department of Surgery, University of Wisconsin,
Madison, WI 53792-7375, USA

Leaper, David, MD
Professor, Professorial Unit of Surgery,
North Tees General Hospital,
Stockton-on-Tees, Cleveland, UK

Lee, James T., MD, PhD, FACS
Professor of Surgery, University of Minnesota,
P.O. Box 11679, Saint Paul, MN 55111, USA

Lee, Seong K., MD
NIH Trauma Research Fellow, Department of Surgery,
San Francisco General Hospital,
University of California, San Francisco, CA 94110, USA

Lipsett, Pamela A., MD, FACS, FCCM
    Associate Professor of Surgery, Anesthesiology,
    Critical Care Medicine, and Nursing, Johns Hopkins
    University Schools of Medicine and Nursing, Block 685,
    600 N Wolfe Street, Baltimore, MD 21287-4685, USA

Lorenz, Wilfried, Prof., MD
    Institute of Theoretical Surgery,
    Philipps University Marburg.
    Baldingerstraße, 35033 Marburg, Germany

Maier, Ronald V., MD, FACS
    Professor and Vice Chair, Department of Surgery,
    University of Washington, Surgeon-in-Chief,
    Harborview Medical Center,
    325 9th Avenue, Box 35-9796, Seattle, WA 98104-2499, USA

Malangoni, Mark A., MD, FACS
    Professor and Vice-Chairman, Department of Surgery,
    Case Western Reserve University School of Medicine,
    Chairperson, Department of Surgery,
    MetroHealth Medical Center, 2500 MetroHealth Drive,
    Cleveland, OH 44109-1998, USA

May, Addison K., MD, FACS
    Associate Professor of Surgery at Vanderbilt University,
    243 Medical Center South, 2100 Pierce Avenue, Nashville,
    TN 37212-3755, USA

Mazuski, John E., MD, PhD
    Associate Professor of Surgery,
    St. Louis University School of Medicine,
    3635 Vista Avenue, P.O. Box 15250, Saint Louis,
    MO 63110-0050, USA

Meakins, Jonathan L., MD, FACS, FRCSC, DSc
    Surgeon-in Chief, Professor and Chair of Surgery,
    Royal Victoria Hospital, Department of Surgery,
    687 Pine Avenue W., Room S10.30, Montreal, Quebec H3A1A1,
    Canada

Moulton, Jonathon F., MD
    Professor of Surgery, Department of Surgery,
    The University of Cincinnati College of Medicine,
    231 Albert Sabin Way, Cincinnati, OH 45267-0558, USA

Mustard Jr., Robert A., MD, FRCS(C), FACS
Assistant Professor of Surgery, University of Toronto,
Toronto, ON M55 1A1, Canada

Nathens, Avery B., MD, PhD, MPH
Assistant Professor of Surgery, University of Washington,
Division of General Surgery and Trauma, Harborview
Medical Center, Department of Surgery,
Box 359796, Seattle, WA 98104, USA

Nyström, Per-Olof, MD, PhD
Associate Professor of Surgery, Department of Surgery,
Jönköping University Hospital,
S-55185 Jönköping, Sweden

Onat, Demirali, MD
Department of Surgery,
Hacettepe University, School of Medicine,
06100 Ankara, Turkey

Paladugu, Ramesh , MD
Vascular Surgery Fellow Michael E. DeBakey,
Department of Surgery, Baylor College of Medicine,
6990 Fannin Suite 1600, Houston, TX-77030, USA

Papia, Guiseppe, MD
Sepsis Research Laboratories,
Toronto General Hospital, University Health Network,
Max Bell Research Centre, 2-934, 101 College Street,
Toronto, ON M5G 2C4, Canada

Parithivel, Vellore, MD, FACS
Associate Chairman, Department of Surgery,
Bronx Lebanon Medical Center, 1650 Selwyn Ave, 4th Floor,
Bronx, NY 10457, USA

Pickleman, Jack, MD, FACS
Professor of Surgery, Chief, Division of General Surgery,
Loyola University Medical Center, Strich School of
Medicine, 2160 South First Avenue, Maywood, IL 60153, USA

Pitcher, Graeme J., MBBCh, FCS (SA)
Senior Pediatric Surgeon, Johannesburg Hospital,
Division of Pediatric Surgery, Senior Lecturer,
University of the Witwatersrand, Medical School,
York Avenue, 2193 Parktown, Johannesburg, South Africa

Polk Jr., Hiram C., MD, FACS
    Ben A. Reid, Sr. Professor and Chairman,
    Department of Surgery, University of Louisville,
    Louisville, KY 40292, USA

Pollock, Allan V., MD, FRCS
    Scarborough Hospital, National Health Service,
    Scarborough, North Yorkshire YO12 6QL, UK

Pruett, Timothy L., MD, FACS
    University of Virginia Health System,
    Department of Surgery,
    P.O. Box 800709, Charlottesville, VA 22906-0709, USA

Pruitt Jr., Basil A., MD
    Editor, Journal of Trauma, UT Health Science Center,
    Department of Surgery,
    7330 San Pedro, Suite 654, San Antonio, TX 78216, USA

Ramsay, Graham, MD
    Professor, Department of Surgery, University of Maastricht,
    6202 AZ Maastricht, Netherlands

Raymond, Daniel P., MD
    Department of Surgery, University of Virginia,
    416 Moseley Charlottesville, VA 22903, USA

Reddy, Yenumala P. , MD
    Department of Surgery, Bronx-Lebanon Hospital Center,
    1650 Selwyn Avenue, Bronx, NY 10457, USA

Redmond, H. Paul, MD, FRCS
    Professor and Head of Surgery, Cork University Hospital,
    Wilton, Cork, Ireland

Richardson, J. David, MD, FACS
    Professor and Vice Chairman, Department of Surgery,
    University of Louisville,
    530 S. Jackson Street, Louisville, KY 40292, USA

Rotstein, Ori D., MD, FACS
    Professor of Surgery, University of Toronto,
    University Health Network, Department of Surgery,
    200 Elizabeth Street, 9EN-232, Toronto, ON M5G2C4, Canada

Saadia, Roger, MD, FRCS (Ed)
  Professor of Surgery, University of Manitoba,
  Health Sciences Center and St Boniface General Hospital,
  Winnipeg, MB R3A1R9, Canada

Sajja, Sai, MD
  Department of Surgery, Bronx-Lebanon Hospital Center,
  1650 Selwyn Avenue, Bronx, NY 10457, USA

Sautner, Thomas, MD
  Associate Professor of Surgery, Vienna General Hospital
  AKH, Department of Surgery,
  Währinger Gürtel 18-20, 1090 Vienna, Austria

Sawyer, Robert G., MD, FACS
  Associate Professor of Surgery,
  University of Virginia Health Systems,
  Department of Surgery, Box 10005,
  Charlottesville, VA 22906-0005, USA

Sayek, Iskender, MD, FACS
  Department of Surgery, Hacettepe University,
  School of Medicine,
  06100 Ankara, Turkey

Schinkel, Christian, MD
  University of Munich, Department of Surgery,
  Marchioninistraße 15, 81377 Munich, Germany

Schöffel, Ulrich, MD
  Professor of Surgery, University of Freiburg,
  Department of Surgery,
  Hugstetter Straße 55, 79106 Freiburg, Germany

Solomkin, Joseph S., MD, FACS
  Professor of Surgery, Department of Surgery,
  The University of Cincinnati College of Medicine,
  231 Albert Sabin Way, Cincinnati, OH 45267-0558, USA

Spain, David A., MD
  Professor of Surgery, Chief of Trauma/Surgical Critical Care,
  Stanford University,
  300 Pasteur Dr H3680, Stanford, CA 94305, USA

Stone, H. Harlan, MD
Professor of Surgery, Phoenix Integrated Surgical Residency
and The University of Arizona College of Medicine
(Phoenix Campus), Suite 619,
1300 North 12th Street, Phoenix, AZ 85006, USA

Tellado, José M., MD
HGU Gregorio Marañon,
Dr. Esquerdo 46, 28007 Madrid, Spain

Vega, Daniel, MD
Hospital Universitario de la Princesa
Diego de Léon, 28006 Madrid, Spain

Veith, Frank, MD, FACS
Professor and Vice Chairman, Department of Surgery,
The William J. von Liebig Chair in Vascular Surgery,
Montefiore Medical Center and Albert Einstein College
of Medicine, 111 East 210 Street,
Bronx, NY 10467, USA

Weissenhofer, Werner, MD
Associate Professor of Surgery, University of Vienna,
c/o Rudolfinerhaus, Billrothstraße 78, 1190 Vienna, Austria

Wacha, Hannes, MD
Professor of Surgery, Department of General Surgery,
University of Frankfurt,
Langestraße 4-6, 60311 Frankfurt, Germany

Wallack, Marc K., MD, FACS
Professor and Chairman Department of Surgery,
Saint Vincents Catholic Medical Centers, Manhattan,
New York Medical College, Chief of Surgery Metropolitan
Hospital Center, New York, NY 10021 USA

Wang, Ping, MD
Professor, Departments of Surgery, Microbiology,
Physiology, and Biophysics, Center for Surgical Research,
The University of Alabama at Birmingham School
of Medicine, Birmingham,
AL 35294-0019, USA

Watters, James M., MD, FRCSC
Department of Surgery, University of Ottawa,
Canada, Ottawa Hospital, Civic Site,
737 Parkdale Avenue, Ottawa, ON K1Y1J8, Canada

West, Michael A., MD, PhD
  Northwestern University, Department of Surgery,
  201 E. Huron, Galter 101-105, Chicago, IL 60611, USA

West, Kristine, MD
  Northwestern University, Department of Surgery,
  201 E. Huron, Galter 101-105, Chicago, IL 60611, USA

Wittmann, Dietmar H., MD
  Professor of Surgery Emeritus,
  990 Gulf Winds Way, Nokomis, FL 34275, USA

Worni, Mathias, MD
  Department of Visceral and Transplantation Surgery,
  University of Bern,
  Inselspital, Freiburgstrasse, 3010 Bern, Switzerland

Yowler, Charles J., MD
  Assistant Professor of Surgery, MetroHealth Medical Center
  Campus of Case Western Reserve University Cleveland,
  OH 41106, USA

1 Introduction

JOHN C. MARSHALL, MOSHE SCHEIN

> As long as surgical infections exist, surgeons must make never-
> ending efforts to control them. It may be described as a time when
> science and art can absolutely prevent bacteria from gaining a foot-
> hold in the human body and can abruptly terminate their activity,
> if they have already become established.
> (*Frank L. Meleney*, 1889-1963).

Most of the interventions that we use in the routine management of infection are recent innovations. Principles of hemodynamic resuscitation and support trace their origins to the work of such pioneers as Alfred Blalock in the early twentieth century, who established that shock reflected an absolute or relative intravascular volume deficit, rather than a severe fright [1]. The antibacterial activity of penicillin was identified by Fleming in the 1920s and agents with antimicrobial activity were used in the treatment of peritonitis during the early decades of the twentieth century [2]. But specific antimicrobial therapy did not become practical until World War II and the ensuing decades [3-5]. Successful modulation of the host response that infection elicits remains a largely unfulfilled dream, – although recent promise has been shown by a variety of strategies [6, 7].

The surgical management of infection dates to antiquity. Evidence of trephination has been identified in skulls that are upwards of 10,000 years old and the management of abscesses and infected wounds was well-codified in the medical practice of the Egyptians, Babylonians, Greeks, and Romans. Ambroise Pare in the fifteenth century undertook the first empiric comparisons of the management of infected wounds and the drainage of intracavitary abscesses had become an accepted practice even before the microorganisms that caused them were identified in the mid-nineteenth century. Incision and drainage of an appendiceal abscess was recorded in 1530, while the first definitive management of appendicitis by appendectomy appears to have been accomplished by Groves in rural Canada in 1883 [8], almost 50 years before the discovery of penicillin.

The Scientific Basis of Surgical Source Control

Source control of infection has a long and enduring history of empiric efficacy, yet it has been little studied in well-designed randomized trials and the principles of its application are implicit, rather than explicit. The reasons for this are many. A large number of medical therapies whose introduction predates the widespread acceptance of clinical research have never been subjected to the rigorous analysis of a randomized, controlled clinical trial. Surgical procedures such as appendectomy or Caesarean section are accepted unquestioningly because they make sense and because clinicians believe, not without reason, that patients benefit from their use. With a few important exceptions deriving from common diseases where the rationale for surgical intervention may be questioned [9, 10], it is unlikely that randomized controlled trials comparing interventional to noninterventional strategies will be undertaken.

However, the formal evaluation of specific approaches to source control is also confounded by the nature of the decisions that must be made [11]. Clinical trials compare populations of patients, but source control decisions must be made for the individual patient, in whom factors such as diagnostic uncertainty, physiological stability, premorbid health status, previous surgical interventions, the surgeon's experience and skills, and the availability of operating time and supportive care combine to create circumstances that are unique to a single patient. The approach to the management of a patient with a diverticular abscess, for example, may well differ in a previously healthy patient with localized findings on physical examination and CT scan when compared to the management of the same problem in a patient who has had a prior renal transplant and a history of peritoneal dialysis. In the former, either percutaneous catheter drainage or resection and primary anastomosis are reasonable options, whereas in the latter, the optimal choice may be a Hartmann procedure. And we hear the voices of those who question this assertion: they only serve to underline the truism that surgical decision making is based on the marriage of evidence from clinical studies, inferences from biology, and the elusive element of surgical experience.

This book, we hope, combines these three elements. We have recruited an international group of authors who are acknowledged leaders in the field of surgical infectious diseases. We have challenged them to integrate evidence with experience and an understanding of biology to create overviews that will help the clinician who must make the difficult decisions. And we have kept them honest by asking a second group of equally eminent commentators to provide supporting or alternative views – in essence to recreate the kind of dialogue that takes place between clinicians discussing a difficult problem.

What Is Source Control?

Constructive dialogue presupposes agreement on the meanings of the words used (Table 1). We have used the phrase "source control" throughout this book for all those physical measures that are undertaken to eliminate a focus of infection, to control ongoing contamination, and to restore premorbid anatomy and function [12]. While many of these interventions are surgical procedures, the scope of source control includes such nonsurgical interventions as the radiologically directed drainage of intracavitary abscesses, the removal of colonized urinary or vascular catheters, and the removal of devitalized tissue through the use of dressing changes.

Table 1. Definition of terms

Source control	All physical measures that are undertaken to eliminate a source of infection, control ongoing contamination, and restore premorbid anatomy and function
Sinus	An abnormal communication to an epithelially lined surface
Fistula	An abnormal communication between two epithelially lined surfaces
Abscess	A fluid-filled collection of tissue fluid, tissue debris, neutrophils, and bacteria, contained within a fibrous capsule
Drainage	The creation of a controlled sinus or fistula
Debridement	The removal of devitalized tissue, foreign bodies, or other adjuvants for bacterial growth

Principles of Source Control

Source control is the applied biology of inflammation. Its foundations lie in the optimal harnessing of the processes of inflammation and tissue repair to expedite the resolution of infection. Its principles are three:

1. Drainage of abscesses
2. Debridement of nonviable or infected tissue
3. Definitive management of the anatomical abnormality responsible for ongoing microbial contamination, so that normal function and anatomy are restored

Drainage

Local activation of inflammation results in a coordinated series of biological responses that serve to bring cells of the innate immune system, predominantly neutrophils, to the site of infectious challenge, and to isolate the resulting melange of microorganisms and host immune cells from the rest of the host. The cardinal manifestations of inflammation – *rubor, tumor, calor, dolor*, and *functio laesa* – reflect local increases in blood flow and in capillary permeability that facilitate the trafficking of neutrophils to the site of injury. Changes in endothelial cell expression of adhesion molecules and reciprocal changes on recruited neutrophils favor neutrophil localization and emigration into the tissues at the site of challenge [13]. Local activation of coagulation, supported by macrophage-derived cytokines, circulating coagulation factors, reduced endothelial anticoagulant activity, and upregulation of tissue factor on local macrophages all serve to convert fibrinogen to fibrin, creating a barrier between the host and the mixture of tissue fluid, neutrophils, bacteria, and cellular debris that reflect the local battle being waged [14]. The result is an abscess, its contents contained within a fibrous capsule. Formation of an abscess effectively isolates the microbial challenge from the systemic circulation. But it also isolates it from the further influx of host immune cells or antibiotics.

Drainage provides egress to the exterior for the contents of the abscess, converting a contained collection to a controlled fistula, if there is internal communication with an epithelially lined surface, or sinus if there is not. Thus the drainage of an abscess is simply the creation of a controlled sinus or fistula. Several self-evident inferences can be made from this observation. First, drainage alone will only be successful in those circumstances when the creation of a controlled sinus or fistula is possible; drainage of the free peritoneal cavity is not possible, nor will drainage alone suffice if the contents of the collection to be drained include solid necrotic tissue in addition to liquid pus. Secondly, the prosthesis used to create the controlled sinus – the drain – must permit free flow of the abscess contents to the exterior; soft Penrose drains maintain a potential space, but they do not produce a well-controlled sinus. Third, if the objective is simply to create a controlled sinus, then the intervention that accomplishes this end with the minimum of risk and physiological derangement to the patient is the best therapeutic option; usually this means an initial attempt at percutaneous drainage. Fourth, with modern imaging techniques, virtually all collections of clinical significance can be visualized preoperatively, and many of them adequately drained. Finally, while it can be difficult to resist the urge to operate, particularly in an unstable and ill patient, the act of surgery itself accomplishes nothing more than the creation of controlled sinuses or fistulae and the removal of dead tissue, and the operation should be limited to this objective.

Debridement

Devitalized tissue and extravasated blood provide an excellent culture medium for microbial growth, protected from circulating phagocytes or antibiotics by virtue of the lack of a blood supply. Similarly, the presence of a foreign body greatly increases the risk of developing an established infection [15]. Debridement is the process of removing nonviable tissue, and, by extension, foreign bodies or devices that promote bacterial growth. Where principles of drainage eliminate the fluid components of an infection, those of debridement are directed against its solid components.

Early in the course of a process that creates tissue injury, the demarcation between viable and nonviable tissue may be far from absolute. Areas of frankly necrotic tissue may be found in larger islands of viable tissue, or tissues may appear ischemic, but be potentially salvageable. The problem of distinguishing viable from nonviable tissue, and the consequences of failing to do so reliably, can create significant clinical dilemmas. When necrotic tissue is on the surface of the wound, and the technique of debridement is gentle (for example the use of wet-to-dry saline dressings) the dilemma is obviated. Surgical debridement of necrotizing soft tissue infections is somewhat more challenging, as the surgeon tries to remove all necrotic tissue, but to minimize the resulting defect and so make reconstruction easier. Bleeding from viable tissues is readily controlled when it occurs in the skin or muscle, and so a decision is generally made to err on the side of removing viable tissues, rather than to fail to debride necrotic material. Serial evaluation and debridement facilitates surgical decision making. The excision of necrotic bowel is more complex again, particularly when the cause of the compromised state is venous thrombosis or a low flow state. The benefits of resection must be weighed against the consequences of loss of bowel length, and are usually best resolved by a planned second-look laparotomy. Finally peripancreatic retroperitoneal necrosis is remarkably well tolerated, while blind exploration in the retroperitoneum carries a significant risk of provoking uncontrollable hemorrhage: delayed debridement has become the preferred management for patients with suspected infected necrosis.

Similar principles underlie the decision to remove an infected foreign body. When the foreign body is a urinary or vascular catheter, the risks are minimal; when it is an infected aortic graft or heart valve, they are not.

Definitive Management

Infections requiring source control measures typically arise because of a definable anatomical lesion – perforation of an appendix or duodenal ulcer, a bullet wound to the esophagus, or a colonized joint prosthesis, for example. The ultimate aim of therapy is to restore function with the least risk and to correct the abnormality that created the infection.

Once again, the optimal decision must weigh the long-term benefits and the short-term risks. Excision of a perforated appendix is a relatively straightforward undertaking, and so removal of the focus of infection by appendectomy is the standard approach to the management of appendicitis. But for the patient with long-standing symptoms and a well-circumscribed appendiceal abscess on CT scan, the safer procedure may be percutaneous drainage, followed at a later date by appendectomy. On the other hand, the physiologically unstable patient with multiple gunshot wounds to the colon is best managed by damage control alone, leaving reconstruction to a later date. Anticipating the long-term needs for reconstruction, and making the appropriate decisions that will ultimately facilitate these, is the hallmark of an experienced surgeon and directs such decisions as the siting of stomas or the placement of incisions.

Time and Mother Nature are the surgeon's two greatest allies, and many a seemingly impossible situation can be converted to one that is merely a challenge by careful patience.

References

1. Blalock A (1930) Experimental shock: the cause of the low blood pressure produced by muscle injury. Arch Surg 20:959
2. Behan RJ (1934) Acute generalized suppurative peritonitis. Treatment by intra-abdominal lavage with ethyl alcohol (reduction of mortality from 50 to 4 percent). Am J Surg 28–34
3. Schweinburg FB, Glotzer P, Rutenburg AM, Fine J (1951) The therapeutic effective of aureomycin in experimental peritonitis in the dog. Ann Surg 134:878–884
4. Schatten WE (1956) Intraperitoneal antibiotic administration in the treatment of acute bacterial peritonitis. Surg Gynecol Obstet 103:339–346

5. Rogers DE (1959) The changing pattern of life-threatening microbial disease. N Engl J Med 261:677–683
6. Bernard GR, Vincent J-L, Laterre PF, LaRosa SP, Dhainaut J-F, Lopez-Rodriguez A, Steingrub JS, Garber GE, Heletrbrand JD, Ely EW, Fisher CJ Jr, for the Recombinant Human Activated Protein C Worldwide Evaluation in Severe Sepsis (PROWESS) Study Group (2001) Efficacy and safety of recombinant human activated protein C for severe sepsis. N Engl J Med 344:699–709
7. Marshall JC (2000) Clinical trials of mediator-directed therapy in sepsis: what have we learned? Intensive Care Med 26:S75–S83
8. Seal A (1981) Appendicitis: a historical review. Can J Surg 24:427–433
9. Crofts TJ, Park KG, Steele RJ, Chung SS, Li AK (1989) A randomized trial of nonoperative treatment for perforated peptic ulcer. N Engl J Med 321:970–973
10. Lo CM, Liu CL, Lai ECS, Fan ST, Wong J (1996) Early versus delayed laparoscopic cholecys-tectomy for treatment of acute cholecystitis. Ann Surg 223:37–42
11. McLeod RS, Wright JG, Solomon MJ, Hu XH, Walters BC, Lossing A (1996) Randomized con-trolled trials in surgery: issues and problems. Surgery 119:483–486
12. Jimenez MF, Marshall JC (2001) Source control in the management of sepsis. Intensive Care Med 27:S49–S62
13. Carlos TM, Harlan JM (1994) Leukocyte-endothelial adhesion molecules. Blood 84:2068–2101
14. McGilvray ID, Rotstein OD (1998) The role of coagulation in systemic inflammation: a review of the experimental evidence. Sepsis 2:199–208
15. Poret HA, Fabian TC, Croce MA, Bynoe RP, Kudsk KA (1991) Analysis of septic morbidity following gunshot wounds to the colon: the missile is an adjuvant for abscess. J Trauma Injury Infect Crit Care 31:1088–1095

Part I: Principles of Source Control

2 The Biological Rationale

David L. Dunn

Key Principles

- Host defenses are occasionally incapable of combating the introduction of microbes and establishment of infection, particularly when a large number of microbes are present or host defenses are diminished, or when an ongoing source of microbial contamination exists.
- Source control consists of:
  a) reduction or eradication of the primary source of microbial inoculation or established infection, and
  b) prevention of the ongoing introduction of microbes.
- Inadequate source control increases morbidity and mortality as much as seven-fold.

General Approach

The nature of the interaction between microbes and the mammalian host has become increasingly well understood. Host defenses are categorized as *physical barrier* (integument, endothelium), *humoral* (antibody, complement), *cellular* [phagocytic leukocytes (polymorphonuclear, macrophages); T and B lymphocytes], and *cytokine*, (molecules which serve as regulatory intercellular signals within the local tissue milieu). Many areas of the body (skin, gut) harbor an extensive microbial flora that is capable of providing an initial microbial inoculum when physical barriers are diminished or breached (for example, during a surgical procedure). Under normal circumstances endogenous host defenses are capable of containing and eradicating substantial numbers of microbes at a site of local tissue invasion or infection. Inability to contain infection or the ongoing introduction of microbes at a local tissue site can result in:

- Local spread of infection
- Metastatic infection at one or more tissue sites (due to hematogenous spread)
- Severe systemic infection associated with widespread activation of host defenses and cytokine release (sepsis syndrome).

Host defenses act to prevent microbial invasion, or, once invasion has occurred, to limit microbial proliferation in an attempt to eradicate, or at least limit, infection to a localized site of disease. The presence of serious infection at a specific body site, however, presents a precarious situation. Large numbers of proliferating microbes, widely breached or diminished host defenses, ongoing introduction of microbes, or all of these factors in concert may result in infection that spreads beyond the confines of the initial site. Thus, control of an existing source of contamination and/or infection is a critical factor in the management of surgical infection. But what is the evidence to support this contention?

The dictum that pus should be drained antedates modern surgery, and for centuries this principle was most commonly applied to obvious subcutaneous abscesses. However, prior to the advent of antimicrobial agents, nineteenth century surgeons (e.g., McBurney, Mikulicz) recognized that intra-abdominal sources of infection due to appendicitis or rupture of a hollow viscus were associated with very high mortality that could be diminished by surgical removal of the inciting source. The surgical treatment of appendicitis in the late nineteenth and early twentieth centuries provides a cogent example of the critical importance of source control, since other treatment modalities (fluid resuscitation, hemodynamic monitoring, antibiotic administration) were not available. As late as the 1930s, emergent operation for appendicitis was not routine in the United States, and it was not infrequent that perforation occurred leading to an uncontrolled source of infection. This process was associated with >15 deaths per 100,000 individuals, and appendicitis was the 15th most common cause of death in the nation. Yet within three to four decades, during which time immediate operation became the standard of care for appendicitis, the attendant mortality had fallen drastically to ~0.7 per 100,000 persons [1].

For some time most surgeons have agreed that effective source control is of paramount importance in fighting surgical infection, and that all other forms of treatment are secondary. Intriguingly, despite the large number of clinical trials performed to examine the impact of antimicrobial agents on the incidence of infection after surgery, until recently little effort has been expended to investigate the impact of effective control of the initial source of infection. Recently, a series of retrospective and prospective clinical trials have been performed observing many different outcome parameters among patients who develop intra-abdominal infection. These studies have served to elucidate the importance of source control in modern therapeutic regimens.

Many of these trials initially provided descriptive information. For example, Grunau and colleagues examined the clinical course of 48 patients who developed postoperative intra-abdominal infection and observed a mortality of 19% among 37 patients in whom infection was eliminated, while mortality was 100% in the subgroup of 11 individuals in whom the source of infection persisted [2]. Similarly, Solomkin et al., noted similar outcomes among patients who were treated for established intra-abdominal infection: regardless of antibiotic regimen, patients in whom source control was not successfully established exhibited significantly higher mortality (45%) compared to those in whom the source of infection was contained or eradicated (6%) [3]. Subsequently, infection-scoring systems have been employed that correlate underlying host diseases, etiology, location, extent, and severity of intra-abdominal infection with clinical outcome. Elimination of the source of infection at the time of surgical intervention has been deemed a "successful operation", and has been shown to closely correlate with survival. Wacha and colleagues showed that source control improved survival in a prospective, multicenter study involving 355 patients ($p < 0.001$) [4]. Similarly, a recent retrospective analysis of 258 patients with diffuse peritonitis indicated that mortality decreased substantially in a subgroup of patients in whom source control was achieved (13%) when compared with a subgroup of patients in whom it was not (26%) [5].

The biological principles underlying source control as the mainstay of therapy for surgical infections have been best demonstrated using experimental animal models of intra-abdominal infection. In most models, established infection is created either by the introduction of microbes in a fibrin clot, or by ligating a portion of bowel that contains large numbers of microbes (e.g., cecal ligation and puncture) (see Chap. 3). Ahrenholz et al. demonstrated that the introduction of microbes into the rodent peritoneal cavity without other substances leads to bacteremia and high mortality within 2-3 days. However, microbial sequestration resulting from implantation of the same number of microbes within a fibrin clot was associated with a lower mortality occurring later (~7-10 days). Mortality was completely prevented by removal of the infected fibrin clot during the incipient stages of infection, that is, by efficient source control [6].

Peritoneal host-microbial interactions have been examined in considerable detail, allowing investigators to extrapolate the sequence of events that occurs during clinical infection, as well as the interplay between host defenses and microbial armaments [7]. For example, after spontaneous perforation of the sigmoid colon during an episode of diverticulitis, large numbers of aerobic and anaerobic bacteria enter the normally sterile peritoneal cavity. Specialized peritoneal diaphragmatic lymphatics on the underside of the diaphragm provide rapid transit from the peritoneal cavity to the bloodstream via the thoracic duct, resulting in bacteremia in some patients. Local or diffuse peritoneal contamination occurs depending on the extent of initial soilage and the ability of resident host defenses to contain the infection. These defenses consist of macrophages, polymorphonuclear leukocytes, and inflammatory fluid that enter the peritoneal cavity as a result of the initial interaction between microbes and microbial cell wall compounds with host complement, immunoglobulin, and resident leukocytes.

Macrophages secrete proinflammatory cytokines such as tumor necrosis factor-α, interleukin-1, interleukin-6, and interleukin-8, all of which enhance the phagocytic and microbicidal properties of other phagocytic cells within the local milieu and recruit additional phagocytic cells to the site of invasion and infection. The protein-rich inflammatory fluid contains fibrinogen and prothrombin, and the latter protein catalyzes fibrinogen polymerization into fibrin, a process that is capable of sequestering large numbers of microbes. Ileus and omental containment also serve to sequester infection. If these defenses are able to prevent ongoing soilage from the gut, the most likely outcome is the appearance of one or more intra-abdominal abscesses. Abscesses, in turn, are associated with bacteremic episodes, inanition, and bowel obstruction. Should ongoing gut soilage or abscess formation take place without mechanical intervention such as surgical exploration or percutaneous drainage, the uncontrolled infection is likely to lead to death. Although some types of trivial local infection (e.g., furuncles, simple cellulitis) may be amenable to antibiotic therapy alone, these remain the exception rather than the rule, and serious infections within a body cavity invariably require effective source control subsequent to diagnosis.

Controversies

Preoperative Preparation

Although the preoperative preparation of the surgical patient prior to operative intervention typically has not been considered a form of source control, some of the maneuvers could be construed as such and therefore should be mentioned. Specifically, preoperative skin preparation using a topical microbicide, mechanical bowel preparation with concurrent administration of intraluminal antimicrobial agents, and immediate preoperative skin preparation of both the operative field and the hands of the surgeon serve to reduce the potential for microbial contamination of the wound once the physical barriers of the integument and/or an endothelial barrier (such as of the gastrointestinal tract) are breached. Initial clinical studies examining surgical site infection rates among patients undergoing elective colonic resection provided evidence that mechanical preparation of the large bowel along with oral antibiotics, which together serve to reduce the intraluminal colonic microflora by 3-5-fold, reduced infection rates from ~40%-60% to ~8% [8]. Thus, certain standard maneuvers can be viewed as a form of source control, in that an attempt is made to reduce the potential initial inoculum prior to host physical barriers being breached.

Nonoperative Treatment of Intra-abdominal Infection

The acceptance of nonoperative management of sigmoid diverticulitis with contained perforation by percutaneous drainage and antibiotic therapy represents a significant change in surgical practice. Previously, many patients who developed these problems underwent two or three separate operations – initial abscess drainage, subsequent resection and creation of a stoma, and finally an operation to restore bowel continuity. It is now well accepted that some patients fare well with initial percutaneous drainage and antibiotic therapy, followed by a one-stage operation with resection and primary colonic anastomosis [9]. However, even with nonoperative intervention, source control remains of paramount importance.

Critical Factors and Decision Making

Surgeons routinely attempt to tip the balance between host defenses and microbial invasion in favor of preventing or treating infection. Control of the initial source of infection and prevention of ongoing contamination is of critical importance, and is clearly associated with improved outcome. Other modalities, albeit important, must represent second-line therapeutic options that will not cure infection without effective source control.

References

1. Wangensteen OH, Wangensteen SD (1978) The rise of surgery: from empiric craft to scientific discipline. University of Minnesota Press, Minneapolis, p 140
2. Grunau G, Heemken R, Hau T (1996) Predictors of outcome in patients with postoperative intra-abdominal infection. Eur J Surg 162:619–625
3. Solomkin JS, Dellinger EP, Christou NV, Busuttil RW (1990) Results of a multicenter trial comparing imipenem/cilastatin to tobramycin/clindamycin for intra-abdominal infections. Ann Surg 212:581–591
4. Wacha H, Hau T, Dittmer, R, Ohmann C (1999) Risk factors associated with intraabdominal infections: a prospective multicenter study. Langenbecks Arch Surg 384:24–32
5. Seiler CA, Brugger L, Forssmann U, Baer HU, Buchler MW (2000) Conservative surgical treatment of diffuse peritonitis. Surgery 127:178–184
6. Ahrenholz DH, Simmons RL (1980) Fibrin in peritonitis. I. Beneficial and adverse effects of fibrin in experimental E. coli peritonitis. Surgery 88:41–47
7. Dunn DL, Barke RA, Knight NB, Humphrey EW, Simmons RL (1985) The role of resident macrophages, peripheral neutrophils, and translymphatic absorption in bacterial clearance from the peritoneal cavity. Infect Immun 49:258–264
8. Bartlett JG, Condon RE, Gorbach SL, Clarke JS, Nichols RL, Ochi S (1978) Veterans Administration Cooperative Study on Bowel Preparation for Elective Colorectal Operations: impact of oral antibiotic regimen on colonic flora, wound irrigation cultures and bacteriology of septic complications. Ann Surg 188:249–254
9. Schoetz DJ Jr (1999) Diverticular disease of the colon: a century-old problem. Dis Colon Rectum 42:703–709

Invited Commentary

Ronald V. Maier

The biological rationale for source control is, indeed, a fascinating and challenging concept. Dr. Dunn in this introductory chapter has concisely iterated the major concepts and beliefs underlying the rationale for efficient and effective source control of infectious processes. A major implication of this overview is that primary surgical source control remains unproven by prospective randomized controlled trials (RCTs) and, as such, is in large part an empiric act of faith. In contrast, as cogently stated, there have been seemingly unlimited prospective randomized trials investigating the impact of improvements in the secondary components of source control, such as antibiotic selection. However, these secondary issues are not the critical issue in most cases. In fact, the ethical acceptability of such trials is based on the presumed near equivalence of expected outcomes. In most cases, adequate surgical debridement or mechanical elimination of infected tissues or contaminated devices will suffice for a cure. Unfortunately, there have been very limited Level I prospective RCTs to clearly define the true contribution and importance of mechanical source control to subsequent morbidity and mortality. In addition, the extent of debridement and approach (e.g., open vs. closed) have been minimally investigated. And, because of the ethical dilemma inherent in the use of a control group when mortality is the end point in these potential trials, they are unlikely to ever be performed.

The importance of source control for surgical infectious disease has been apparent empirically for millennia. While definitive supporting data are limited, there are even fewer to make us question our beliefs. In addition, recent investigations into the immunologic and inflammatory response of the host to infectious challenges have identified the biological basis underlying the subsequent host morbidity and mortality. In animal models, source control by removal of the infectious focus in toto is the treatment that best modifies the host's pathophysiologic response to the disease process and improves survival. Similarly, the infectious source and deleterious host response can rarely be controlled by antibiotics alone, while surgical or mechanical intervention is frequently curative. While the size of the inoculum is important, and correlates directly with risk for infectious progression, more important is the speed and completeness of mechanical control of both inoculum source and duration of inoculum exposure, as the critical components for both minimizing the biological response and improving survival of the host. For example, survival from a transmural colon injury varies greatly depending upon the efficiency and expediency with which control of soilage and repair of the injury to prevent persistent or recurrent contamination is achieved. Currently, our focus is on the diagnosis or recognition of a potential exposure to an infectious process with either a preemptive or expedient total or near-total eradication of the bacterial load. With this tenet achieved, along with assistance from fastidious hygiene and a plethora of antibiotic combinations, the deleterious biological processes involving the host's endogenous innate immunity can be controlled to provide the lowest morbidity and best chance for survival.

Thus, *surgical or mechanical control of the infectious focus, while itself nonbiological, determines the extent of the host's biological response to the disease*. Importantly, the concept is not one of operation versus non-operation, but of the mechanical resolution of the focus involved, whether this be: an extensive operative debridement and drainage; a minimally destructive laparoscopic procedure; a percutaneous closed evacuation of the infectious focus; or merely an opening of wounds to drain and cleansing of contaminated tissues. The principle is to eradicate all disease where the bacterial inoculum has gained the upper hand in overcoming host resistance for further tissue invasion or systemic dissemination.

While not mentioned explicitly, the major remaining challenges in the application of source control are how to construct experimental and clinical protocols to best define the biological response to infection and how to achieve adequate but not excessive, functionally destructive source control. Future research needs to address the following unanswered issues in source control:

- How do we determine the appropriate extent of what is frequently very destructive excisional therapy? The challenge is to provide adequate removal of infected tissue while minimizing functional loss; e.g., treatment of necrotizing fasciitis without major tissue loss or amputation. When is closed drainage via intervention radiology or laparoscopy adequate to avoid the morbidity of open surgery; e.g., treatment of infected ischemic pancreatitis without major organ resection?

- How do we best use our secondary adjuncts for therapy? Which antibiotics are best and for which condition? How important are tissue levels? Does prevention of toxin production or toxin neutralization require different antibiotic doses or drugs (e.g., antibodies to toxins)? Do select antibiotics or inadequate doses of antibiotics potentially increase the release of bacterial breakdown products and toxins, causing an enhanced host pathologic response and increased morbidity and mortality? Are other pharmacologic approaches focused on controlling the host immuno-inflammatory response equally important as antibiotic bactericidal activity?
- And we need to develop methodology for on line monitoring of the host immuno-inflammatory state as a critical determinant in outcome. Using survival as our sole determinant is no longer appropriate and excessively delayed. We need techniques to monitor the host's immediate biological response to intervention to optimally guide therapy; e.g., critical markers are selected cytokine levels or the activation state of the cells of innate immunity, namely, macrophages and neutrophils. With better markers of the host's biological response, we will be best able to define the optimal combination of surgical and nonsurgical intervention for control of the infectious challenge. While the remaining challenges are great, the rewards are unlimited.

Editorial Comment

Dr. Dunn mentions preoperative bowel preparation with antimicrobials as a "source control" measure. He does so within the section on controversies but does not discuss it as a controversy. However, the value of *mechanical* colonic preparation has never been scientifically proven and not a few recent prospective randomized trials showed that nonpreparation might be associated with a better outcome than mechanical preparation [1]. The North American enthusiasm for administering intraluminal antimicrobial agents to decrease the concentration of colonic bacteria is based on studies which compared intraluminal antibiotics to no antibiotics at all in the control group [2], or compared intraluminal antibiotics to an inadequate, narrow spectrum agent given to the controls [3]. In a European trial one-dose prophylaxis with an adequate systemic agent proved superior to intraluminal erythromycin and neomycin [4]. Currently, British and European surgeons omit intraluminal antibiotics.

We agree with Dr. Dunn that "nonoperative management of sigmoid diverticulitis with contained perforation by percutaneous drainage and antibiotic therapy represents a significant change in surgical practice" but wish to stress that small peridiverticular abscesses [5], as well as appendicular abscesses [6] will completely respond to antibiotic therapy – not necessitating a surgical intervention for source control at all.

As both Dr. Dunn and Dr. Maier emphasize, the control of an active source and evacuation of contained and noncontained pus are life-saving measures. But within the immense continuum of conditions, which represent varying degrees of surgical contamination and infection, there are entities which should be best treated with the knife "on hold" – as discussed in the individual chapters of this book.

References

1. Platell C, Hall J (1998) What is the role of mechanical bowel preparation in patients undergoing colorectal surgery? Dis Colon Rectum 41:875–882
2. Clarke JS, Condon RE, Bartlett JG, Gorbach SL, Nichols RL, Ochi S (1977) Preoperative oral antibiotics reduce septic complications of colon operations: results of prospective, randomized, double-blind clinical study. Ann Surg 186:251–259
3. Condon RE, Bartlett JG, Nichols RL, Schulte WJ, Gorbach SL, Ochi S (1979) Preoperative prophylactic cephalothin fails to control septic complications of colorectal operations: results of controlled clinical trial. A Veterans Administration cooperative study. Am J Surg 137:68–74
4. Weaver M, Burdon DW, Youngs DJ, Keighley MR (1986) Oral neomycin and erythromycin compared with single-dose systemic metronidazole and ceftriaxone prophylaxis in elective colorectal surgery. Am J Surg 151:437–442
5. Ambrosetti P, Morel P (1998) Acute left-sided colonic diverticulitis: diagnosis and surgical indications after successful conservative therapy of first time acute diverticulitis. Zentralbl Chir 123:1382–1385
6. Nitecki S, Assalia A, Schein M (1993) Contemporary management of the appendiceal mass. Br J Surg 80:18–20

3 Experimental Models of Source Control

Ping Wang, Irshad H. Chaudry

Key Principles

- Various animal models such as for endotoxemia, endotoxic shock, or bacteremia have been used to study the pathobiology of sepsis, and such models provided useful information regarding the mechanism of cell and organ dysfunctions under those conditions. However, those models do not permit control of the source of infection.
- A number of investigators have used cecal ligation and puncture (CLP) in various species to produce polymicrobial sepsis. The CLP model of sepsis mimics many features of clinical peritonitis, including the progressive changes in cardiovascular responses (i.e., an early hyperdynamic phase followed by a late hypodynamic phase).
- The CLP model of sepsis is associated with cellular dysfunction (such as hepatocellular depression) and upregulation of proinflammatory cytokines (such as TNF). Furthermore, the ligated and punctured cecum can be excised at various intervals to serve as a source control model of sepsis. Such a model can be used for testing pharmacological agents in the management of sepsis.

General Approach

The complex pathophysiology of sepsis is becoming better understood as more studies are being reported [1-6]. Through such studies, information might be forthcoming which will lead to better management of the septic patient.

Various animal models of such conditions as endotoxemia, endotoxic shock, or bacteremia have been used to study the pathobiology of sepsis and such models provide useful information regarding mechanisms of cell and organ dysfunction under conditions of systemic challenge [4-6]. However, those animal models may not simulate the progressive cardiovascular changes of polymicrobial sepsis – an early hyperdynamic phase followed by a late hypodynamic phase – which often occur in the clinical setting. The model of cecal ligation and puncture (CLP) produces polymicrobial sepsis [4, 5, 7-9], that mimics many features of clinical peritonitis [4, 5, 7, 10, 11]. Various species of animals have been used for producing sepsis by CLP, including the rat [7], mouse [12], sheep [13] and dog [14]. In the rat, CLP with two punctures in the ligated cecum with an 18-gauge needle, followed by crystalloid resuscitation is associated with an early hyperdynamic phase (characterized by increased cardiac output, increased tissue perfusion, decreased vascular resistance, and increased oxygen delivery and consumption), followed by a late hypodynamic phase (characterized by decreased cardiac output, reduced tissue perfusion, increased vascular resistance, and decreased oxygen delivery) [7, 11, 15]. The early hyperdynamic phase of sepsis occurs 2-10 h after CLP, while the late hypodynamic phase of sepsis occurs 16 h or later after CLP [7, 11, 15]. Thus, the CLP model of sepsis permits one to study animals during both the hyperdynamic and hypodynamic phases, and to study the mechanism responsible for the transition one to the other. This model of sepsis is associated with a mortality of 94 % at 48 h after CLP [7]. Although the typical model of CLP produces acute sepsis, a chronic state of sepsis can be induced by reducing needle size for punctures and/or the number of punctures in the ligated cecum, or by providing chronic fluid resuscitation [8]. CLP results in immediate and constant drainage of cecal bacteria into the peritoneal cavity in the presence of devitalized tissue and thus bears an obvious resemblance to disorders such as perforated appendicitis and diverticulitis. The CLP model of sepsis in small animals such as the rat and mouse is simple and inexpensive. Moreover, the ligated and punctured cecum can be excised after the onset of sepsis to serve as a source control model.

Hepatocellular depression occurs as early as 1.5 h after CLP and persists up to 20 h despite the maintenance of normotension [11, 16]. The depression observed during the early stage of sepsis does not appear to be due to a reduction in hepatic blood flow or to alterations in the hepatic microcirculation [11]. The association of elevated circulating levels of proinflammatory cytokines such as TNF with hepatocellular dysfunction [11, 16] during early hyperdynamic sepsis may suggest a cause and effect relationship between the two events. This is further supported by the finding that infusion of TNF at a dosage which does not decrease cardiac output and mean arterial pressure, produces significant depression in hepatocellular function with a marked elevation in plasma IL-6 levels [17]. Thus, observations derived from a clinically relevant animal model such as CLP suggest that TNF may be responsible for the depression in hepatocellular function observed during early sepsis.

Controversies/Limitations

Severe hypotension follows the administration of a large dose of endotoxin; however, CLP is characterized by biphasic cardiovascular response – an early hyperdynamic stage followed by a late hypodynamic stage of sepsis. The mortality of CLP can be reduced by using a smaller needle or by puncturing the ligated cecum only once [7]. Continuous intravenous fluid administration prolongs survival time and reduces the mortality rate to 40 % at 5 days after CLP [8]. Moreover, the ligated and punctured cecum can be excised at specific intervals following CLP, after which the peritoneal cavity can be irrigated with warm saline to remove/control the site of infection. Furthermore, transgenic animals devoid of a particular cytokine gene can be used for discerning the contribution of a specific mediator during sepsis. Since intestinal flora is dependent on types of diet, one can modify the septic responses by changing the cecal flora, for example by the use of meat rather than grain diets. Young rats have been used to investigate the impact of maternal milk following CLP or during endotoxemia. The results indicate that while the

Table 1. Other experimental models of surgical infection

Reference	Species	Nature of the model	Comments
Ozmen V et al. (1993) [20]	Rats	Peritoneal implantation of gelatin containing different quantities of a premixed slurry of filtered human fecal materials	Irrigation with normal saline, saline-cephalothin or ozonated saline can be used as source control
Ahrenholz DH, Simmons RL (1980) [21]	Rats	Peritoneal implantation of bovine fibrin clots containing *E. coli* (2×10^8). Operative debridement of the fibrin completely eliminated abscess formation in surviving rats	Radical peritoneal debridement ay reduce the septic complications of peritonitis and thus serves as source control
Nelson JL et al. (1999) [22]	Rats	Peritoneal implantation of a bacteria-filled osmotic minipump for continuous release of bacteria	Due to the nature of the ongoing peritoneal sepsis, this model may not be used for source control
Kinasewitz GT et al. (2000) [23]	Baboons	Fibrin clot containing $1.9-6.7 \times 10^{11}$ CFU/kg was introduced into the peritoneal cavity	The cardiovascular, hemostatic and immunological responses of baboons with sepsis exhibit a variable course that resembles the clinical manifestations of Gram-negative sepsis in humans
Fink MP, Heard SO (1990) [4]	Various	Intravascular infusion of bacteria	This model does not permit source control.
Mela-Riker L et al. (1988) [24]	Rats	Subcutaneous injection of *E. coli* (10^9 colony-forming units)	This model produces sustained, hyperdynamic sepsis. Excision of the subcutaneous abscess can be used as source control

maternal milk protected animals after CLP, it did not protect animals following endotoxemia [18]. It should be also pointed out that although complete neutralization of TNF by its antibodies reduces endotoxin-induced lethality, the blockade of TNF prior to CLP does not protect animals after CLP [19].

The CLP model of sepsis uses healthy animals whereas patients typically become septic following traumatic injury or other diseases. To model the development of sepsis in a compromised host, one can induce insults such as trauma and hemorrhage prior to the onset of sepsis. The two-hit model of trauma-hemorrhage, and subsequent sepsis has been utilized for assessing the susceptibility to septic challenge following trauma-hemorrhage and resuscitation. Typically antibiotics are not administered to the experimental animals before and after CLP in order to avoid the release of toxins by dying bacteria. The CLP model of sepsis produces persistent, rather than episodic bacteremia, and the model can be further refined by the use of antibiotics at varying time intervals after the experimental insult.

Critical Factors and Decision Making

CLP is the most commonly used model of sepsis-peritonitis. This model in the rat and other species offers numerous advantages for studying the pathophysiology of sepsis, and can be used as a preclinical model in identifying potentially effective pharmacological agents (Table 1). It resembles common intra-abdominal infectious processes such as perforated diverticulitis and appendicitis, and allows one to examine not only the progressive change in cardiovascular responses but also changes in cell and organ functions during the hyperdynamic stage and hypodynamic stage of sepsis. Furthermore, the punctured cecum can be excised and the peritoneal cavity irrigated in order to control the source of infection.

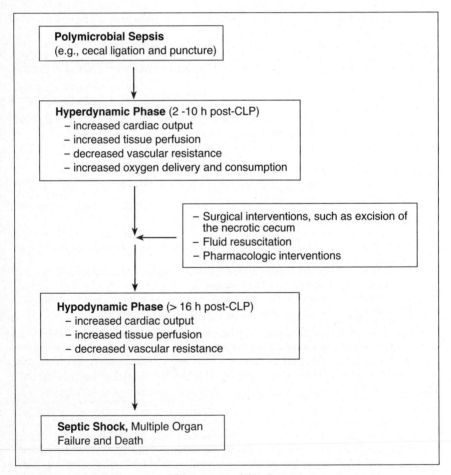

Diagram 1. A schematic summary of the content of this chapter

References

1. Baue AE, Durham R, Faist E (1998) Systemic inflammatory response syndrome (SIRS), multiple organ dysfunction syndrome (MODS), multiple organ failure (MOF): are we winning the battle? Shock 10:79–89
2. Tracey KJ, Abraham E (1999) From mouse to man: or what have we learned about cytokine-based anti-inflammatory therapies? Shock 11:224–225
3. Teplick R, Rubin R (1999) Therapy of sepsis: why have we made such little progress? Crit Care Med 27:1682–1683
4. Fink MP, Heard SO (1990) Laboratory models of sepsis and septic shock. J Surg Res 49:186–196
5. Deitch EA (1998) Animal models of sepsis and shock: a review and lessons learned. Shock 9:1–11
6. Wang H, Bloom O, Zhang M, Vishnubhakat JM, Ombrellino M, Che J, Frazier A, Yang H, Ivanova S, Borovikova L, Manogue KR, Faist E, Abraham E, Andersson J, Andersson U, Molina PE, Abumrad NN, Sama A, Tracey KJ (1999) HMG-1 as a late mediator of endotoxin lethality in mice. Science 285:248–251
7. Wichterman KA, Baue AE, Chaudry IH (1980) Sepsis and septic shock: a review of laboratory models and a proposal. J Surg Res 29:189–201
8. Yang S, Hauptman JG (1994) The efficacy of heparin and antithrombin III in fluid-resuscitated cecal ligation and puncture. Shock 2:433–437
9. Hadjiminas DJ, McMasters KM, Robertson SE, Cheadle WG (1994) Enhanced survival from cecal ligation and puncture with pentoxifylline is associated with altered neutrophil trafficking and reduced interleukin-1b expression but not inhibition of tumor necrosis factor synthesis. Surgery 116:348–355
10. Chaudry IH, Wichterman KA, Baue AE (1979 Effect of sepsis on tissue adenine nucleotide levels. Surgery 85:205–221
11. Wang P, Chaudry IH (1996) Mechanism of hepatocellular dysfunction during hyperdynamic sepsis. Am J Physiol 270:R927–R938
12. Ayala A, Chaudry IH (1996) Immune dysfunction in murine polymicrobial sepsis: mediators, macrophages, lymphocytes and apoptosis. Shock 6 [Suppl]:S27–S38
13. Fox GA, Lam CJ, Darragh WB, Neal AM, Inman KJ, Rutledge FS, Sibbald WJ (1996) Circulatory sequelae of administering CPAP in hyperdynamic sepsis are time dependent. J Appl Physiol 81:976–984
14. Stahl TJ, Alden PB, Ring WS, Madoff RC, Cerra FB (1990) Sepsis-induced diastolic dysfunction in chronic peritonitis. Am J Physiol 258:H625–H633
15. Yang S, Cioffi WG, Bland KI, Chaudry IH, Wang P (1999) Differential alterations in systemic and regional oxygen delivery and consumption during the early and late stages of sepsis. J Trauma 47:706–712
16. Wang P, Ba ZF, Chaudry IH (1995) Hepatocellular dysfunction occurs earlier than the onset of hyperdynamic circulation during sepsis. Shock 3:21–26
17. Wang P, Ayala A, Ba ZF, Zhou M, Perrin MM, Chaudry IH (1993) Tumor necrosis factor-a produces hepatocellular dysfunction despite normal cardiac output and hepatic microcirculation. Am J Physiol 265:G126–G132
18. Witek-Janusek L, Ratmeyer JK (1991) Sepsis in the young rat: maternal milk protects during cecal ligation and puncture sepsis but not during endotoxemia. Circ Shock 33:200–206
19. Remick D, Manohar P, Bolgos G, Rodriguez J, Moldawer L, Wollenberg G (1995) Blockade of tumor necrosis factor reduces lipopolysaccharide lethality, but not the lethality of cecal ligation and puncture. Shock 4:89–95
20. Ozmen V, Thomas WO, Healy JT et al (1993) Irrigation of the abdominal cavity in the treatment of experimentally induced microbial peritonitis: efficacy of ozonated saline. Am Surg 59:297–303
21. Ahrenholz DH, Simmons RL (1980) Fibrin in peritonitis. I. Beneficial and adverse effects of fibrin in experimental E. coli peritonitis. Surgery 88:41–47
22. Nelson JL, Alexander JN, Mao JX et al (1999) Effect of pentoxifylline on survival and intestinal cytokine messenger RNA transcription in a rat model of ongoing peritoneal sepsis. Crit Care Med 27:113–119

23. Kinasewitz GT, Chang AC, Peer GT et al (2000) Peritonitis in the baboon: a primate model which stimulates human sepsis. Shock 13:100
24. Mela-Riker L, Bartos D, Vlessis AA et al (1988) Chronic hyperdynamic sepsis in the rat. Circ Shock 25:231–244

Invited Commentary

MALCOLM R. KELL, H. PAUL REDMOND

Animal models provide a useful adjuvant when investigating human disease. In the case of surgical sepsis, animal models have provided invaluable insights into the dynamics of immune dysfunction following septic challenge. These models are divided into two groups: infectious models of sepsis such as CLP or non-infectious models of sepsis, such as bacterial product infusion.

Septic models mimic certain aspects of human disease following pathogen challenge. However, they have limitations. CLP is infamous for the variability between study groups and inter-study differences in mortality. In addition many factors that modify the course of sepsis in humans are not included in CLP models – antibiotics, age, metabolic disease, cardiovascular status, concurrent injury – to name a few. CLP more closely resembles an animal model of perforated appendicitis, albeit with a mortality of greater than 90 %. The perfect model of mixed sepsis would have to be easy to reproduce, relevant to human disease, and atraumatic in initiation, and it should have a microbiology similar to that encountered in human sepsis. These factors must be considered when drawing comparisons between animal sepsis models and human disease. CLP is still the best model of mixed polymicrobial sepsis currently used as it allows investigation of either a primary septic response or as a second-hit phenomenon.

Aseptic models of sepsis are commonly used since they allow ease of crossover between in vivo and in vitro work. The primary fault of aseptic models is that they tend to include only one bacterial product. Endotoxin is the most commonly investigated bacterial product. Neither infusion or bolus experiments accurately model human disease, since endotoxin levels in human disease are varied and there is no clear level that correlates with outcome. In addition, since mixed sepsis is the rule in surgical sepsis, the use of only a single bacterial product may be misleading. Lipopolysaccharide, bacterial lipoprotein, bacterial superantigen, and other bacterial wall products have a synergistic effect in human disease that is not reflected in a model of challenge with a single product. In addition, the question of the most appropriate mode of delivery has not been clearly answered: surgical sepsis represents ongoing exposure to bacterial products with surgical intervention resulting in a peak of bacterial product. Clearly neither bolus nor infusion can accurately mimic human disease.

Experimental models of sepsis use one strain of syngeneic animals. This provides insight into the immune response of this particular animal. Clearly the immune response of the inbred rodent, though similar in many respects, differs in important respects from that of humans. Human innate responses are much more sensitive to the effects of endotoxin, and the adaptive response to superantigen is vastly more toxic than in animal models. In addition, syngeneic animal models do not reflect genetic variability and cytokine polymorphisms in the much broader genetic pool surgeons encounter when treating patients with sepsis.

Much animal work has investigated the concept that the gut acts as an "undrained abscess" that can drive immune activation [1]. Supporting this concept, critically ill patients develop pathologic GI colonization that can precede signs of systemic inflammation by the same organisms [2]. Most research has focused on endotoxin, as the bacterial product that can mediate this effect. Endotoxin was initially identified through Coley's work on bacterial toxins in the treatment of malignancy [3]. Carswell then identified tumor necrosis factor as the link between endotoxin and tumor cachexia [4]. From this point hence endotoxin has been considered a key bacterial product involved in the innate immune activation that occurs in the systemic inflammatory response syndrome (SIRS). However, this concept has been questioned: in humans there is no clear link between endotoxin, gut barrier function, systemic cytokine levels, and outcome [5, 6].

It is essential that we recognize the limitations of the models employed in research, and that we incorporate more clinically relevant variables when designing experiments that mimic surgical sepsis.

References

1. Marshall JC, Christou NV, Meakins JL (1993) The gastrointestinal tract. The "undrained abscess" of multiple organ failure. Ann Surg 218:111–119
2. Marshall JC, Nathens AB (1996) The gut in critical illness: evidence from human studies. Shock 6:S10–S16
3. Coley WB (1893) The treatment of malignant tumours by repeated inoculations of erysipelas; with a report of ten original cases. Am J Med Sci 105: 487–490
4. Carswell EA, Old LJ, Kassel RL, Green S, Fiore N, Williamson B (1975) An endotoxin-induced serum factor that causes necrosis of tumors. Proc Natl Acad Sci USA 72:3666–3670
5. Kanwar S, Windsor AC, Welsh F, Barclay GR, Guillou PJ, Reynolds JV (2000) Lack of correlation between failure of gut barrier function and septic complications after major upper gastrointestinal surgery. Ann Surg 231:88–95
6. Kelly JL, O'Sullivan C, O'Riordain M, O'Riordain D, Lyons A, Doherty J, Mannick JA, Rodrick ML (1997 Is circulating endotoxin the trigger for the systemic inflammatory response syndrome seen after injury? Ann Surg 225:530–543

Editorial Comment

Dr. Wang and Dr. Chaudry have made extensive use of CLP models in their study of the biology of sepsis. As Drs. Kell and Redmond mention, mortality with CLP is quite variable. While a model of CL plus puncture with an 18-G needle had substantial mortality in Chaudry's hands, it carried no mortality at all in our rats [1]. In fact, to obtain a mortality of 40 % we had to excise the tip of the ligated cecum.

Thus, each group of investigators has to develop, calibrate and validate their own CLP model. Neither the authors nor the commentators mention Nichols's model of intra-abdominal infection, which implants a standardized capsule of feces-barium mixture into the peritoneal cavity [2].

Although the above-mentioned models mimic "clinical sepsis" with its "cold" and "warm" components and have contributed to our understanding of its local and systemic biology, they are a far cry from human intra-abdominal infection. Wang and Chaudry claim that "antibiotics are not administered to the experimental animals before and after CLP. The primary reason for this is to avoid the release of a large amount of toxins by killing bacteria by antibiotics when administered after the onset of sepsis." But in fact the administration of antibiotics immediately after CLP typically prevents the early death in these animals. And animals that survive the first 48-72 h after CLP tend to survive altogether: the intraperitoneal abscesses (discovered at autopsy later on) are well tolerated, often resolve spontaneously, and allow a prolonged survival [3].

In reality, while the rodent models of peritonitis described in this chapter mimic many aspects of the biology of sepsis, they are poor models for the evaluation of source control, because they do not incorporate the adjuvant interventions typically employed in the management of peritonitis in humans. Large animal models using sheep or pigs circumvent some of these limitations. Nonetheless it is a deficiency of the current literature that the role of source control measures has not been systematically defined. What, for example, is the influence of the time to intervention on survival or on the expression of pro-inflammatory mediators?

References

1. Schein M, Maeder S (1991) The open management in experimental peritonitis: no beneficial effect on early mortality. Surg Res Comm 10:127–132
2. Nichols RE, Smith JW, Balthazar ER (1978) Peritonitis and intra-abdominal abscess. An experimental model for evaluation of human disease. J Surg Research 25:129–134
3. Cheadle WG, Hershman MJ, Pietsch JD, Logan WA, Polk HC (1988) The natural history of murine intra-abdominal abscess formation. Arch Surg 123:1342–1346

4 Drainage

GYU I. GANG, JONATHAN F. MOULTON, JOSEPH S. SOLOMKIN

Key Principles

- Percutaneous abscess drainage (PD) is the preferred option in most cases.
- Operative intervention is indicated for failure of PD or when there are absolute contraindications to PD.
- PD can temporize, permitting delayed definitive management of an infectious focus.

For Either Approach

- The choice of drain size is determined primarily by the viscosity of the fluid to be drained.
- There is no limit on the number of drains that can be placed.
- The abscess cavity should be evacuated as completely as possible.
- Catheters can be removed when criteria for abscess resolution are met, including clinical signs and symptoms of infection (fever, leukocytosis), decrease in daily drainage to less than 10 ml, and a change in the character of the drainage from purulent to serous.
- Contrast studies can aid in evaluating resolution of the abscess cavity and closure of underlying gastrointestinal leaks.

General Approach

Contemporary management of patients with suspected intra-abdominal infection relies heavily on imaging studies to define the pathology and its anatomic extent. Exceptions to this principle include early acute appendicitis and clinically obvious diffuse peritonitis. The sensitivity and specificity of currently available imaging techniques for diagnosing intra-abdominal infection exceeds clinical judgment. Moreover, CT scanning or ultrasonography can be used to guide the percutaneous drainage of pus, at significantly less physiologic cost to the patient.

The major philosophical change wrought by experience with percutaneous drainage is the recognition that abscess cavities do not need to be externalized to be resolved. In the past, standard surgical practice was to use multiple latex drains with large drain tracts. The success of percutaneous drainage with small nonreactive catheters is in large part due to the efficacy of currently available antibiotics in clearing residual microorganisms left in abscess walls and inflamed tissue.

Percutaneous drainage is usually successful if the following criteria are met:
- There is a well-established, unilocular fluid collection
- A safe percutaneous route of access is available
- The patient is jointly evaluated by a surgeon and a radiologist so that correct judgments and decisions are made
- There is immediate operative backup available in case of failure or complications

The indications for open surgical drainage are:
- Inability to perform percutaneous drainage safely
- Failure of percutaneous drainage
- The presence of a pancreatic or carcinomatous abscess
- An association with a high output bowel fistula
- Involvement of the lesser sac
- The presence of multiple, isolated interloop abscesses

Occasionally, exploration and open drainage are undertaken when an abscess is suspected clinically, but cannot be localized by CT or ultrasound. Abscesses in the pelvis are usually drained directly through the rectum or vagina, obviating the need for either percutaneous drainage or an abdominal operation.

Critical Factors and Decision Making

Decision making is more complex for community-acquired intra-abdominal abscesses arising as a consequence of inflammatory visceral disease, for example appendicitis, or Crohn's disease with extensive bowel inflammation, interloop abscesses, and fistulae. Definitive therapy may be postponed, and percutaneous drainage used as a temporizing measure, until the patient can tolerate a more extensive operative procedure.

The decision to perform an extirpative operative procedure is based on recognition that deleterious host responses, including organ failure, are driven as much by the presence of necrotic tissue as by the presence of microorganisms. The decision to evacuate necrotic or inflamed tissue may be deferred in favor of percutaneous drainage of any identifiable collections, aggressive antibiotic therapy, and a brief period of observation. The absence of a clear-cut improvement in 48-72 h strongly suggests the need for operative intervention.

Techniques for Percutaneous Drainage

The choice of catheter size is determined primarily by the viscosity of the fluid to be drained. In the majority of cases, 8 to 12 French drains are sufficient. Larger drains may be needed for collections containing tissue debris or more viscous fluid. Drains of larger caliber can be placed, if needed, by exchange over a guide wire. There is no absolute limit on the number of drains that can be placed percutaneously. While most abscesses can be drained with a single catheter, there should be no hesitation in placing as many drains as are needed to effectively evacuate the abscess(es).

Following catheter placement, the cavity should be evacuated as completely as possible and irrigated with saline until the fluid is clear. Initial manipulation of the catheter(s) and irrigation should be done as gently as possible to minimize the induction of bacteremia. Immediate imaging determines the need for repositioning the catheter, placing a large-bore catheter, or for placing additional drains. For cavities that are completely evacuated at the initial drainage and for which there are no abnormal communications to viscera, simple gravity drainage generally suffices. For larger or more viscous collections and those with ongoing output due to fistulous connections, suction drainage with sump catheters is more effective. Thoracic drains should always be placed connected to water-seal suction.

Drains should be checked regularly to monitor the volume and nature of the output, ensure adequate function and clinical response, and recognize and correct any catheter-related problems. Most authorities recommend periodic irrigation of the drains, once or several times per day, with sterile saline to prevent occlusion of the catheter with fibrin. Irrigation may be performed by either physicians or trained nurses. In general, irrigation with proteolytic agents (e.g., acetylcysteine) or antibiotics is of little value, although fibrinolytic agents may be useful for evacuation of fibrinous or hemorrhagic collections. Repeat imaging studies, in particular contrast studies performed through the catheter are used to document abscess resolution and to identify problems. Occasionally, it may be necessary to replace or reposition tubes or add additional catheters. The need for follow-up imaging studies should be determined on a case-by-case basis by monitoring clinical progress and drainage output.

Catheters should be removed when criteria for abscess resolution are met. *Clinical criteria* of success include resolution of symptoms and indicators of infection (fever, leukocytosis). *Catheter-related criteria* include a decrease in daily drainage to less than 10 ml and a change in the character of the drainage from purulent to serous. *Radiographic criteria* include documentation of abscess resolution and closure of any fistulous communications. If catheters are maintained until these criteria are satisfied, the likelihood of recurrence of the abscess will be minimized. Although some authorities recommend gradual catheter removal over several days, we usually remove the drain in one step and have had no significant problem with recurrence. For sterile fluid collections, the drain should be removed as soon as possible, generally within 24-48 h, to minimize the risk of superinfection.

Recognition of Failure

Specific indications for percutaneous abscess drainage have expanded significantly over the past decade and now include many conditions previously thought undrainable, such as multiple and/or multiloculated abscesses, abscesses with enteric communication, and infected hematomas. These conditions have higher failure rates than seen with single abscesses.

The causes of failure of percutaneous drainage include fluid that is too viscous for drainage or the presence of phlegmonous or necrotic debris. Technical modifications such as increasing the drain size and the use of irrigation can occasionally overcome these problems. Recognition of phlegmonous or necrotic tissue on follow-up imaging studies may lead to cessation of attempts at percutaneous drainage or a modification of the expected goal. Successful drainage of multiloculated collections and multiple abscesses can be accomplished by the use of an adequate number of catheters, and by mechanical disruption of adhesions using a guide wire. Fistulous communications, either unrecognized or persistent, are yet another potential cause of failure, as is drainage of a necrotic tumor mistakenly diagnosed as an abscess. Recognition of a significant soft-tissue component and the use of percutaneous biopsies can minimize this risk. Suspicious fluid also may be sent for cytology.

Selection of Drains for Operatively Managed Infections

Similar considerations apply to the selection and management of intraoperatively placed drains. The number, size and type of drain should be determined by the abscess size and the characteristics of the abscess contents. Operatively placed drains should be monitored and removed when signs and symptoms of infection have been resolved. In the event of a slow resolution of clinical signs of infection, imaging can be used to define the adequacy of drainage and to diagnose any reaccumulation of infected fluid.

Nonreactive drains should be used except when there is a deliberate decision to create a drain tract. Siliconized and nonreactive drains form such tracts poorly and after removal no egress path will exist for any fistulous drainage.

In general, infected *lesser sac collections* associated with *acute necrotizing pancreatitis* respond poorly to percutaneous drainage, although percutaneous drainage may be used to temporize critically ill patients who might not survive open intervention. However, management of pancreatic abscesses continues to evolve, and the trend is toward less invasive strategies. In most centers, pancreatic abscesses and infected peripancreatic necrosis are approached directly through an upper abdominal incision. Debridement is carried out with both blunt and sharp dissection, removing as much necrotic tissue as can be excised without excessive bleeding. Drains are placed dependently and exteriorized through the laterally placed wounds; sump suction drains are preferred if no fistula is suspected (see Chap. 17).

Interloop abscesses are explored through a midabdominal incision. Each abscess cavity is thoroughly debrided, but drains are not generally used. Confirmation of the presence of pus is obtained by direct vision or by needle aspiration. All of the abscess contents should be evacuated by suction. The cavity should be thoroughly explored digitally and all loculations within it broken down to create a single residual space. The cavity is irrigated and debrided of nonviable tissue. Drains are not needed if the abscess cavity communicates freely with the peritoneal cavity. Otherwise, drains should be brought from the abscess cavity to the exterior as directly as possible.

For abscesses complicating *diverticulitis*, percutaneous drainage usually permits stabilization and allows time to prepare the patient for operative therapy. Subsequent operation is required in most, but not all, patients and can generally

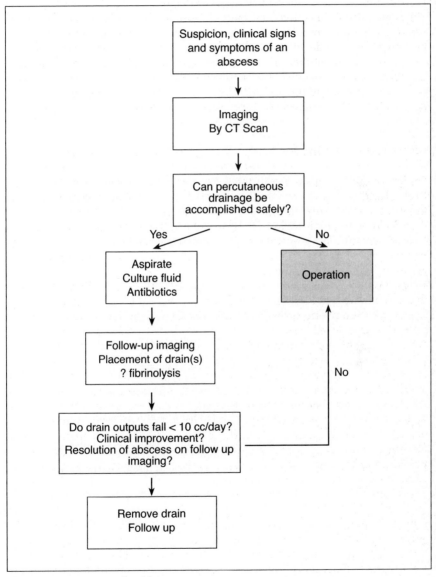

Diagram 1. Management algorithm

be accomplished as a one-step procedure. In high-risk patients who remain asymptomatic following drainage, subsequent sigmoid resection may be avoided. It is important to perform follow-up radiographic studies to exclude the possibility of a perforated neoplasm. Initial concerns regarding persistent fecal fistulas have not been borne out by clinical experience (see Chap. 12).

The results of percutaneous drainage for abscesses complicating *Crohn's disease* are less positive. Patients without fistulous communications to the bowel are usually cured, whereas those with fistulae generally required bowel resection. Among patients requiring operation, initial percutaneous drainage usually leads to significant clinical improvement and permits performance of a one-stage operation.

Low pelvic abscesses in contact with the rectum or vagina may be treated surgically by incision and drainage through these organs. This approach can be facilitated by sonographic guidance. Experience with ultrasound-guided transrectal and transvaginal drainage is growing, and these procedures appear to be effective and well tolerated. Success also has been achieved in the management of tuboovarian abscesses complicating pelvic inflammatory disease that are refractory to medical management. In many cases, the need for hysterectomy and oophorectomy has been obviated.

The management of *appendiceal abscess* depends upon the duration of illness and the ability of the host to withstand operation. In young patients with a short history of symptoms, a modest operative procedure will resolve both the abscess and the appendiceal source with safety and a high probability of success. Older patients with well-defined abscess cavities and less physiologic reserve benefit from percutaneous drainage, and do not require subsequent appendectomy (see Chap. 14).

Reading List

1. Altemeier WA, Culbertson WR, Fullen WD, Shook CD (1973) Intraabdominal abscess. Am J Surg 125:70–79
2. Swenson RM, Lorber B, Michaelson TC, Spaulding EH (1974) The bacteriology of intraabdominal infections. Arch Surg 109:398–399
3. Polk HC Jr, Shields CL (1977) Remote organ failure: a valid sign of occult intraabdominal infection. Surgery 81:310–313
4. Fry DE, Garrison RN, Heitsch RC, Calhoun K, Polk HC (1980) Determinants of death in patients with intraabdominal abscess. Surgery 88:517–523
5. JR, Alfidi RJ, Havrilla TR, Cooperman AM, Seidelmann FE, et al (1977) CT detection and aspiration of abdominal abscesses. AJR 128:465–474
6. Solomkin JS, Reinhart HH, Dellinger EP, Bohnen JM, Rotstein OD, et al (1996) Results of a randomized trial comparing sequential intravenous/oral treatment of ciprofloxacin plus metronidazole to imipenem/cilastatin for intraabdominal infections. The Intra-Abdominal Infection Study Group. Ann Surg 223:303–315
7. Lambiase RE (1991) Percutaneous abscess and fluid drainage: a critical review. Cardiovasc Intervent Radiol 14:143–157
8. Lambiase RE, Deyoe L (1992) Percutaneous drainage of 355 consecutive abscesses: results of primary drainage with 1-year follow-up. Radiology 184:167–179
9. Stain SC, Yellin AE, Donovan AJ, Brien HW (1991) Pyogenic liver abscess: modern treatment. Arch Surg 126:991–996
10. Mueller PR, Ferrucci JT Jr, Butch RJ, Simeone JF, Wittenberg J (1985) Inadvertent percutaneous catheter gastroenterostomy during abscess drainage: significance and management. AJR 145:387–391

11. Solomkin JS, Moulton JS, Luchette FA (1999) Diagnosis and management of intra-abdominal sepsis. In: Irwin RS, Cerra FB, Rippe JM (eds) Intensivecare medicine, 4th edn. Lippincott Williams & amp; Wilkins, Philadelphia, pp 109–124
12. van Sonnenberg E, Wing VW (1984) Temporizing effect of percutaneous drainage of complicated abscesses in critically ill patients. AJR 142:821–826
13. Martin EC, Karlson KB, Fankuchen EI, Cooperman A, Casarella WJ (1982) Percutaneous drainage of postoperative intraabdominal abscesses. AJR 138:13–15
14. Lambiase RE, Cronan JJ, Dorfman GS, Paolella LP, Haas RA (1989) Postoperative abscesses with enteric communication: percutaneous treatment. Radiology 171:497–500
15. Lahorra JM, Haaga JR, Stellato T, Flanigan T, Graham R (1993) Safety of intracavity urokinase with percutaneous abscess drainage. AJR 160:171–174
16. Vogelzang RL, Tobin RS, Burstein S, Anschuetz SL, Marzano M, Kozlowski JM (1987) Transcatheter intracavitary fibrinolysis of infected extravascular hematomas. AJR 148:378–380
17. Haaga JR, Nakamoto D, Stellato T, Novak RD, Gavant ML (2000) Intracavitary urokinase for enhancement of percutaneous abscess drainage: phase II trial. AJR 174:1681–1685
18. Baril NB, Ralls PW, Wren SM, Selby RR, Radin R, et al (2000) Does an infected peripancreatic fluid collection or abscess mandate operation? Ann Surg 231:361–367

Invited Commentary

ROBERT E. CONDON

Optimal source control requires elimination of the source of intra-abdominal contamination. Open procedures to accomplish resection, or closure of a perforation, are the usual primary means of source control. Drainage plays an important *secondary* role in the management of the abscesses that often follow peritoneal contamination, and has an occasional *primary* role in the management of a low volume fistula occurring in the absence of obstruction.

The change in surgical practice during the 1980s from open to percutaneous drainage of intra-abdominal abscesses, via catheters placed under radiological guidance, was a major advance in management. This chapter is an excellent review of the features of effective catheter drainage. The indications for placement of catheters for drainage are straightforward; the indications for catheter removal are a little less intuitive. The authors neatly outline the pre-conditions that guide catheter removal, which deserve emphasis by repetition: any fistula has closed, fever and leukocytosis have resolved, drainage has become serous and its volume is minimal, and complete collapse of the abscess cavity around the catheter has been documented by contrast injection. If all these criteria are met, I agree with the authors that the catheter need not be shortened progressively but can be pulled at once.

Check for the Collapse of the Abscess Cavity

Unfortunately, abscess drainage catheters are sometimes removed without first documenting obliteration of the abscess. Most of the time nothing untoward ensues. But in those circumstances in which an abscess space persists because of the unyielding structure of the surrounding tissues, catheter removal prior to complete collapse of the abscess cavity frequently results in persistence of the abscess and the need for another round of treatment. The collapse of the cavity around the drainage catheter should always be demonstrated by contrast injection prior to catheter removal.

Interloop Abscesses

Multiple interloop abscesses generated by an episode of widespread peritonitis are a vexing problem. Finding safe routes for multiple catheter placement to all the purulent collections often is impossible or impractical; open debridement and drainage is usually the more efficient maneuver. In managing this problem, the role of a "second look" and the utility of the temporary closure device introduced by Wittmann [1] in facilitating such management needs to be kept in mind.

Periappendiceal Abscess

Treatment of a well-established periappendiceal abscess, the so-called appendix mass, by percutaneous drainage without immediate appendectomy is very effective, particularly in patients at the extremes of life. Of course, if the history is relatively long and indolent, the mass not particularly tender, and the patient anemic, then the possibility of carcinoma needs to be entertained. A needle aspiration of the mass and cytological examination prior to drainage catheter placement will help to sort out this uncommon circumstance.

Interval Appendectomy?

Opinion varies about the need for interval appendectomy after resolution of an appendix mass. Recurrent appendicitis occurs in only one patient in six. But in the elderly the consequences of recurrent disease are potentially more serious than in young children. There is no reliable test available to identify the continuing presence of chronic inflammation or of fecal concretions in the retained appendix. My view is, all things being equal, that older patients should have a planned appendectomy about 2 months after resolution of an appendix mass treated successfully by catheter drainage.

Prophylactic Drains?

Although the focus of this superb chapter, and indeed of this entire textbook, is on the abdomen already contaminated, I am impelled to remind readers of the pitfalls associated with the most common reason for placement of drains in current surgical practice. That is, the placement of a drain into a clean abdominal cavity in an attempt to prevent a complication of the operative procedure. Typically, such "prophylactic" drains are placed near a bowel anastomosis or closure with the thought that should there be a leak then the material will have a path out of the abdominal cavity. The futility of draining the general peritoneal cavity was demonstrated years ago by Yates [2]. The equal futility of prophylactic drain placement was shown by Nora [3] and others [4, 5]. Such drains are promptly walled off; if a leak occurs, it does not follow the drain. Prophylactic drainage is not only ineffective but is positively deleterious! The incidence of anastomotic leakage is higher after prophylactic drain placement than if no drains are placed. The reason is that the drain, acting as a foreign body, impairs healing of the adjacent anastomosis, thus increasing the risk of a leak.

References

1. Wittmann DH (1998) Operative and nonoperative therapy of intraabdominal infections. Infection 26:335–341
2. Yates JL (1905) An experimental study of the local effects of peritoneal drainage. Surg Gynec Obst 1:473–492
3. Nora PF, Vanecko RM, Bransfield JJ (1972) Prophylactic abdominal drains. Arch Surg 105:173–176
4. Agrama HM, Blackwood JM, Brown CS, Machiedo GW, Rush BF (1976) Functional longevity of intraperitoneal drains: an experimental evaluation. Am J Surg 132:418–421
5. Lewis RT, Goodall RG, Marien B, Park M, Lloyd-Smith W, Wiegand FM (1990) Simple elective cholecystectomy: to drain or not. Am J Surg 159:241–245

Editorial Comment

An abscess by definition is a confined structure enclosed by an inflammatory wall and possessing a viscous interior. In contrast, free-flowing, contaminated or infected peritoneal fluid or loculated collections, which lack a wall, represent not an abscess, but a phase in the spectrum-continuum of peritoneal contamination/ infection.

A classification of abdominal abscesses, which may need drainage, is offered in the following table.

Classification	Examples
Visceral vs. nonvisceral	Hepatic vs. subphrenic
Primary vs. secondary	Splenic vs. appendiceal
Spontaneous vs. postoperative	Diverticular vs. perianastomotic
Intraperitoneal vs. retroperitoneal	Tubo-ovarian vs. psoas
Simple vs. complex	Complex: Multiple (liver), Multiloculated Communication with bowel (leaking anastomosis) Associated with necrotic tissue (pancreatic) Associated with cancer
Anatomical	Subphrenic, subhepatic, lesser sac, paracolic, pelvic, interloop, perinephric, psoas

(Modified from *Schein's Common Sense Abdominal Surgery*, Springer Verlag, 2000)

Considerations in selecting the percutaneous versus open surgical drainage are the following:

	PC drainage	Open drainage
Surgically accessibility	"Hostile abdomen"	Accessible
PC accessibility	Yes	No
Source controlled	Yes	No
Location	Visceral	Interloop
Number of abscesses	Single	Multiple
Loculated	No	Yes
Communication with bowel	No	Yes
Associated necrosis	No	Yes
Associated malignancy	No	Yes
Contents	Thin	Thick, debris
Invasive radiologist	Available	Not available
Severity off illness	"Stable"	Critically ill
Failed PC drainage	No	Yes

(Modified from *Schein's Common Sense Abdominal Surgery*, Springer Verlag, 2000)

About one-third of intra-abdominal abscesses are not suitable for percutaneous drainage and require an open operation. A few practical dilemmas exist:

Exploratory Laparotomy Versus "Direct" Surgical Approach

A "blind" exploratory laparotomy to search for abscess, a common procedure in the past, is rarely necessary. A "direct" approach that spares the previously un-involved peritoneal spaces and avoids bowel injury and wound complications is almost always possible for spontaneous abscesses, if well defined on CT. However, these abscesses usually respond to percutaneous drainage. Although postoperative abscesses are readily localized by CT, those which fail percutaneous drainage are usually "complex," and so are often not amenable to a "direct" approach (e.g., interloop abscess) or also require the control of the intestinal source. Criteria for making the choice of the approach are summarized below:

	Exploratory laparotomy	"Direct" open drainage
Abscess accurately localized on CT	No	Yes
Early postoperative phase	Yes	No
Late postoperative phase	No	Yes
Single abscess	No	Yes
Multiple abscesses	Yes	No
Lesser sac abscess	Yes	No
Interloop abscess	Yes	No

	Exploratory laparotomy	"Direct" open drainage
Source of infection uncontrolled	Yes	No
Subphrenic/subhepatic	No	Yes
Gutter abscess	No	Yes
Pelvic	No	Yes

(Modified from *Schein's Common Sense Abdominal Surgery*, Springer Verlag, 2000)

Direct Approach: Extraperitoneal Versus Transperitoneal

There are no significant differences in overall mortality and morbidly between the two approaches; the transperitoneal route is, however, associated with a higher incidence of injury to the bowel. It logical to suggest that the extraperitoneal approach should be utilized whenever anatomically possible. Subphrenic and subhepatic abscesses can be approached extraperitoneally through a subcostal incision or, if posterior, thorough the bed of the 12th rib. Older surgeons are still familiar with these techniques, which have largely been replaced by percutaneous drainage. Pericolic, appendicular, and other retroperitoneal abscesses are best approached through a loin incision. Also, late-appearing pancreatic abscesses can be drained extraperitoneally – from the flank – occasionally needing a bilateral approach. Pelvic abscesses are best drained through the rectum or vagina.

When Is Drainage Not Necessary?

Traditionally, multiple hepatic abscesses, which are not amenable to drainage, are treated with antibiotics, with a variable response rate. Some recommend non-operative treatment, with prolonged administration of antibiotics, for children who develop abdominal abscesses following an appendectomy for acute appendicitis. The problem with such "successes" is that the alleged "abscesses," which were imagined on ultrasound or CT, were never proven as such. Instead, they probably represented sterile collections, the majority requiring no therapy at all.

In Conclusion

Abdominal abscesses should be drained; when an "active" source exists it should be dealt with – antibiotic treatment is of marginal value. We wish to stress the old credo that it is impossible to effectively drain the free peritoneal cavity. In addition to producing a false sense of security, drains can erode into intestine or blood vessels and promote infective complications. Drains should be reserved for the evacuation of an established abscess, to allow escape of potential visceral secretions (e.g., biliary, pancreatic) and to establish a controlled intestinal fistula when the bowel cannot be exteriorized. Drains should be removed as soon as they have fulfilled their purpose.

5 Debridement and "Peritoneal Toilet"

JOHN BOHNEN

Key Principles

- The degree of peritoneal contamination correlates with the severity of infection and outcome.
- The host responds to peritoneal infection by absorbing pathogens into the bloodstream and by mounting a local peritoneal inflammatory reaction; both responses kill bacteria but affect the host adversely.
- The goal of peritoneal toilet is to remove mechanically as many contaminants as possible to reduce the severity of infection and limit adverse host responses.
- Surgically aggressive forms of peritoneal debridement may remove more contaminating material, but at the cost of increased resources and adverse effects. Their value is controversial.

Introduction

"Peritoneal debridement" refers to the mechanical removal of foreign and devitalized material from the peritoneal cavity. Although "peritoneal toilet" is a more general term that refers to any method that cleans out the peritoneal cavity, such as placement of a drain, the terms "debridement" and "toilet" will be used interchangeably. The measures by which surgeons achieve peritoneal toilet represent a continuum of aggressiveness from conventional operation to serial, planned explorations of the peritoneal cavity (Table 1). Conventional operation consists of a single procedure that removes free (i.e., not adherent to peritoneal surfaces), grossly infected and nonviable material from the peritoneal cavity with simple mechanical means such as suction and lavage, with or without the addition of antimicrobial agents to the lavage fluid [1]. Continuous peritoneal, lavage refers to

Table 1. Degree of aggressiveness in achieving peritoneal toilet

Conventional	Single operation with manual debridement, suction and lavage
	Single operation as above, plus antibiotic lavage
	Continuous postoperative lavage, with or without antibiotic
	Radical peritoneal debridement
	Open peritoneal drainage without planned reoperation
Most aggressive	Scheduled reoperation (including "staged abdominal repair")

fluid instillation (and drainage) through catheters into the peritoneal cavity for the purpose of infusing and removing simultaneously large volumes (e.g., liters per hour) of crystalloid solution postoperatively [2]. Radical peritoneal debridement describes suction and irrigation plus the meticulous removal of all solid material such as fibrin and contaminants that have adhered to the viscera and other peritoneal surfaces [3, 4]. In open peritoneal drainage, also called "laparostomy", the surgeon does not close either the abdominal fascia or skin, leaving the viscera and other peritoneal contents covered with dressings but relatively exposed to environmental air [5]. Scheduled reoperation refers to planned, serial operative explorations of the peritoneal cavity [6, 7].

Infectious Challenge to the Host

> The degree of peritoneal contamination correlates with the severity of infection and outcome.

The degree of physiologic derangement, measured by the Acute Physiology and Chronic Health Evaluation or a similar scoring system, correlates with the probability of death from peritoneal infection [8]. The physiologic changes that contribute to such scores reflect both the host response to infection and the severity of the infection itself. Animal and clinical studies in a variety of infectious conditions have demonstrated the intuitively obvious fact that larger numbers and concentrations of contaminating microbial pathogens lead to more severe infections. In human patients with peritonitis, fecal peritonitis carries a higher mortality rate [9], and severe contamination of the surgical wound results in a higher incidence of surgical site infection [10].

Thus, the density of the infecting bacterial inoculum correlates with the severity of infection and determines, along with patient co-morbidities, host defenses and treatment, the ultimate outcome. In secondary bacterial peritonitis, the contaminants include not only the microbial pathogens, but also nonviable "adjuvant" substances, that increase the severity of infection [11] – from the contaminating fluid (blood, bile, food, feces), the host (necrotic tissue, blood, fibrin), or the radiologist (barium).

Since the severity of the infection depends on the degree of peritoneal contamination with microbial pathogens and adjuvant substances, an important goal of the surgical management of intraperitoneal infection is to remove or neutralize the contaminants to the greatest extent possible.

Host Response to Infection

> The host responds to peritoneal infection by absorbing pathogens into the bloodstream and by mounting a local peritoneal inflammatory reaction; both responses kill bacteria but affect the host adversely.

The host responds to peritoneal contaminants in two ways: absorption of bacteria into the bloodstream via lymphatics, and acute local peritoneal inflammation

[11]. Systemic absorption of microorganisms from the peritoneal cavity enables the host to kill microbial pathogens through the actions of centrally located phagocytic cells, especially hepatic macrophages (Kupffer cells), while preserving normal peritoneal anatomy and physiology. Absorption from the peritoneum is mediated by lymphatics and occurs within minutes of peritoneal contamination. This mechanism can contain small bacterial inocula such as from minor intestinal leaks that occur intraoperatively, without leading to exaggerated peritoneal inflammatory responses. However, the systemic absorption of large microbial inocula leads to intense physiologic derangement, caused by the actions of molecular products of Kuppfer and other host defense cells.

Since large microbial inocula could overwhelm systemic responses if absorbed completely, the host benefits from the second response, peritoneal inflammation, which kills intraperitoneal bacteria locally in the abdominal cavity and traps them in fibrin deposits [11]. Such fibrin trapping probably prevents microorganisms from eliciting overwhelming systemic responses to the infection. Entrapment in fibrin functionally exteriorizes the bacteria from the body (ultimately as abscesses) and limits their growth. However, this process sequesters the bacteria from killing by antimicrobial agents and from their removal by host phagocytic cells or surgical drainage. Fibrin trapping of microorganisms is a double-edged sword that contributes beneficially to host defenses in the absence of therapeutic measures, but may frustrate conventional operative and adjunctive antibiotic therapy by protecting the pathogens on the surfaces of the peritoneal membranes.

The clinical outcome depends on the balance between the microbial pathogens and the cellular and molecular host defenses within and remote from the peritoneal cavity.

Rationale for Peritoneal Debridement

> The goal of peritoneal toilet is to remove mechanically as many contaminants as possible to reduce the severity of infection and limit adverse host responses.

Peritoneal toilet functions as a surgical adjunct to controlling the initial, proximate source of peritoneal infection. Proximate source control fixes the cause and prevents further leakage of contaminants into the peritoneal cavity; peritoneal toilet removes the microbial load and adjuvant substances already encountered at operation. To offer the most benefit to the patient, peritoneal toilet must remove the greatest possible density of pathogens and adjuvant-substances without causing further damage to host tissues.

Aggressive methods of peritoneal toilet (i.e., procedures that exceed simple suction and peritoneal lavage) derive from the premise that microbial inoculum density influences clinical outcome. Their rationale relies on the assumption that aggressive procedures do indeed reduce the number of contaminants at the end of an operative procedure; that the benefit of achieving a lower bacterial density at the end of an operation is sustained beyond the immediate postoperative period; that reducing the concentration of contaminants improves clinical outcome directly or by enhancing the effects of antimicrobial agents; and that any benefit of removing more contaminants outweighs the costs related to adverse effects and resource utilization. None of these assumptions has been studied adequately to prove or disprove them.

Aggressive Peritoneal Debridement

> Surgically aggressive forms of peritoneal debridement may remove more contaminating material, but at the cost of increased resources and adverse effects. Their value is controversial.

The most commonly used and reported modalities of aggressive peritoneal toilet have been continuous postoperative lavage, radical peritoneal debridement, open packing of the peritoneal cavity ("laparostomy") and scheduled reoperation. Unfortunately, most clinical trials of these treatment methods have not stratified patients by severity of illness, or adjusted the results according to the adequacy of proximate source control (i.e., "closing the leak"). Only in the last decade or so have patients in clinical trials been stratified according to severity of infection as reflected by physiologic changes. Thus, the earlier studies cited below have had serious methodological limitations in their failure to ensure that treatment groups have had equivalent severities of infection. Further, published reports have not compared the long-term effects and full costs of standard vs. aggressive forms of achieving peritoneal toilet.

Continuous postoperative lavage has had several champions who found favorable results in clinical trials [2], although these studies were not stratified according to patient severity, and did not use concurrent controls or prospective randomization. Other studies have found no benefit to continuous lavage [12]. The technique is labor intensive, and has largely fallen out of favor. Radical peritoneal debridement yielded spectacular results in an uncontrolled, unstratified study of patients who were described as having advanced peritonitis [3]. The rationale for this procedure makes some sense because the debridement of all contaminants and fibrin deposits on peritoneal surfaces should reduce the numbers of intraperitoneal bacterial pathogens. However, the only randomized controlled trial of radical debridement showed no benefit compared to standard therapy [4]. It must be noted that this study was dominated by patients with appendicitis, i.e., patients whose outcomes one would not expect to be improved significantly by aggressive surgery, and was not stratified for severity of illness or proximate source control. A larger randomized, controlled trial of radical debridement in patients with severe peritonitis, stratified appropriately, would determine its efficacy.

Laparostomy similarly has come into and out of favor, with some promising results [5], and discouraging outcomes [13]. The rationale for the procedure is to treat the peritoneal cavity as an "abscess", to be drained as a single entity. The price to pay for lack of coverage of the viscera is the risk of incisional hernia and intestinal fistulas for which management is difficult in the absence of an intact abdominal wall [14].

Scheduled reoperation for severe peritonitis seeks to accomplish what radical debridement and laparostomy do, i.e., aggressive peritoneal toilet while maintaining an intact abdominal wall. Another theoretical advantage is that scheduled reoperation enables the surgeon to detect new sources and foci of infection in the abdomen, which may develop after the initial surgical procedure. Scheduled reoperation has been described in two distinct circumstances. At times the abdominal wall cannot be closed primarily without undue tension because of edema of intra-abdominal structures due to longstanding or very severe intraperitoneal infection, or to loss of abdominal fascia due to previous ventral hernia or fascial infection. In such cases, temporary abdominal closure at the skin level with towel clips or plastic sheet, or fascial closure with prosthetic mesh, is followed by closure of the abdominal wall once the underlying infection has resolved [15]. In those situations, the scheduled reoperation is indicated to reconstruct the abdominal wall.

The other indication for scheduled reoperation is to treat severe abdominal infection. Besides providing repeated entrance into the abdomen to remove residual contaminants, planned reoperations can identify other, unexpected sources of contamination. In scheduled reoperation the abdominal wall is closed with a prosthetic device such as nonabsorbable mesh, to facilitate multiple reentries into the abdomen [6, 7]. As will be discussed in subsequent chapters, some promising evidence has accumulated to support the use of scheduled reoperation for severe peritonitis, but results from the published literature are contradictory. Potential adverse outcomes are intestinal fistula [14] and incisional hernia. Scheduled reoperation is labor intensive, and therefore, costly. Whether the costs and adverse effects are outweighed by better clinical outcomes has not been studied in a properly designed prospective randomized clinical trial.

Controversies

Controversy has developed around the practice of achieving peritoneal toilet because of two general issues: the results associated with the procedures themselves and the research methodologies used to study those procedures. Compared to standard methods of achieving peritoneal toilet, more aggressive measures, from antibiotic lavage to scheduled reoperation, have achieved mixed results in clinical trials. Therefore, despite theoretical advantages, aggressive peritoneal toilet has its strong proponents but generally has not become accepted practice. To settle the controversy would require a prospective, randomized clinical trial. Unfortunately, clinical trials of therapy in abdominal infections face challenges not found in most other types of clinical research.

Patients with abdominal infections present for treatment with a variety of underlying etiologies, and differing degrees of severity of infection, coexisting health problems, diagnostic delay, and inadequacy of resuscitation, all of which are critical determinants of outcome. It is difficult to balance these outcome determinants among treatment groups in clinical trials of therapy. Although this problem has been overcome to some extent by stratifying patients according to the degree of physiologic change before treatment, peritonitis trials have not yet been controlled for the other key determinant of outcome, the success of control of the proximate source of contamination ("source control"). Difficulties in balancing treatment groups according to the efficacy of source control include the heterogeneity of possible sources of infection within patient treatment groups, the variety of methods surgeons use to achieve source control and lack of accepted definitions for successful source control [16].

These methodological difficulties have led to a growing list of treatment options based on theoretical rationales, without clear evidence of success for any of them.

Critical Factors and Decision Making

> The critical factors for decision making will be considered for scheduled reoperation because of its theoretical advantages and promising results in some studies.

Despite a lack of clear guidance from the published literature, the surgeon must make decisions about therapy that aim to save patients from acute peritoneal infections, while minimizing adverse effects and costs. Before considering individual patients, surgeons must decide beforehand whether scheduled reoperation is feasible in their practice setting – is it worth the costs and the risks of multiple operations, ventral hernias, and intestinal fistulas?

Decisions regarding feasibility must consider the availability of human and physical resources and the acceptance by the hospital administration and perioperative services that include nursing, anesthesia, and intensive care. The consideration of the worthiness of scheduled reoperation depends on the surgeon's interpretation of the published literature and clinical experiences. If the answer is "yes, scheduled reoperation has a place in my practice," the surgeon must then decide when to use it by answering two questions for each patient with peritonitis: "Can I close the abdominal fascia and maintain a safe intra-abdominal pressure?" and "Is the infection so severe that I should consider scheduled reoperation?" If the surgeon cannot close the fascia primarily because of tissue edema and intestinal dilatation, or if such closure would lead to abdominal compartment syndrome due to increased pressure in the abdomen [17], temporary abdominal closure can achieve coverage of the viscera. In that case the scheduled reoperation is used to establish permanent abdominal closure as described above [15].

Several situations might compel the surgeon to think that the infection is so severe that scheduled reoperation should be considered. Perhaps the initial degree of peritoneal contamination was overwhelming. At the end of the operation, the surgeon might not have been satisfied that proximate source control had been achieved, e.g., because of ongoing intestinal ischemia or the possibility of anastomotic leak. Perhaps the surgeon was not convinced that all existing loci of infection had been dealt with because of technical challenges or because the patient was hemodynamically unstable on the operating table. In such situations the surgeon would use scheduled reoperation to ensure source control and achieve peritoneal toilet.

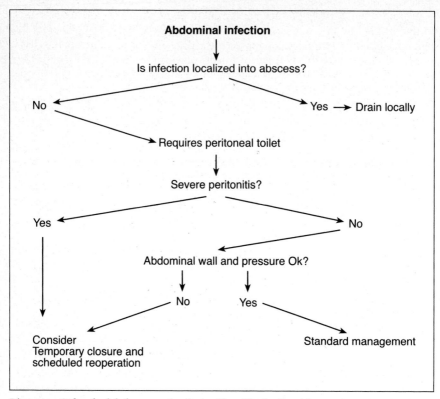

Diagram 1. Only scheduled reoperation is considered in the algorithm

References

1. Schein M, Saadia R, Decker G (1988) Intraoperative peritoneal lavage Surg Gynecol Obstet 166:187–195 (Collective review of antibiotic lavage of the peritoneal cavity.)
2. Stephen M, Loewenthal J (1979) Continuing peritoneal lavage in high-risk peritonitis. Surgery 85:603–606 (Early study that strongly supported continuous postoperative lavage; not stratified for severity of illness; no concurrent control group.)
3. Hudspeth AS (1975) Radical surgical debridement in the treatment of advanced generalized bacterial peritonitis. Arch Surg 110:1233–1236 (Uncontrolled study that showed zero mortality for radical debridement for abdominal infection.)
4. Polk HC, Fry DE (1980) Radical surgical debridement in the treatment for established peritonitis. The results of a prospective randomized clinical trial. Ann Surg 192:350–355 (Controlled trial that found no benefit from radical debridement, challenging Hudspeth's findings.)
5. Steinberg D (1979) On leaving the peritoneal cavity open in acute generalized suppurative peritonitis. Am J Surg 137:216–220 (Early study showing benefit of laparostomy.)
6. Teichmann W, Wittmann DH, Andreone PA (1986) Scheduled reoperations (Etappenlavage) for diffuse peritonitis. Arch Surg 121:147–152 (Promising results from scheduled reoperation.)
7. Wittmann DH, Aprahamian C, Bergstein JM (1990) Etappenlavage: advanced diffuse peritonitis managed by planned multiple laparotomies utilizing zippers, slide fastener, and Velcro

analogue for temporary abdominal closure. World J Surg 14:218–226 (Promising results again, discussion of technique.)

8. Bohnen JMA, Mustard RA, Oxholm SE et al (1988) APACHE II score and abdominal sepsis: a prospective study. Arch Surg 123:225–229 (Physiologic alterations correlate with probability of death from abdominal infection.)

9. Stephen M, Loewenthal J (1978) Generalized infective peritonitis. Surg Gynecol Obstet 147:231–234 (Fecal peritonitis was associated with greater mortality.)

10. National Academy of Sciences-National Research Council (1964) Postoperative wound infections: the influence of ultraviolet irradiation of the operating room and of various other factors. Ann Surg 160[Suppl 2]:1–132 (Classic paper showing that heavier wound contamination is associated with greater wound infection rates.)

11. Hau T, Ahrenholz DH, Simmons RL (1979) Secondary bacterial peritonitis: the biologic basis of treatment. Curr Probl Surg 16:1–65 (Seminal paper that integrated the biology, clinical presentation, and principles of management of intra-abdominal infection.)

12. Leiboff AR, Soroff HS (1987) The treatment of generalized peritonitis by closed postoperative peritoneal lavage. Arch Surg 122:1005–1010 (Summary of work on postoperative lavage cast doubt on its value.)

13. Kinney EV, Polk HC (1987) Open treatment of peritonitis: an argument against. Adv Surg 21:19–28 (Argument against laparoscopy, highlighting complications.)

14. Schein M, Decker GAG (1990) Gastrointestinal fistulas associated with large abdominal wall defects: experience with 43 patients. Br J Surg 77:97–100 (Large series of dreaded complications from open management of abdominal infections.)

15. Moore EE, Burch JM, Franciose RJ, Offner PJ, Biffl WL (1998) Staged physiologic restoration and damage control surgery. World J Surg 22:1184–1191 (Method of achieving abdominal closure in stages when inadvisable or impossible at first laparotomy.)

16. Bohnen JMA, Marshall JC, Fry DE, Johnson SB, Solomkin JS (1999) Clinical and scientific importance of source control in abdominal infections: summary of a symposium. Can J Surg 42:122–126 (Surgical Infection Society symposium on the definition and importance of source control in abdominal infection.)

17. Schein M, Wittmann DH, Aprahamian CC, Condon RE (1995) The abdominal compartment syndrome: the physiological and clinical consequences of elevated intra-abdominal pressure. J Am Coll Surg 180:745–753 (Comprehensive review.)

Invited Commentary

HIRAM C. POLK JR., DAVID A. SPAIN

The title of this chapter, "Debridement and Peritoneal Toilet", has erroneous connotations that are difficult to eliminate from a surgeon's mind. The principles of surgical management are almost always drainage, diversion, and debridement. Debridement in the peritoneal cavity is, in essence, excision. We were fascinated originally by the report of Hudspeth [1], but our attempt to emulate his work was unsuccessful; we could not confirm its advantages. While our work has been widely quoted [2], it may be that by lumping our observations we are also guilty of a serious interpretational error. It is clear that radical peritoneal debridement, as we practiced it, may have contributed to the small excessive mortality rate in elderly patients. Conversely, its benefit in younger patients who were well able to withstand the trauma of such an operative undertaking may have been understated. It seems unlikely that this clinical experiment will ever be repeated, and it is important that these caveats be recognized.

Parenteral nutrition permits more facile management of intestinal fistulas, and, therefore, reduces some of the obligatory problems of peritoneal debridement and the open abdomen approach to both sepsis and damage control. Laparostomies for trauma are more tolerable than they were in the past. Notwithstanding that, enterocutaneous fistulas continue to carry a significant mortality rate and are unacceptable treatment options in this scenario. It must be said that the lessons of the trauma surgeon in managing the concept of staged or damage control laparostomies have been extraordinarily helpful. The early facile and inexpensive closure of the abdomen with an intravenous fluid bag, in lieu of expensive temporary prosthetic devices, has been a major improvement. Furthermore, the concept of timing, in terms of reoperation, elimination of edema, and sequential full-thickness abdominal wall closure, is also extremely helpful [3].

The fundamental issue of when such a concept should be applied to advanced peritoneal infection remains as unclear today as it was when Hudspeth [1] first described it and when my former associate, Ed Kinney, and I attempted to properly position it in the late 1980s. Notwithstanding the advances made in fluid control, abdominal wall substitution, and staged reoperation, a remaining critical factor is the material available to protect the often exposed small bowel. Ultimate intraoperative and postoperative judgment is essential in this situation, and it may be that devices such as nonabsorbable mesh may have some role in protecting the exposed small bowel. Three or four cases we have so treated have certainly turned out better than we would have expected.

Mortality is the most important outcome to be avoided in peritonitis and, as stated by the authors in the accompanying chapter, there is no persuasive evidence that any one of these approaches achieves a better outcome than the other. The proper emphasis on the considerable antibiotic resistance and the overwhelming cost of ongoing intraperitoneal antibiotic lavage will preclude it ever being repeated in North America in any current reader's lifetime. It still may be that this is a valuable form of therapy. The extreme unlikelihood of definitive trials may mean that the proper analysis will be in the animal laboratory. In the meantime, surgeons will have to use those skills that have been most helpful in the past: discerning judgment, meticulous technique, and attentive overall support of the surgical patient.

References

1. Hudspeth AS (1975) Radical surgical debridement in the treatment of advanced generalized bacterial peritonitis. Arch Surg 110:1233–1236
2. Polk HC Jr, Fry DE (1980) Radical surgical debridement in the treatment for established peritonitis: the results of a prospective randomized clinical trial. Ann Surg 192:350–355
3. Fabian TC, Croce MA, Pritchard FE, et al (1994) Planned ventral hernia. Staged management for acute abdominal wall defects. Ann Surg 219:643–650

Editorial Comment

Although cosmetically appealing and popular with surgeons, there is no evidence whatsoever that intraoperative peritoneal lavage – as compared to a combination of sucking out and swabbing or mopping – reduces mortality or infective complications in patients receiving adequate systemic antibiotics [1, 2]. Obsessive irrigators should be aware that leaving saline or Ringer's behind may interfere with peritoneal defenses by "diluting the macrophages" [3]. (Bacteria swim perhaps better than macrophages!)

Aggressive methods of source control and "toilet" are further discussed in Chaps. 41 and 42.

References

1. Schein M, Saadia R, Decker G (1988) Intraoperative peritoneal lavage. Surg Gynecol Obstet 166:187–195
2. Platell C, Papadimitriou JM, Hall JC (2000) The influence of lavage on peritonitis. J Am Coll Surg 191:672–680
3. Dunn DL, Barke RA, Ahrenholz DH, Humphrey EW, Simmons RL (1984) The adjuvant effect of peritoneal fluid in experimental peritonitis: mechanism and clinical implications. Ann Surg 199:37–43

6 Device Removal

Victor Lazaron, Gregory J. Beilman

Key Principles

- Make sure diagnosis of infection is secure.
- Determine whether device removal would pose significant risk.
- Assess complicating factors (virulence of infection, debilitation or immuno-suppression of patient, etc.) and history (has an attempt at conservative therapy failed?)
- When in doubt, take it out.

The management of device-related infections presents a unique set of challenges for source control – primarily of the relative merits of device removal versus extended antibiotic therapies. The gold standard of therapy in the setting of serious infection remains the removal of foreign bodies. However, a number of devices cannot be removed without serious medical consequences. Few high-quality data exist to guide the surgeon in making these judgments. A structured approach to this clinical problem is presented.

The spectrum of implantable devices runs the gamut from those absolutely necessary for life such as the ventricular assist devices to those that are easily removed, for example, temporary central venous catheters (Table 1). Standard therapy for central venous catheter infection includes device removal [1, 2]. However, when the surgeon contemplates the removal of other devices, the risk to the patient of device removal must be balanced against the benefit gained in treating infection. There are no randomized, controlled studies demonstrating the optimal therapy for these more difficult cases. However, many case series demon-

Table 1. Implantable devices in decreasing order of medical necessity

Ventricular-assist devices (LVAD, RVAD, BiVAD)
Implantable pacemaker/defibrillator
Orthopedic hardware
Ventriculoperitoneal shunt
Hemo/peritoneal dialysis catheter
Peritoneovenous shunt
Long-term venous access device (Portacath, Hickman, etc.)
Short-term venous access device

strate that infections may sometimes be cleared without removal of the most vital devices [11-13]. A systematic approach should be employed in treating the patient with suspected implantable device-associated infection utilizing the key principles outlined above.

General Approach

Accurate diagnosis is the first step and the cornerstone of treatment. Most patients with implantable devices in situ are suspected of having infection because of fever, with or without leukocytosis. However, dependence on such nonspecific signs as an indication of infection can lead to the unnecessary removal of uninfected devices. Studies of intravascular catheters removed for such "suspected infection" demonstrate that rates of infection may be as low as 15 % [3, 4]. Therefore, it is important to establish a specific diagnosis of catheter-related infection. Techniques of diagnosis vary with device type. Vascular access catheters may be assessed by culturing the catheter lumen at the hub, and the skin site, and by drawing quantitative blood cultures through the port [5, 6]. Negative cultures have a 96 % negative predictive value for device-associated infection. Temporary catheters may be exchanged over a guide wire and the catheter tip cultured quantitatively [7]. Portacath-type reservoir catheters and ventriculoperitoneal shunts may be accessed for obtaining cultures. Implanted pacemakers, defibrillators, and orthopedic hardware are typically not accessible for obtaining cultures. However, imaging studies may reveal peri-device fluid collections that can be sampled under radiologic guidance [8]. Pacemaker lead infection is diagnosed by blood cultures and transesophageal echocardiography [9]. Ventricular assist device(VAD)-related infection can be diagnosed by blood cultures and by imaging using labeled-leukocyte scintigraphy [10].

The second step is the assessment of the medical difficulties posed by device removal, and the underlying patient risk factors which would prompt a less conservative approach. You will not, of course, remove an LVAD, whereas you have already removed a temporary triple lumen catheter by this point. It is the cases between the extremes where judgment is required. The list of devices in Table 2 is a rough guide, but patient factors may significantly alter your judgment. A functioning hemodialysis catheter in a dialysis patient with absolutely no other percutaneous options for access is more essential than an ankle screw. Such judgments generally should be made in conjunction with other specialists, and always, of course, with the patient in question.

Next, assess the clinical characteristics of the current infection in this particular patient. How is the patient doing? Treatment of the patient with signs of systemic inflammatory response syndrome (SIRS) and a potentially infected device is likely to require a more aggressive approach than of the patient with only a low-grade fever. Similarly, the patient on steroids or who has systemic immunosuppression from AIDS or transplantation may not demonstrate the systemic response of an otherwise healthy patient. He or she, too, will need a more aggressive work-up and treatment plan. What infection are you dealing with? Cultures are helpful in planning treatment. Many clinicians will attempt a con-

Table 2. Case series describing treatment of device-associated infection without device removal

Device	Treatment	Reference
Pacemaker/ Implantable defibrillator	Device removal mandatory	
Orthopedic hardware	Long-term antibiotics	19
	Antibiotic therapy	20
Ventriculoperitoneal Shunt	Device removal mandatory	
Hemodialysis catheter	Antibiotic therapy plus antibiotic "lock"	21, 22
Peritoneal dialysis catheter	Antibiotic therapy +/–	
	IP urokinase	23
	Revision of catheter tract	24
Peritoneovenous shunt	Antibiotic therapy[a]	25
Long-term venous catheter	Antibiotic therapy	26, 27

[a] For treatment of peritonitis or wound infection, but not bacteremia which requires device removal.

servative course of therapy for a coagulase-negative staphylococoal infection in a healthy patient, leaving a needed device in place, whereas *S. aureus, Candida,* or Gram-negative infection would prompt early device removal.

Finally, if a trial of conservative therapy has been attempted without success or if infection has recurred, device removal is indicated.

Specific antibiotic therapy can be tailored to the infection and the patient. Many clinicians treat coagulase-negative Staphylococcal infections by device removal alone, although there are no reliable data to support this practice, or indeed to support any specific duration of antibiotic therapy in other catheter-related infections. Our current practice is 3-7 days of intravenous vancomycin (quinupristin/dalfopristin or linezolid may also be options in selected patients). Interestingly, removal of intravascular devices is not required in order to clear coagulase-negative staphylococoal bacteremia. However, leaving the device in situ is associated with a 20 % recurrence rate during the same hospitalization versus a 3 % recurrence rate if the device is removed [13]. *Staphylococcus aureus* bacteremia should be treated for a minimum of 7-10 days, and for at least 4 weeks if endocarditis or septic thrombosis is suspected. Device removal is associated with decreased recurrence and mortality and is strongly encouraged [14]. Candidemia likewise mandates device removal because of its persistence and increased mortality if the device is left in place. Systemic therapy with fluconazole for susceptible *Candida albicans*, given for 7-14 days, may be appropriate treatment in selected patients [15, 16]. A course of amphotericin B should be strongly considered for patients with serious device-related infections (ICU, endocarditis), those not responding to fluconazole, or those with concomitant immunosuppression. Gram-negative device-related infections are unusual, but should be treated with device removal and 7 days of intravenous antibiotics. Leaving the device in situ increases treatment failure and recurrence rates [17, 18].

Controversies

Removal of the infected device remains the gold standard for the treatment of device-related infections. However, the growing use of a wide variety of implantable devices is prompting clinicians to attempt treatment of infection without device removal. Attempts at salvage of life-sustaining infected devices, such as dialysis catheters or LVADs, is controversial. Numerous case series suggest that the strategy can be used successfully, but the only controlled study unequivocally demonstrating safety and efficacy is for central venous catheter-associated coagulase-negative Staphylococcal bacteremia. Several case reports and series describing the techniques for treating device-associated infection *without device removal* are listed in Table 2. We can expect more series, and perhaps controlled studies, in this area in the future.

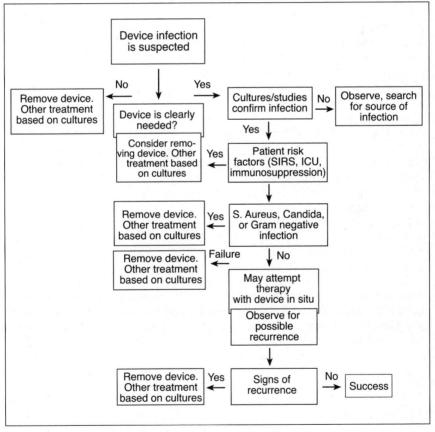

Diagram 1. Decision-making algorithm

Critical Factors and Decision Making

To summarize, the critical factors in making treatment decisions are:

1. Accurate diagnosis of infection with culture and sensitivity data when possible
2. An understanding of the medical difficulties posed by device removal
3. Patient and infection-specific factors which may bias the clinician towards removal versus an attempt at treatment with the device in place

A device which is no longer needed should always be removed.

Device removal is strongly recommended in patients with documented infection with *S. aureus, Candida,* or Gram-negative organisms, and in critically ill patients with SIRS and a strongly suspected device-related infection. Treatment of device-associated infection without device removal requires sound clinical judgment, balancing the relative risks and benefits of device retention and removal.

References

1. Wilson MA, Garrison NR (1995) Infections of intravascular devices in surgical infections. In: Fry DE (ed) Surgical infections. Little Brown, Boston
2. Sitges-Serra A, Girvent M (1999) Catheter-related bloodstream infections World J Surg 23:589–595
3. Bozzetti F, Terno G, Bonfanti G, et al (1983) Prevention and treatment of central venous catheter sepsis by exchange via a guidewire: a prospective controlled trial. Ann Surg 198:48–52
4. Padberg FT Jr, Ruggieor J, Blackburn GL, et al (1981) Central venous catheterization for total parenteral nutrition. Ann Surg 193:264–270
5. Cercenado E, Ena J, Rodriquez-Creixems M, et al (1990) A conservative procedure for the diagnosis of catheter-related infections. Arch Intern Med 139: 1417–1420
6. Capdevilla JA, Planes AM, Palomar M, et al (1992) Value of differential quantitative blood cultures in the diagnosis of catheter-related sepsis. Eur J Clin Microbiol Infect Dis 11:403–407
7. Maki DG, Weise SJ, Sarafin HW (1977) A semi-quantitative method for identifying intravenous catheter-related infection. N Engl J Med 296:1305–1315
8. Eustace S, Shah B, Mason M (1998) Imaging orthopedic hardware with an emphasis on hip prostheses. Orthop Clin North Am 29:67–84
9. Voet JG, Vandekerckhove YR, Muyldermans LL, et al (1999) Pacemaker lead infection: report of three cases and review of the literature. Heart 8:88–91
10. de Jonge KC, Laube HR, Dohmen PM, et al (2000) Diagnosis and management of left ventricular assist device valve-endocarditis: LVAD valve replacement. Ann Thorac Surg 70:1404–1405
11. Lee JH, Geha AS, Rattehalli NM, et al (1996) Salvage of infected ICDs: management without removal. Pacing Clin Electrophysiol 19: 437–442
12. Abbey DM, Turner DM, Warson JS, et al (1995) Treatment of postoperative wound infections following spinal fusion with instrumentation. J Spinal Disord 8:278–283
13. Raad I, Davis S, Khan A, et al (1992) Catheter removal affects recurrence of catheter-related coagulase-negative staphylococci bacteremia (cRCNSB). Infect Control Hosp Epidemiol 13:215–221
14. Dugdale DC and Ramsey PG (1990) *Staphylococcus aureus* bacteremia in patients with Hickman catheters. Am J Med 89:137–141

15. Rex JH, Bennett JE, Sugar AM, et al (1994) A randomized trial comparing fluconazole with amphotericin B for the treatment of candidemia in patients without neutropenia. N Engl J Med 331:1325–1330
16. Nguyen MH, Peacock JE, Tanner DC, et al (1995) Therapeutic approaches in patients with candidemia: evaluation in a multicenter, prospective observational study. Arch Intern Med 155:2429–2435
17. Elting LS, Bodey GP (1990) Septicaemia due to *Xanthomonas* species and non-aeruginosa *Pseudomonas* species: increasing incidence of catheter-related infections. Medicine 60:196–206
18. Benezra D, Kiehn TE, Gold GWM, et al (1988) Prospective study of infections in indwelling central venous catheters using quantitative blood cultures. Am J Med 85:495–498
19. Stein A, Bataille JF, Drancourt M, et al (1998) Ambulatory treatment of multidrug-resistant Staphylococcus-infected orthopedic implants with high-dose oral co-trimoxazole (trimethoprim-sulfamethoxazole). Antimicrob Agents Chemother 42:3086–3091
20. Abbey DM, Turner DM, Warson JS, et al (1995) Treatment of postoperative wound infections following spinal fusion with instrumentation. J Spinal Disord 8:278–283
21. Boorgu R, Dubrow AJ, Levin NW, et al (2000) Adjunctive antibiotic/anticoagulant lock therapy in the treatment of bacteremia associated with the use of a subcutaneously implanted hemodialysis access device. ASAIO J 46:767–70
22. Shah J, Feinfeld DA (2000) Use of 'locked-in' antibiotic to treat an unusual gram-negative hemodialysis catheter infection. Nephron 85:348–350
23. Gadallah MF, Tamayo A, Sandborn M, et al (2000) Role of intraperitoneal urokinase in acute peritonitis and prevention of catheter loss in peritoneal dialysis patients. Adv Perit Dial 16:233–236
24. St Laurent M, Surendranath C, Saad T, et al (1998) A new salvage procedure for peritoneal dialysis catheters with exit site infections. *Am Surg* 64:1215–1217
25. Prokesch RC, Rimland D (1983) Infectious complications of the peritoneovenous shunt. Am J Gastroenterol 78:235–240
26. Atkinson JB, Chamberlin K, Boody BA (1998) A prospective randomized trial of urokinase as an adjuvant in the treatment of proven Hickman catheter sepsis. J Pediatr Surg 33:714–716
27. Malanoski GJ, Samore MH, Pefanis A, Karchmer AW (1995) Staphylococcus aureus catheter-associated bacteremia: minimal effective therapy and unusual infectious complications associated with arterial sheath catheters. Arch Intern Med 155:1161–1166

Invited Commentary

Lori L. Burrows

This chapter describes the basic principles to be followed when the removal of a medical device is contemplated. The use of medical devices of increasing levels of complexity and with a range of exposure to nonsterile areas or exit sites has risen exponentially in the past several decades. Regardless of site, infection remains the major complicating factor in medical device usage. While scrupulously introduced, totally implanted devices are less prone to infection, when infection occurs, it has much more serious repercussions. The authors correctly advise that the decision to remove a device must be balanced with the effect of its loss on the health of the patient, but the golden rule remains "If in doubt, take it out."

The difficulty associated with treatment of medical device infection arises in part from changes in physiology of the colonizing or infecting organisms that occur following their attachment to a surface. Microorganisms attached to surface form "biofilms," slow-growing accretions of cells within polysaccharide matrices that exhibit significantly enhanced resistance to host defenses and antimicrobial therapy compared with their free-swimming counterparts [1-3]. Their increased resistance to antibiotics often leads to incomplete clearance of infection, sometimes with concomitant selection of resistant mutants. Problems can also arise from chronic indolent biofilm infections with organisms of low virulence. Although these microbes may not cause acute febrile episodes, they may continuously stimulate a low-grade inflammatory response that can, for example, erode device/tissue junctions or anastomoses [4].

The authors caution that a correct diagnosis of infection is essential to an educated decision regarding device removal. The input of infectious disease specialists with medical device infection experience can be helpful in directing therapy and aiding in the choice of whether to remove the infected device. In cases where no organism can be cultured, either because empiric therapy has been started or because the organism has fastidious growth requirements, it is now possible to apply molecular diagnostic techniques such as 16S rDNA polymerase chain reaction and DNA sequencing to identify the etiologic agent [5-8].

As the authors note, depending upon the infecting organism, stage of the infection, and type of device, aggressive and prolonged medical therapy can often allow salvage of the device. Some antibiotics have proven more useful than others for this application, possibly because they are more effective at penetrating biofilm matrices and at killing slow-growing organisms. In general, however, medical failures will eventually necessitate removal of the device. The authors mention Gram-negative bacteria, *Staphylococcus aureus* and *Candida albicans* in particular as etiological agents of medically recalcitrant medical device infections and cite improved outcomes upon device removal.

To reduce or prevent biofilm-related infections, it is necessary for surgeons to be vigilant in handling devices in a completely aseptic manner when introducing or replacing them. Perioperative antimicrobial treatment of the patient, as well as the device, is helpful. The past decade has seen the introduction of temporary medical devices such as intravenous and urinary catheters and stents either coated or impregnated with a variety of antimicrobial agents, including antibiotics, antiseptics such as chlorhexidine, or silver compounds [9-14]. While the nominal value of these devices is in prophylaxis, they may also have considerable utility in reducing de novo biofilm formation if it is necessary to remove and immediately replace an infected device at a proximal site. The antimicrobial agent will reduce or prevent biofilm formation on the new surface while any infection of the surrounding tissues is resolved with more conventional therapy. With future developments in biomaterials engineering, these surface treatments may be incorporated into more complex and more completely implanted devices, giving added assurance that any organisms that manage to gain access to the device surface will not be able to survive.

References

1. Costerton JW, Stewart PS, Greenberg EP (1999) Bacterial biofilms: a common cause of persistent infections. Science 284:1318–1322
2. Davey ME, O'Toole G A (2000) Microbial biofilms: from ecology to molecular genetics. Microbiol Mol Biol Rev 64:847–867
3. Doyle RJ (1999) Biofilms. Methods Enzymol 6:310
4. Holzheimer RG, Dralle H (2001) Antibiotic therapy in intra-abdominal infections – a review on randomised clinical trials. Eur J Med Res 6:277–291
5. Relman DA (1999) The search for unrecognized pathogens. Science 284:1308–1310
6. Wagar EA (1996) Direct hybridization and amplification applications for the diagnosis of infectious diseases. J Clin Lab Anal 10:312–325
7. Wagar EA (1996) Defining the unknown: molecular methods for finding new microbes. J Clin Lab Anal 10:331–334
8. Fredricks DN, Relman DA (1999) Application of polymerase chain reaction to the diagnosis of infectious diseases. Clin Infect Dis 29:475–488
9. Burrows LL, Khoury AE (1999) Issues surrounding the prevention and management of device-related infections. World J Urol 17:402–409
10. Bassetti S, Hu J, D'Agostino RB Jr., Sherertz RJ (2001) Prolonged antimicrobial activity of a catheter containing chlorhexidine-silver sulfadiazine extends protection against catheter infections in vivo. Antimicrob Agents Chemother 45:1535–1538
11. Collin GR (1999) Decreasing catheter colonization through the use of an antiseptic-impregnated catheter: a continuous quality improvement project. Chest 115:1632–1640
12. Darouiche RO, Smith JA Jr, Hanna H, et al (1999) Efficacy of antimicrobial-impregnated bladder catheters in reducing catheter-associated bacteriuria: a prospective, randomized, multicenter clinical trial. Urology 54:976–981
13. Pugach JL, DiTizio V, Mittelman MW, Bruce AW, DiCosmo F, Khoury AE (1999) Antibiotic hydrogel coated Foley catheters for prevention of urinary tract infection in a rabbit model. J Urol 162:883–887
14. Raad I, Hanna H (1999) Intravascular catheters impregnated with antimicrobial agents: a milestone in the prevention of bloodstream infections. Support Care Cancer 7:386–390

7 Definitive Versus Temporizing Therapy

Donald E. Fry

Key Principles

- The principle objective in the surgical management of intra-abdominal infection is to control the anatomic source of the infection, and not necessarily to fully treat the underlying disease process responsible for the infection.
- Surgical choices at the time of achieving source control may require that the procedure be *temporizing* with the knowledge that a subsequent procedure will be required, or the choice may be *definitive* with the procedure designed to both control the source but also manage the underlying disease.
- The judgment to select a temporizing versus a definitive procedure requires an integrated assessment of
  1. the surgeon's knowledge about the underlying disease,
  2. systemic host factors, and
  3. the severity of the local inflammatory response.

The principal objective in the initial surgical management of the patient with intra-abdominal infection is source control. Stemming the flow of contamination is essential for antimicrobial and systemic supportive management to be effective in the clinical outcome of the patient. However, for each primary disease entity that may cause intra-abdominal infection, there are multiple management options available to the surgeon. For example, in perforative appendicitis the most common choice for source control is appendectomy. Removal of the diseased appendix is a safe option for most patients and is *definitive management*. Appendectomy not only eliminates the source of contamination – the hole in the appendix – but it also removes the condition responsible for the secondary peritonitis – the diseased appendix itself. Infrequently, other options may need to be chosen. With perforation and associated severe appendiceal abscess, the perforated appendix may not be readily identified. In this circumstance, external drainage alone may be the prudent option since attempts at finding and removing the appendix risk injury to bowel structures that are severely inflamed within the wall of the abscess cavity. *Temporizing management* means that control of the source may require another procedure at a future time for definitive management. In the example of the appendiceal abscess, interval appendectomy may be required at a future date, although this is controversial [1]. The temporizing strategy accepts that a future procedure may be required, but does so because pursuit of definitive management places the patient at increased risk. Temporary management achieves immediate control of the source and leaves definitive management for another day.

Table 1. Choices for source control in common scenarios of acute secondary peritonitis

Disease	Temporizing choice	Definitive choice
Perforated peptic ulcer	Omental patch closure	Vagotomy and pyloroplasty, or vagotomy and gastrectomy
Perforated benign gastric ulcer	Omental patch closure	Excision of ulcer and vagotomy/pyloroplasty; or gastrectomy
Perforated gastric cancer	None	Gastric resection
Perforated gallbladder with subhepatic abscess	External drainage of abscess	Drainage of abscess and cholecystectomy
Perforated gallbladder with common duct stones	Cholecystectomy with T-tube drainage of common duct	Cholecystectomy and common bile duct exploration; or choledochoduodenstomy?
Perforated cecum from right colon cancer	Right hemicolectomy and ileostomy	Right hemicolectomy and ileotransverse colostomy
Perforated sigmoid colon secondary to diverticulitis	Resection of perforated segment and colostomy	Resection and primary anastomosis
Perforated colon cancer	Resection and colostomy	Colectomy and primary anastomosis

Definitive Versus Temporizing Management

There are numerous temporizing and definitive choices. Table 1 identifies examples of temporizing and definitive management choices for common diseases that cause intra-abdominal infection. A definitive choice for the disease may still be a temporizing choice relative to reconstruction (e.g., perforated colon). The choice of a definitive or temporizing strategy is obviously influenced by the completeness of information that the surgeon may have about the patient's clinical circumstances. The specific choice of definitive management or not is dictated by:
- *Knowledge of the disease* being managed
- *Systemic risk factors* that are present in the patient at the time of management
- *Local factors* within the peritoneal cavity that are encountered at the time of surgical intervention for source control

Knowledge of the Disease

Is the perforation due to a malignancy? This question is vitally important in the selection of a definitive operation, and may preempt systemic and local factors that might otherwise favor the choice of a temporizing strategy. Perforation of a gastric lesion is an example of the cancer conundrum. Local excision, closure, and vagotomy and pyloroplasty are logical (among other choices) for the management of a perforated benign gastric ulcer. The surgeon accepts this choice knowing that it may not prove to be definitive (when compared to gastric resection) for the patient's disease [2]. However, a perforated gastric cancer requires gastrectomy, even though local inflammatory changes or the overall conditions of the patient might favor a more expedient and less risky management strategy [3].

Perforation of a sigmoid mass can be managed by limited resection if the cause is diverticular disease. If the perforation is from colon cancer, then resection of a longer segment of colon with its mesentery is necessary. The surgeon will commonly not have a definitive diagnosis, and the choice may be dictated by the management option of the worst case situation (i.e., assume that it is cancer) [4]. The highly contentious, second decision needs to be made about primary anastomosis or colostomy [5]. Intraoperative preparation of the colon with anastomosis would be advocated by some, while colostomy would be advocated by most. Other systemic and local factors may affect the clinical decision (see Chap. 12).

Other situations may dictate changes in the surgical strategy. Ileocecal perforation secondary to Crohn's disease would favor more limited resection of the bowel than if the cecal perforation is a result of adenocarcinoma [6]. Cholecystectomy alone for a perforated gallbladder may seem prudent, but knowledge of choledocholithiasis may require the temporizing strategy of using a T-tube. Knowledge of the patient's disease enforces the concept that the choice of temporizing versus definitive management is never absolute, but rather, surgical judgment must be modified as the clinician understands more clinical variables.

Systemic Factors

Patient factors commonly affect the decision process. Such systemic factors may reflect preexisting clinical conditions, or may be acquired circumstances due to systemic responses to the intra-abdominal infection.

Preexistent protein-calorie malnutrition and hypoalbuminemia, chronic renal failure or hepatic cirrhosis, or chronic corticosteroid management are common co-morbid conditions. These systemic factors result in poor wound healing, favor temporizing choices that anticipate less efficient wound healing, and may reduce surgical wound morbidity from the procedure. Patients with unstable or decompensated cardiac disease, and or severe preexistent pulmonary disease will likely have poor tissue perfusion and oxygenation, which favors avoiding anastomoses or other definitive measures.

Intra-abdominal infection itself produces acute systemic derangements that favor temporizing strategies. Hypovolemia and sepsis generally result in conditions that favor brevity in the length of operation and of general anesthesia. Respiratory distress syndrome, hepatic failure, renal failure, and coagulopathy as component parts of evolving organ failure similarly favor the temporizing choice. On the other hand, for patients without either preexistent or acquired systemic factors, definitive intervention is favored.

Local Factors

The intensity of inflammation within the peritoneal cavity is the most consistently cited variable influencing the decision for temporizing versus definitive strategies. Inflammation affects attempts to suture intestinal structures, since the tensile strength of tissues that are approximated is compromised when tissues are severely edematous. While the inflammatory process initially results in increased bulk perfusion to the area of injury, the consequences of sustained and destructive inflammation yield increased tissue hydrostatic pressure and relative ischemia to the area.

The magnitude of inflammation is highly variable in intra-abdominal infection, requiring the surgeon to make a subjective assessment about its consequences for surgical repair. The duration of peritonitis is one variable that affects the severity of inflammation. Delays in seeking medical attention, or delays because of uncertainty about the diagnosis, result in increased local inflammatory changes. In one study of peritonitis [7], local symptoms of peritonitis had commonly been present for 3 days before operation was undertaken. A perforated appendix or perforated diverticulum which has been present for this long will be associated with a more severe local inflammatory response than that which is seen within 12-24 h of perforation. The density of bacterial contamination is yet another variable that affects the inflammatory response. No culturable bacteria are identified in acute perforated peptic ulcers [8], while sigmoid perforations have 10^{10} microorganisms per gram of colonic contaminant. The effects of the bacteria are augmented by adjuvant factors from the perforation. Bile acids promote inflammation. Activated pancreatic enzymes in the contaminants from the duodenum or proximal jejunal perforations will enhance the inflammatory response. Free hemoglobin, necrotic tissue, and biologic debris within human stool will also enhance the inflammatory response generated by the microbial contaminant.

Making the Decision

Surgical judgment at the time of the source control procedure is required to make the choice regarding the extent of the operation (see Diagram 1). When technical ease allows removal of the disease (e.g., appendectomy for perforative appendicitis), then definite procedures are favored. Catastrophic situations with distorted anatomic detail from massive contamination and extensive inflammation favor the limited intervention to achieve control of the source, including eradication of pus, exudate, and necrotic tissue. There are many "gray" areas that fall between these two extremes. When systemic and local factors are sufficiently severe that the surgeon has second thoughts about proceeding with definitive management, then temporizing strategies are preferred. However, even when making the temporizing choice, appropriate control of the source of contamination is always required and cannot be compromised.

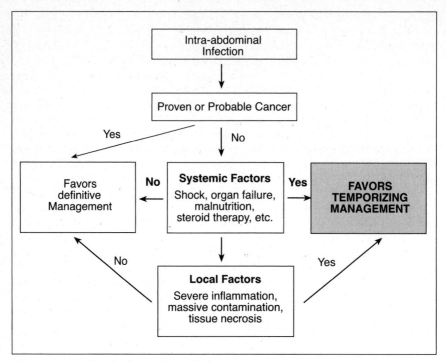

Diagram 1. Algorithm for the selection of definitive versus temporizing choices when operations for source control are being performed in patients with intra-abdominal infection

References

1. Strom PR, Turkleson ML, Stone HH (1983) Safety of incidental appendectomy. Am J Surg 145:819–822
2. Jordan PH Jr, Marrow C (1988) Perforated peptic ulcer. Surg Clin N Am 68:315–329
3. Stechenberg L, Bunch RH, Anderson MC (1981) The surgical therapy for perforated gastric cancer. Am Surg 47:208–210
4. Khan S, Pawlak SE, Eggenberger JC, et al (2001) Acute colonic perforation associated with colorectal cancer. Am Surg 67:261–264
5. Farkouh E, Hellou G, Allard M, Atlas H (1982) Resection and primary anastomosis for diverticulitis with perforation and peritonitis. Can J Surg 25:314–316
6. Talamini MA (1998) Crohn's disease of the small bowel. In: Cameron JL (ed) Current surgical therapy, 6th edn. Mosby, St Louis, pp 131–135
7. Mosdell DM, Morris DM, Voltura A, Pitcher DE, Twiest MW, Milne RL, Miscall BG, Fry DE (1991) Antibiotic treatment for surgical peritonitis. Ann Surg 214:543–549
8. Boey J, Wong J, Ong GB (1982) Bacteria and septic complications in patients with perforated duodenal ulcer. Am J Surg 143:635–639

Invited Commentary

EDWIN A. DEITCH

The chapter by Dr. Fry provides a clear and well-balanced approach to the surgical management of patients with intra-abdominal infections due to common surgical diseases. Several important concepts are stressed, including the concept that in most patients with peritonitis definitive therapy that both controls the source of the infectious process as well as its manifestations is the best option. However, there are some patients in whom source control either *cannot be achieved* or in whom it *should not be attempted*. This concept too is well articulated by Fry and is summarized for common causes of secondary peritonitis in Table 1, as well as outlined in an algorithm focusing on the choice between definitive versus temporizing therapy. The notion that the principle objective in the initial surgical management of the patient with intra-abdominal infection is source control whenever possible is well covered. Since adequate source control is so important in limiting morbidity and optimizing patient survival, it is important to discuss the *shades of gray* that may exist in obtaining "source control" in patients with intra-abdominal infections as well as to point out those circumstances in which surgical source control may not be the optimal initial therapy. Thus, my commentary will focus on these issues building upon the foundation laid in the previous chapter.

The "Difficult" Source Control

There are several groups of patients in whom source control and definitive therapy are most difficult. These include the trauma patient (Chap. 32), the patient with postoperative peritonitis (Chaps. 35 and 42), the patient with necrotizing pancreatitis (Chap. 17) and ICU patients, especially those with organ failure or dysfunction. For example, diagnosing an intra-abdominal infection in the patient after abdominal surgery is frequently difficult, since the standard signs we rely on to diagnose an intra-abdominal process, such as pain, fever, or leukocytosis, are unreliable. In fact, the first clear sign of an intra-abdominal infection may be the development of hemodynamic instability or organ failure. Likewise, in the trauma patient, where peritonitis may occur secondary to a missed injury or break down of an anastomosis, diagnosis may be difficult [1]. Once a diagnosis of intra-abdominal infection is made, the next decision is whether or not the patient is an immediate candidate for surgery. In this respect, it is important to classify patients according to whether they have a localized walled-off abscess or diffuse peritonitis. Patients with localized fluid collections are candidates for percutaneous drainage, while patients with generalized peritonitis require prompt laparotomy, debridement of necrotic tissue, and when possible, control of the source of intraperitoneal contamination. Furthermore, in the high-risk patient, definitive source control may not be possible due to extensive inflammation or peritoneal contamination limiting the ability of the surgeon to safely remove the diseased tissue or perform an anastomosis.

In planning the approach to intra-abdominal infection in these high-risk patients, understanding the response of the peritoneal cavity to infection is critical. Under normal circumstances, the peritoneal cavity is relatively resistant to a bacterial challenge. However, in the presence of adjuvant substances, such as fibrin, hemoglobin, and necrotic tissue, bacteria can evade the normal host defenses, and cause an intra-abdominal infection. Conceptually, it is useful to view the various types of abdominal sepsis (peritonitis, phlegmon, abscess) as a continuum. This point can be illustrated by considering what occurs when a colonic anastomosis leaks or a diverticulum ruptures. First, the peritoneal host defenses attempt to isolate the site of bacterial contamination from the rest of the peritoneal cavity. This is accomplished by the induction of a local inflammatory response with the resultant influx of neutrophils and the deposition of fibrin to trap the invading bacteria and to help seal the site of perforation. If the locally deposited fibrin, with the aid of the omentum and surrounding viscera, can wall off the colonic leak, a generalized peritonitis does not occur. Instead, a phlegmon or abscess develops, which may require debridement or drainage. In fact, in some circumstances (phlegmon and/or small abscesses), local host defenses in conjunction with antibiotics can lead to resolution of the inflammatory process without surgery. On the other hand, attempts to remove diseased tissue in a hostile abdomen in an overly aggressive attempt to achieve definitive source control may only make matters worse. Thus, in some patients, temporizing measures and surgical moderation rather than definitive therapy should be the goal.

In summary, in addition to the concepts outlined in the chapter by Dr. Fry, consideration of the stage of the intra-abdominal process (peritonitis, abscess, or phlegmon) as well as the local conditions within the abdomen and the degree of bacterial contamination are important factors in deciding whether definitive source control can or should be attempted.

Reference

1. Deitch EA, Livingston DH, Hauser CJ (1999) Septic complications in the trauma patient. New Horizons 7:158–172

Editorial Comment

The precise selection of a *definitive* versus *temporizing* source control procedure in the emergency surgical patient is crucial for survival. Both doing "too little" or doing "too much" may kill the patient. How to arrive at the "correct" decision requires experience and often a sixth sense: it is easier to mechanically cut, resect, and stitch up than decide exactly what to do – it requires judgment – which Drs. Fry and Deitch shared above with us.

As Dr. Fry stressed, the choice of operation should be tailored to the condition of the patient (systemic factors), the disease (i.e., the source), and its local consequence (i.e., local factors). It is only logical (but never scientifically proven) that operations of a lesser magnitude are safer in compromised hosts. Using objective scores to measure the severity of acute illness (and chronic health), such as the APACHE II, may aid in tailoring the procedure to the patient. "Fit" patients (i.e., APACHE II scores below 10) can tolerate any operation, while in the sicker (i.e., APACHE II scores above 15) less done may be better [1].

As Dr. Deitch discussed, there are conditions for which the source control is difficult. There are also sources which are easy to control – and there are those for which there is *no need for an operative source control*. The addition of modern CT scanning to well-developed clinical acumen allows the surgeon to pursue selective nonoperative management in a growing spectrum of conditions. Lack of systemic toxicity, localized abdominal findings, accurate CT diagnosis of the source – coupled with absent or a minimal amount of free air or contrast extravazation – predicts that an operation may not be necessary in conditions such as perforated peptic ulcers [2], colonoscopic colonic injuries [3], and post-ERCP perforations of the duodenum [4].

One can view the surgical patient who requires source control as being *inflamed,* locally and systematically, by a myriad of inflammatory mediators generated by the primary disease process, be it inflammatory, infectious or traumatic. The greater the inflammation, the sicker the patient, and higher is the expected mortality and morbidity. A too big operation, inappropriately performed, and too late, just adds wood to the inflammatory fire. The philosophy of treatment underlined here by weathered surgeons such as Fry and Deitch is that in order to effectively cure or minimize the inflammatory processes the management should be accurately tailored to the individual patient's disease. The punishment should fit the crime.

References

1. Schein M, Gecelter G, Freinkel W, Gerding H (1990) APACHE II in emergency operations for perforated ulcers. Am J Surg 159:309–313
2. Crofts TJ, Park KG, Steele RJ, Chung SS, Li AK (1989) A randomized trial of nonoperative treatment for perforated peptic ulcer. N Engl J Med 320:970–973
3. Lo AY, Beaton HL (1994) Selective management of colonoscopic perforations. J Am Coll Surg 179:333–337
4. Stapfer M, Selby RR, Stain SC, Katkhouda N, Parekh D, Jabbour N, Garry D (2000) Management of duodenal perforation after endoscopic retrograde cholangiopancreatography and sphincterotomy. Ann Surg 232:191–198

8 Deciding on the Extent of Surgical Therapy

Giuseppe Papia, John C. Marshall

Key Principles

- The extent of source control intervention is guided by the nature of the infection and the stability of the patient, and tempered by an awareness of what will be required in the future.
- The fundamental principles of source control include the *drainage* of abscesses or localized collections of infection, debridement of devitalized and necrotic tissue, and *definitive management* of foci of ongoing contamination.
- The first priority in planning the extent of source control is to ensure adequate infection control; the second, to eliminate a source of ongoing contamination; and the third, to minimize the morbidity associated with future intervention.
- The more extensive the initial intervention, the greater the challenge of subsequent reconstruction: the optimal intervention is that which accomplishes the source control objectives in the simplest manner.

A 63-year-old man is hospitalized with left lower quadrant pain and tenderness, in association with fever and leukocytosis. The CT scan reveals extensive diverticulitis of the sigmoid colon, with a 7-cm peridiverticular abscess containing fluid and air. What is the optimal treatment? Antibiotics and expectant observation? Surgical drainage with a proximal diverting colostomy? Surgical drainage by resection of the involved colon, with or without an anastomosis? Or percutaneous drainage?

There are numerous options for source control in complex infections; selecting the optimal strategy for a particular clinical situation is often difficult. Multiple factors must be considered in making a decision, including the site and extent of the infection, its associated complications, the physiologic stability of the patient, the duration of the disease process, the preceding surgical history, the availability of resources for imaging or interventional radiology, and the experience of the surgeon and the availability of assistance. While generic guidelines can be offered for the management of a particular infection, the large number of variables that may influence the final decision in an individual patient effectively precludes a single approach, and management must be tailored to the specific clinical circumstances. The clinical variability present in patients with a particular infection, and the inherent complexity of the decision-making process poses a significant impediment to the design and conduct of clinical trials to compare therapeutic strategies [1]. Nonetheless, principles can be articulated that should guide a final decision.

Physiologic Stabilization

Resuscitation and physiologic stabilization of the unstable patient takes precedence over source control, and in almost all circumstances, intervention should be delayed at least long enough to stabilize the patient hemodynamically, and to institute appropriate monitoring. The exception is the rare circumstance where infection is accompanied by exsanguinating hemorrhage and surgery is undertaken as a heroic measure to control bleeding, such as might occur, for example, following erosion of a focus of infection into a major blood vessel such as the aorta. Whether planned source control will necessitate a trip to the interventional radiology suite or to the operating room, transport of an unstable patient is hazardous, monitoring in the radiology department is invariably suboptimal, and the induction of anesthesia is accompanied by peripheral vasodilatation. Prior stabilization minimizes the risks of intervention. When infection is accompanied by significant physiologic instability, resuscitation and stabilization is best accomplished in the intensive care unit.

Imaging

High-resolution computed tomography (CT) has provided the clinician with a rapid, and highly effective diagnostic tool that can not only establish the need for intervention, but can also provide valuable information to aid in planning that intervention. For most patients in whom source control measures are contemplated, radiographic delineation of the problem prior to planned intervention greatly facilitates decision making, and the role of urgent surgical intervention, guided by signs and symptoms alone, is diminishing. There are of course obvious exceptions – the patient with diffuse peritonitis and intra-abdominal free air on X-ray examination, the patient in whom ischemia poses an immediate threat to intestinal viability, the patient with a rapidly spreading soft-tissue infection, or the patient with clinically apparent acute appendicitis – however, if accurate anatomic delineation of the underlying problem will aid in choosing between therapeutic options, appropriate radiographic investigations should be performed.

Treatment

Source control measures can be classified into those directed towards the drainage of a discrete focus of infection (thereby creating a controlled sinus or fistula), those undertaken to *debride* devitalized and infected tissue or to remove colonized devices, and those performed with the objective of *definitively correcting* a locus of ongoing microbial contamination [2]. In general, the best management option is the one that accomplishes its objective with a minimum of intervention, and thus with the least risk to the patient, both now and in the future.

Drainage

The least morbid approach to drainage involves the percutaneous placement of a small bore drain under CT or ultrasound guidance [3, 4]. Although the technique is most applicable to unilocular abscesses, more complex collections can be drained with the use of multiple drains. And even if percutaneous drainage does not provide definitive control of a focus of infection, it may often permit the clinician to temporize, transforming an emergent situation with a significant risk of morbidity into a more elective one. For example, percutaneous drainage in the unstable or high-risk patient with acute cholecystitis will usually result in resolution of the acute inflammatory process, permitting subsequent laparoscopic or open cholecystectomy on an elective basis. Laparoscopic drainage of abscesses within the peritoneal cavity [5] and mediastinum [6] has been described. Although experience is anecdotal, minimally invasive approaches offer many of the advantages of percutaneous drainage, and may also be attractive for the control of infection by debridement (see below) in anatomically challenging locations, such as the retroperitoneum of patients with infected peripancreatic necrosis [7]. Operative intervention is generally reserved for patients in whom less invasive procedures have been unsuccessful, or in whom additional intervention is contemplated to achieve definitive management of the source of bacterial contamination. A midline abdominal incision permits the widest access to the peritoneal cavity, and maximizes the potential sites for stoma placement should one be needed. However, if the infectious process is localized, a lateral incision such as a subcostal or flank incision may be more appropriate. The success of percutaneous techniques has largely rendered obsolete the classical posterior extraserous approach to the subphrenic space, through the bed of the 12th rib [8].

Debridement

Debridement is the physical removal of dead or devitalized tissue or colonized foreign bodies. Devitalized tissue provides an excellent culture medium for bacteria, and protects them from antibiotics and host phagocytic cells, consequently its removal is desirable. However, at least in the early stages of an infection, a zone of partially viable tissue is typically present between that tissue which is clearly viable and that which is clearly not. Debridement can result in significant bleeding and when that bleeding occurs in a relatively inaccessible site such as the retroperitoneum, it can present a significant threat to the patient. In general, debridement of necrotic skin and subcutaneous tissues, and of muscle in patients with myonecrosis, should be undertaken aggressively and without delay [9, 10]. On the other hand, tissue necrosis in the retroperitoneum does not pose an imminent threat to life, and for patients with infected pancreatic necrosis, debridement may be better delayed until demarcation of tissue planes has occurred, typically at least 3 or 4 weeks after the onset of the disease [11]. The decision to remove a colonized foreign body must weigh the benefits of device removal against the risks of intervention; for deep-seated devices, a trial of anti-biotic therapy is almost always warranted.

Definitive Management

The need for definitive management of the pathologic process causing infection has become one of the major indications for operative intervention in patients requiring source control. Such interventions may include the resection of a necrotic or perforated tumor or the excision of the sigmoid colon in patients with diverticulitis or an inflamed organ such as the gallbladder or appendix. Recent reports suggest that resection and primary anastomosis is at least as good as, and perhaps superior to, resection and colostomy, for the patient with perforated diverticulitis [2, 12]. Not only is the risk of major morbidity with the primary operation relatively small, but anastomosis obviates the often underestimated morbidity that accompanies reconstructive procedures such as colostomy closure [13, 14].

The need for subsequent intervention must be carefully and explicitly addressed by the surgeon at the time of the initial intervention, and may well change as developments in nonsurgical therapy occur. For example, although definitive antiulcer therapy (a vagotomy and drainage procedure, with or without a gastric resection) can be safely performed in many patients undergoing operation for perforated peptic ulcer, proton pump inhibitors, and an understanding of the role played by *H. pylori* in the pathogenesis of acid pepsin disease have largely elimi-nated the need for surgical management, and most patients can be managed with patch closure only, followed by medical therapy – or even without operative in-tervention.

Late Reconstructive Procedures

Surgical intervention to control infection raises the probability that the patient will require subsequent reconstructive procedures before returning to optimal health. Such procedures commonly include the closure of stomas and the repair of abdominal wall hernias; abdominal fistulae are less common, although their treatment typically commits the patient to a prolonged course away from work and normal activities of daily living. It is important for the surgeon to consider the need for such subsequent reconstructive procedures in devising a therapeutic plan at the time of the initial intervention.

The morbidity of complex infection arises not only during the initial infectious episode, but also during subsequent reconstructive interventions [15]. This late morbidity can be minimized if the surgeon consciously plans for the future at the time of the initial intervention. Stomas, when created, should be sited so that their closure is facilitated. Bringing both ends of defunctioned intestine out through the same stoma site can greatly facilitate subsequent stoma closure.

Alternatively, a proximal loop ileostomy protecting an anastomosis is substantially easier to close than the end colostomy and pelvic pouch created during a Hartmann procedure.

Selection of Procedure

The primary objective of source control intervention is to eliminate the potential for a focus of infection to serve as a portal of entry for bacteria and bacterial products. Excision or exteriorization of the focus of infection will generally accomplish this goal, and the optimal choice is the one that is the simplest and safest – typically percutaneous drainage or superficial debridement. An infectious process that is poorly localized, or inaccessible to percutaneous techniques, will be best managed surgically. Similarly, soft-tissue infections with a virulent course call for immediate and aggressive surgical debridement.

Once the focus of infection has been controlled, definitive management of the source of contamination can be approached in a more deliberate, and even elective, manner. Percutaneous drainage of an appendiceal abscess, for example, usually controls the infectious process and permits the surgeon to plan delayed therapy in the form of an interval appendectomy. When control of the infection is accomplished operatively, these definitive procedures should be undertaken simultaneously, if inflammation is minimal, and the physiologic status of the patient permits a longer procedure. If there is extensive inflammation, definitive therapy may carry a higher risk of complications such as anastomotic leak.

Summary

These principles can be used to guide the decision-making process for the patient presented at the beginning of the chapter. Resuscitation and stabilization is the most urgent priority, superseding any consideration of source control intervention. This has been accomplished, and we have been able to characterize the problem anatomically with a CT scan, that shows diverticulitis and a diverticular abscess. While expectant observation with antibiotics is a possible option here, it is not the best, for it will be slow, and carries the risk that the abscess may rupture into the free peritoneal cavity. A much better option in a stable patient is percutaneous drainage of the abscess, followed later by an elective sigmoid resection with primary anastomosis. Resection is another option, but requires immediate surgical intervention with its potential risks in a sick patient, and may result in contamination of the peritoneal cavity. On the other hand, if the clinical or radiographic findings suggest that the infectious process is not localized to the left lower quadrant, operative intervention with sigmoid resection will be more effective in achieving source control than percutaneous drainage.

References

1. Christou NV, Barie PS, Dellinger EP, Waymack JP, Stone HH (1993) Surgical Infection Society intra-abdominal infection study. Prospective evaluation of management techniques and outcome. Arch Surg 128:193–198
2. Jimenez MF, Marshall JC (2001) Source control in the management of sepsis. Intensive Care Med 27:S49–S62
3. Gerzof SG, Robbins AH, Johnson WC, Birkett DH, Nabseth DC (1981) Percutaneous catheter drainage of abdominal abscesses: a five year experience. N Engl J Med 305:653–657
4. vanSonnenberg E, Wittich GR, Goodacre BW, Casola G, D'Agostino HB (2001) Percutaneous abscess drainage: update. World J Surg 25:362–372
5. Kok KY, Yapp SK (2000) Laparoscopic drainage of postoperative complicated intra-abdominal abscesses. Surg Laparosc Endosc Percutan Tech 10:311–313
6. Lin JC, Hazelrigg SR, Landrenau RJ (2000) Video-assisted thoracic surgery for diseases within the mediastinum. Surg Clin North Am 80:1511–1533
7. Pamoukian VN, Gagner M (2001) Laparoscopic necrosectomy for acute necrotizing pancreatitis. J Hepatobiliary Pancreat Surg 8:221–223
8. Spain DA, Martin RC, Carrillo EH, Polk HC, Jr (1997) Twelfth rib resection: preferred therapy for subphrenic abscess in selected surgical patients. Arch Surg 132:1203–1206
9. McHenry CR, Piotrowski JJ, Petrinic D, Malangoni MA (1995) Determinants of mortality for necrotizing soft-tissue infections. Ann Surg 221:558–565
10. Elliott DC, Kufera JA, Myers RAM (1996) Necrotizing soft tissue infections – risk factors for mortality and strategies for management. Ann Surg 224:672–683
11. Mier J, Leon EL, Castillo A, Robledo F, Blanco R (1997) Early versus late necrosectomy in severe necrotizing pancreatitis. Am J Surg 173:71–75
12. Umbach TW, Dorazio RA (1999) Primary resection and anastomosis for perforated left colon lesions. Am Surg 65:931–933
13. Edwards DP, Leppington-Clarke A, Sexton R, Heald RJ, Moran BJ (2001) Stoma-related complications are more frequent after transverse colostomy than loop ileostomy: a prospective randomized clinical trial. Br J Surg 88:360–363
14. Shellito PC (1998) Complications of abdominal stoma surgery. Dis Col Rect 41:1562–1572
15. Hackam DJ, Rotstein OD (1995) Stoma closure and wound infection: an evaluation of risk factors. Can J Surg 38:144–148

Invited Commentary

RHONDA S. FISHEL, ADRIAN BARBUL

> Come gather around surgeons wherever you roam
> And admit that your treatment options have grown
> And accept that surgery does not stand alone
> There is a battle for your patient and it's ragin'
> The decision to cut is no longer cast in stone
> Because the times, they are a changin'
> *(With apologies to Bob Dylan)*

As the opportunities to use our manual prowess as surgeons have declined, the need for superior judgment has been enhanced. Although our patient care goals remain the same, the means to get there are continuously evolving. To the extent that we embrace this concept, our role in patient care will be maintained. Naturally, there are still patients for whom surgery is the first line of treatment. Further, we serve often to correct complications or salvage treatment failures of other modalities. Nonetheless, the more limited role for surgery in the management of many inflammatory and infectious processes has occurred because of advancement in several areas.

Diagnostic Advancements

"The skin should never stand between you and the diagnosis." These words, passed from generation to generation of surgeons, must now be modified. The field of radiology, with its expanding armamentarium of studies, has offered increasing accuracy in the diagnosis of infection and inflammation. In addition to plain films (with or without fluoroscopy), we have ultrasound, magnetic resonance imaging (MRI), tagged white blood cell scans, and of course computerized tomography (CT). CT is available in most locations, day or night, work day or holiday, with images a surgeon can read and that can be electronically sent to the home of the radiologist. The studies provide information that heretofore was only available by laparotomy. CT scan is exquisitely sensitive in demonstrating free intra-abdominal air, as well as showing pancreatitis, mesenteric stranding, intestinal leakage, bowel obstruction, and gas-containing soft-tissue collections in the abdomen and beyond. CT scan is reasonably, but not completely, accurate in separating phlegmon from drainable abscess. As with other effective, readily available techniques, CT scan is highly overused. "If you build it, they will come" has never been more true. We worry that CT scan has come to replace a good physical examination and evaluation using simpler studies. For example, a patient with a rigid abdomen and free air under the diaphragm does not need a confirmatory abdominal CT. Likewise, a young man with diffuse abdominal pain localizing to the right lower quadrant, fever, McBurney's point tenderness, and an elevated white blood count, might be able to go to the operating room without a scan. A flocculent abscess from skin popping an illicit substance is just that, and can be drained based on exam alone.

Percutaneous Drainage

"There is no body cavity that cannot be reached with a number 14 needle and a good strong arm" – The Fat Man, *House of God* [1]. Of course we would scoff today at the Braille-like approach of the Fat Man. First described in the mid-1970s, percutaneous drainage of infection has virtually supplanted open drainage of loculated deep collections [2-4]. This technique is generally effective for single or multiple abscesses, may be used in the abdomen, chest, retroperitoneum, or pelvis, and is performed via either CT or ultrasound guidance. In some cases, aspiration alone will suffice; however, if the collection is large, or associated with an ongoing source of leakage, a catheter will be left in place. It is most interesting that, in many circumstances, this technique alone provides adequate treatment of an abscess. This goes in the face of the long held surgical principle of abscess drainage which states that the infected cavities need to be opened widely and kept packed until they heal from the bottom up.

Percutaneous Drainage Is Particularly Useful in Several Circumstances

An abscess is present following the perforation of a piece of bowel such as a diverticular process (as discussed by the authors in this chapter) or an appendiceal abscess. Assuming the process is localized, percutaneous drainage allows the process to cool down, and surgery to take place electively rather than emergently. As Drs. Papia and Marshall note, this would permit a one stage procedure for the treatment of diverticulitis with primary anastomosis, likely obviating the need for a colostomy. In the case of a critically ill patient, percutaneous drainage, even if only providing temporary control of infection, can be performed using local anesthetic which is better tolerated than the general or regional anesthetic required for surgery. A postoperative patient with an abscess from an ongoing bowel leak benefits from percutaneous drainage to allow localization of the process and adequate control of the infection/inflammation by creating a controlled fistula. The alternative to this would be to return to the operating room at a time when the abdomen will show pronounced inflammation. The risk of further bowel injury in that setting is not insignificant, nor is the potential for heavy blood loss. Urgent operative intervention would thus be limited to the patient with diffuse peritonitis.

Improved Understanding of the Behavior of Certain Disease Processes

"Oh, they ask the same questions every year, it is just that the answers change." – preparing residents to take the Board Exams. For the most part, we are treating the same surgical inflammations and infections as we have done for years, it is the role of surgery in this process that has evolved. Pancreatitis is a case in point. Surgeons have had a love/hate relationship with this disease for years. The pendulum has swung from never operating, to the notion that everyone benefits from surgery, to the daily look and debridement (with or without zipper), to the wait and see approach [5]. This latter strategy involves such frequent trips to CT scan, that there are often grooves carved in the floor between the patient's bed and the scanner. As abscesses are found they are drained percutaneously. If abundant pancreatic tissue becomes necrotic, a one-time necrosectomy is performed, although now some surgeons are advocating surgical debridement only if the necrotic collection is infected [6]. If the disease has changed it is only in the context that ICU care has generally allowed us to keep even the sickest pancreatitis patient alive. We appreciate the raging fire and subsequent smoldering of the process better. We realize that we do not have much of a hose, just the ability for support, prevention of treatable causes such as gallstones, and clean up. Does this mean that the surgeon should abdicate his or her role in the management of pancreatitis? Not at all, we just have to be more cognizant of when we should use the weapons that we have.

There remains a crucial role for surgery to play in the management of inflammatory processes and infection. The role has two arms, which we think are equally important. The first and perhaps most obvious is the ongoing need for surgical intervention. At least today, the treatment of diffuse peritonitis is still surgical exploration, generally via laparotomy, though in selected cases the use of laparoscopy may be sufficient and efficacious. Simple appendicitis, chronic diverticulitis, and cholecystitis should, under most circumstances, be treated operatively and definitively. The risk of infarcted small bowel from obstruction, volvulus, or mesenteric ischemia merits surgical exploration as there is no diagnostic test which is specific and sensitive for these diagnoses. Obvious soft-tissue abscesses, fasciitis, and myonecrosis are certainly best managed surgically. Many a life and limb have been lost by prolonged antibiotic management in the absence of surgical intervention. Although the operation required is frequently dramatic, such as amputation, it may well be life saving. We have all witnessed the elaborate dance with the latest technology that takes place before some of our medical colleagues will call us to care for a clearly surgical problem.

The second arm of our role in the management of these patients is sometimes more subtle and has to do with judgment. Each disease process occurs in the context of a patient complete with co-morbidities of varying significance, which forces us to consider every case individually. The enthusiasm for the big operation for the big problem becomes tempered over time as we care for the calamities we create. We occasionally have to accept the standby position while methods less invasive are utilized, and be prepared to intervene if these are unsuccessful or attendant with complications. (While the invasive radiologists have been most helpful to us, their procedures may be complicated by bleeding or bowel perforation which they cannot repair.) The reward becomes the outcome and not the operation. If we acknowledge that uncontrolled infection and/or inflammation results in the release of cytokines and other mediators which will instigate organ dysfunction and potentially organ failure, it would follow that rapid, decisive control of infection would be desirable. We believe that the surgeon remains the ideal physician to manage this process. We are most adept at aggressive resuscitation which is often crucial in these patients, and we can act decisively when warranted. We can recognize most quickly the success or failure of a treatment modality, and can provide the big fix if necessary and deal with its sequelae. Although our role has changed in character, it remains ever important.

References

1. Shem S (1978) The house of God. Dell Publishing, New York
2. Gerzof SG, Robbins AH, Johnson WC, Birkett DH, Nabseth DC (1981) Percutaneous catheter drainage of abdominal abscesses: a five year experience. N Engl J Med 305:653–657
3. Boland GW, Meuller PR (1996) An update on abscess drainage. Semin Inter Rad 25:27–34
4. Ferruci JT, Meuller PR (1985) Catheter drainage of abdominal abscesses and fluid collections: indications, technique and instrumentation. In: Ferruci JT, Wittenberg J, Mueller PR (eds) Interventional radiology of the abdomen, 2nd edn. William & Wilkins, Baltimore, pp 109–139
5. Baron TH, Morgan DE (1999) Acute necrotizing pancreatitis. N Engl J Med 340:1412–1417
6. Büchler MW, Gloor B, Müller CA, Friess H, Seiler CA, Uhl W (2000) Acute necrotizing pancreatitis: treatment strategy according to the status of infection. Ann Surg 232:619–626

9 Consequences of Failed Source Control

Philip S. Barie, Soumitra R. Eachempati

Key Principles

- Failure of source control is more important than "antibiotic failure" in defining the outcome of surgical infections in general and intra-abdominal infections in particular.
- Source control of an intra-abdominal infection may fail because of a poor choice of operation, or the correct operation performed poorly or with poor timing.
- Leaving the abdomen open is a viable (and often necessary) adjunct to surgical management of recurrent intra-abdominal infection.
- Systemic consequences of failed source control include nosocomial infections, nutritional and metabolic disorders, and multiple organ dysfunction syndrome.

Introduction

Failure of source control is a particular problem in those infections, for example intra-abdominal infections and necrotizing soft tissue infections, where a surgical procedure of some kind (e.g., celiotomy, debridement, percutaneous drainage) is central to the management of the infection. Some clinical features of failed source control are generic to the problem of sepsis and a dysregulated host response, whereas other features are specific complications of the underlying infection.

Hypovolemia, carbohydrate intolerance, and organ dysfunction are examples of generic adverse consequences, whereas abdominal compartment syndrome, enterocutaneous fistula, and amputation are examples of specific consequences. Some complications may be interrelated, such as organ dysfunction related to abdominal compartment syndrome, or necrotizing fasciitis that develops in an abdominal incision. Considering that the large majority of cases of failed source control will occur in the treatment of complicated intra-abdominal infections, this discussion is oriented toward the peritoneal cavity.

General Approach to Failed Source Control: Intra-abdominal Infection

It is fortunate that surgical intervention for intra-abdominal infection is usually successful, because the consequences of failure are grave, and include the possibility of death [1]. Some complications arise from the recurrent infection itself, whereas others are clearly iatrogenic. The magnitude of the morbidity of failed source control may also be related to the timeliness of reintervention, which, in turn, is dependent upon a high index of suspicion and rapid diagnosis.

Uncontrolled infection will spread and the progression can sometimes be rapid, because coincident tissue ischemia is commonplace. An infection may become generalized within the peritoneal cavity because of the combined effects of failure of peritoneal host defenses [2], and proteases elaborated by pathogens, or because of an initial source control procedure that contaminates previously uninfected loci. Contamination can occur as a result of open procedures or percutaneous drainage; for example, with the latter, the catheter may inadvertently transit an adjacent hollow viscus, or may rupture a thin-walled collection as it is being punctured. Similarly, leakage may occur along the tract of the catheter.

Infection can invade natural tissue planes, but it may also take advantage of surgically created planes, for example, a contiguous surgical incision. The *surgical incision* is invariably contaminated by bacteria after an abdominal operation for infection; depending on the type and extent of the infection and whether the incision is closed completely, the infection rate may be 30 % or higher [3]. A surgical site infection therefore is not necessarily a manifestation of failed source control. Conversely, however, failure of source control, with the potential for ongoing contamination of the wound, is a risk factor for the development of necrotizing infection of the wound. Necrotizing soft tissue infection is a devastating complication, because the need for surgical debridement may result in tissue loss sufficient to preclude wound closure even after the infection itself is controlled. Both patient and surgeon must then contend with all of the potential complications of an open abdomen, including fluid and protein losses, gut dysmotility, enterocutaneous fistula, and evisceration (early), or herniation (late, after skin grafting has closed the wound) [4].

Rarely an uncontrolled infection can *erode into other intra-abdominal structures*. Examples include cholecystic abscess eroding into the liver, peritoneal intracavitary abscess eroding into an adjacent hollow viscus, and infection (especially from enzyme-rich purulent fluid in necrotizing pancreatitis) that erodes into a splanchnic vessel, causing sudden, massive hemorrhage. Although a gallbladder infection may involve the liver prior to initial presentation, it is rare for erosion of a viscus or major vessel to occur unless the infection was missed or mismanaged. Exceptions include localized infection caused by a perforated tumor, for example, a carcinoma of the colon, or an inflammatory process such as sigmoid diverticulitis that erodes into the bladder or vagina.

Perforation can occur from progressive disease within the inciting focus, or from erosion of adjacent structures (which may become adherent as a result of attempts at self-containment). Perforation may also occur after the failure of an intestinal anastomosis, or as a result of an iatrogenic injury to bowel sustained during surgery. If the perforation occurs freely within the peritoneal cavity, generalized peritonitis is the result, whereas a contained perforation usually causes an abscess. A fistula is more likely to occur when an infected hollow viscus perforates into an adherent hollow viscus than from erosion of an intermediary abscess.

The *surgical procedures necessary to regain control of an infection have numerous inherent complications*. Percutaneous drainage procedures can rupture an abscess, leading to bacteremia or generalized peritonitis [5]. Drainage may be inadequate, or the catheter may puncture another organ during insertion. If a perforation communicates freely with the abscess, a fistula may result along the track of the catheter. Also, infection may persist until devitalized tissues are debrided or resected. However, the complications of percutaneous drainage are generally fewer and less severe than those of formal open drainage, so percutaneous drainage is reasonable to undertake should circumstances permit.

Open drainage usually requires a formal transabdominal approach. Selected cases, such as liver abscess or psoas abscess, or other types of retroperitoneal abscess (except for peripancreatic infections) may be amenable to a localized extraperitoneal surgical approach. Otherwise, a transperitoneal approach will be necessary, with the consequence that catabolism, insulin resistance [6], and third-space fluid losses will be accentuated. Usually, the original incision will need to be reopened, and extensive debridement of the wound may be necessary. Intra-abdominal dissection may be extensive and difficult, and the risk of hemorrhage and iatrogenic intestinal injury is increased [7]. An intestinal stoma may be necessary to protect a tenuous anastomosis, or divert the fecal stream when resection or anastomosis is not possible. At best, stoma creation requires yet another operation to restore gut continuity, but stomas have their own complications. If perfusion or healing is poor they may retract, dehisce, or infarct. Retraction or nearby hardware (e.g., retention sutures) may result in an ill-fitting appliance, continuous wound soilage, and persistent infection. Peristomal hernias are common; stricture at the level of the fascia is possible. Ileostomies are prone to fluid and electrolyte derangements and local skin irritation.

It may not be possible or desirable to close the abdomen at the conclusion of an open drainage procedure, although the use of open abdomen approaches remains controversial. If the fascia is closed, the closure may fail, resulting in dehiscence or evisceration, or intra-abdominal hypertension may lead to *abdominal compartment syndrome* [8, 9]. Normal intra-abdominal pressure is less than 5 cm H_2O, and can be measured easily by instillation of 50 ml saline into the bladder. When intra-abdominal pressure exceeds 20-25 cm H_2O, which may occur secondary to edema or packing, renal vein obstruction can lead to oliguria and an elevated diaphragm can cause decreased lung volumes and compliance. Uncorrected, overt renal or respiratory failure may ensue. Correction may be achieved as simply as paracentesis (if tense ascites is the cause), but often the incision must be reopened.

The *open abdomen* poses several challenges, including maintaining the right of domain of the viscera, preventing evisceration and dessication, promoting drainage and peritoneal toilet, and minimizing fluid and protein losses [4]. These goals may conflict, since an artificial barrier of some sort is necessary to keep the viscera in place. If the barrier is impermeable, fluid retention is enhanced but toilet may be impaired. Many variations of permeable (mesh) and impermeable barrier dressings may be employed with or without suction. The general principles are to keep adherent surfaces such as gauze or permanent mesh away from serosa to minimize injury, to maintain peritoneal toilet without undue disturbance of the underlying viscera, and to avoid closing the abdomen prematurely so as to avoid recreation of the conditions that required the abdomen to be opened in the first place. An abdominal wall hernia is a certain consequence if the abdomen must be left open for more than a week or two, and is likely even if early closure is possible.

Ileus and intestinal obstruction may occur with either an open or closed abdomen. Ileus can result from exposure, repeated handling, or fluid/electrolyte abnormalities, especially low serum potassium, calcium, or magnesium concentrations, while obstruction is caused by inflammatory adhesions or adhesions to abdominal wall prostheses. Either will make patients intolerant of enteral feedings and increase the risk of bacterial overgrowth, possible bacterial translocation, and aspiration of gastric contents.

General Approach to Failed Source Control: Soft Tissue Infection

Necrotizing soft tissue infections present insidiously but often progress rapidly, making timely diagnosis and therapy (surgical debridement and antibiotics) a challenging imperative [10, 11]. Initial debridement must extend to ostensibly normal tissue, and reoperations with daily wound inspections are necessary until the progression has been arrested. Whereas local wound care is paramount, the surgeon must also be alert to the possibility of an intra-abdominal source. For example, soft tissue infections caused by *Clostridium septicum* may result from an occult perforation of a colon carcinoma [12], whereas a retroperitoneal perforation of a colon tumor may present as a necrotizing infection of the thigh if the infection extends along an iliopsoas muscle. Progression of a soft tissue infection invariably results in increased tissue loss, and may necessitate amputation. Physical deformity and functional disability are highly likely, if the patient survives (see Chap. 22).

Nonspecific Consequences of Failed Source Control

Systemic Inflammatory Response Syndrome

The common manifestation of inadequate source control is persistence or recurrence of signs of infection. The systemic inflammatory response syndrome (SIRS) may persist for a few days after successful surgical intervention for intra-abdominal infection, [13]. Indeed, the resolution of fever and leukocytosis is a time-honored (albeit controversial) end point for the duration of antibiotic therapy [14]. However, suspicion should be high for persistence or recurrence of uncontrolled infection when SIRS is present more than 96 h after the initial source control procedure. Persistent SIRS is associated with increased morbidity and mortality from multiple organ dysfunction syndrome (MODS) [13]. This association may be a result of the adverse consequences of persistent fever and tachycardia in patients with coronary artery disease. Alternatively, it has been hypothesized that the development of a compensatory anti-inflammatory response syndrome (CARS) [15] may lead to an increased risk of subsequent nosocomial infection.

Hypovolemia, Ischemia, and Reperfusion

Cytokine-mediated interactions between neutrophils and endothelial cells lead to increased microvascular permeability, with tissue exudation and fluid accumulation both systemically and locally in the peritoneal cavity. Similar mechanisms result in systemic vasodilatation and left ventricular dysfunction. In aggregate, hypovolemia can be pronounced, and delayed resuscitation may lead to tissue ischemia. Organs that are especially susceptible to ischemia are the kidneys and the gastrointestinal viscera, including the liver, gallbladder, pancreas, and colon, although cardiac and skeletal muscle are also susceptible. Resuscitation reintroduces oxygen to the ischemic microenvironment and can superimpose an oxidant injury [16].

The consequences of large-volume fluid resuscitation include hypoalbuminemia, anemia, tissue edema sufficient to preclude wound closure, compartment syndrome (abdominal or extremity), and fluid overload with cardiopulmonary dysfunction. Compartment syndromes require surgical decompression. Fluid overload syndromes may require diuretic therapy with the risk of hypokalemia, alkalosis, hypovolemia, and ototoxicity; or renal replacement therapy, risking vascular access complications, hemodynamic instability, and neurotoxicity.

Nutritional/Metabolic Complications

Although hypoalbumenia is partly dilutional and partly due to downregulation of albumin synthesis as part of the acute phase response, and therefore not a valid marker of nutritional compromise, malnutrition and metabolic derangements are commonplace. Patients with severe peritonitis, an open abdomen, or a gastrointestinal fistula may be intolerant of tube feedings. Moreover, sepsis syndrome and elective surgical interventions are associated with insulin resistance. Hyperglycemia may result in hypovolemia from osmotic diuresis, and in severe cases, ketoacidosis or decreased mental status. Hyperglycemia may also be associated with an increased incidence of nosocomial infection.

Nosocomial Infection

Nosocomial infection may develop at the surgical site or the remote site. Patients with inadequate source control are at particular risk because the surgical site will be disrupted by the reintervention, or a new surgical site will be created. Each time a natural epithelial barrier such as the epidermis is disrupted, the risk of infection is increased. For the same reason central venous catheters and endotracheal tubes pose an increased risk of nosocomial infection.

Nosocomial infections at an abdominal surgical site may be caused by the original infecting pathogen, or by nosocomial flora such as methicillin-resistant *S. aureus,* multidrug resistant enteric Gram-negative bacilli (e.g., *Enterobacteriaceae, Pseudomonas aeruginosa*), enterococci, and yeast. Superinfection of necrotizing soft tissue infections by opportunistic organisms may also occur, particularly if the exposed soft tissue is extensive and wound care is challenging (see Chap. 28).

The patient with inadequate source control is also at risk for nosocomial infection remote from the surgical site. Pneumonia is common, and is related to the duration of mechanical ventilation and to previous antibiotic use. In general surgical ICUs in the United States, the incidence of ventilator-associated pneumonia is more than 14 cases per 1,000 ventilator-days [3, 17]. S. aureus is the most prevalent pathogen (20 %), and methicillin-resistant strains cause one-half of the cases. P. aeruginosa causes nearly as many nosocomial pneumonias as do staphylococci. Mortality ranges from 35 % to 70 %, depending on the pathogen and its susceptibility. Catheter-related bloodstream infections are less common but equally dangerous. The incidence of catheter-related bloodstream infections in US surgical ICUs is more than 5 cases per 1,000 indwelling catheter-days [3]. The most common pathogen is S. epidermidis (85 % methicillin-resistant), S. aureus, and enterococci (25 % vancomycin-resistant). Mortality ranges from 30 % to 40 %.

Tertiary (nosocomial) peritonitis is another manifestation of failed source control that deserves mention [18]. Some investigators consider tertiary peritonitis to be a failure of peritoneal host defense mechanisms with colonization of the peritoneal cavity rather than an invasive infection [19], although inadequate source control almost invariably contributes to its development. Adhesions are extensive, but fluid collections are walled-off poorly. Individual loops of bowel may be so matted together as to be indistinct, and exposure of solid viscera may be very difficult. The fluid is often serosanguineous rather than purulent, white blood cell function is impaired, and exudate cannot form. Isolated organisms include opportunistic pathogens such as S. epidermidis, P. aeruginosa, enterococci, and yeast. Antimicrobial therapy may be less important than the restoration of peritoneal toilet, which must be accomplished mechanically. Rather than repetitive opening of the incision, it may be advantageous to leave the incision open and provide daily peritoneal toilet at the bedside under intravenous analgesia and sedation [19] (see Chap. 35).

A common risk factor for all nosocomial infections is antibiotic use. Each subsequent course of antibiotics increases the risk of a drug-resistant superinfection, making prompt recognition and intervention, and minimization of antibiotic treatment the cornerstones of successful therapy. Antibiotics that have been associated with the emergence of multidrug resistant pathogens include metronidazole [20, 21], third-generation cephalosporins (especially ceftazidime) [22-24], and vancomycin [24]; it is especially important to use these drugs sparingly.

Clostridium difficile-associated colitis typically develops as a result of antibiotic therapy, and may cause systemic inflammation and toxicity. The diagnosis can be difficult because diarrhea may be absent, presenting signs may be nonspecific, or the disease may be mistaken for worsening of the infection being treated initially. For example, antibiotic-associated colitis that complicates the nonoperative management of diverticulitis can appear to be worsening of the diverticulitis. Severe antibiotic-associated colitis can lead to colonic necrosis and perforation, with superimposed bacterial peritonitis.

Multiple Organ Dysfunction Syndrome

Almost every patient with failed source control will have some degree of multiple organ dysfunction syndrome (MODS), and death from uncontrolled infection is invariably associated with MODS. The pathogenesis of MODS is complex and incompletely understood, but certain features are relevant to the consequences of failed source control. It is likely that several different mechanisms interact synergistically to produce organ injury. Ischemia/reperfusion can contribute to both local and remote organ injury [25]. Activation of the proinflammatory response mediated by cytokines, chemokines, eicosanoids, adhesion molecules, coagulation factors, and reactive oxygen and nitrogen intermediates can disrupt and occlude the microcirculation [26]. Disrupted signal transduction and deranged intercellular communications may lead to dysautonomia and pathologic responses to hypovolemia, shock, and resuscitation. Regardless of the precise mechanism the response is characteristic and somewhat stereotypical, although it does not manifest identically in each patient. Although there are many methods to quantify MODS, the manifestations are fairly consistent, in varying degrees one or more of hemodynamic instability (cardiovascular), stupor/coma (central nervous system), thrombocytopenia (coagulation), cholestasis (hepatic), hypoxemia (pulmonary), and azotemia (renal). The risks of prolonged hospitalization, recurrent nosocomial infections, and death are directly related to the numbers of organs affected, and especially high-grade dysfunction of several organs [27]. It is difficult to interdict organ dysfunction once established even by regaining source control. Organ dysfunction can be progressive even in patients in whom source control has been achieved [28]. The best treatment is prevention in the form of timely and effective resuscitation and rapid resolution of the SIRS response by initial, definitive source control.

References

1. Christou NV, Barie PS, Dellinger EP, et al (1993) Surgical Infection Society intra-abdominal infection study. Prospective evaluation of management techniques and outcome. Arch Surg 128:193–198
   This prospective, open, consecutive, nonrandomized trial examined management techniques and outcome in 239 patients with severe peritonitis and an APACHE II score greater than 10. Forty-six patients underwent one reoperation; 15, two reoperations; 10, three reoperations; five, four reoperations; and seven, five reoperations. Seventy-seven patients (32%) died. Reoperation had a 42% mortality rate (35 of 83 patients died) compared with a 27% mortality rate (42 of 156 died) in patients who did not undergo reoperation. There was no difference in mortality between patients treated with a "closed-abdomen technique" (31% mortality) and those treated with variations of the "open-abdomen" technique (44% mortality). A low serum albumin level, youth, and a high APACHE II score were independently associated with reoperation, whereas a high APACHE II score, low serum albumin concentration, and high New York Heart Association cardiac function status were independently associated with death.
2. Solomkin JS, Wittman DH, West MA, Barie PS (1999) Intra-abdominal infections. In: Schwartz SI, Shires GT, Spencer FC, et al (eds) Principles of Surgery, 7th edn. McGraw-Hill, New York, pp 1515–1550
   This is a current and comprehensive review of the pathophysiology and management of intra-abdominal infections.)

3. National Nosocomial Infections Surveillance (NNIS) (1999) System report, data summary from January 1990 to May 1999, issued June 1999. Am J Infect Control 27:520–532
   These data are updated annually, and represent infectious isolates from more than 320 American hospitals of various types. The database is managed by the Centers for Disease Control and Prevention.
4. Kriwanek S, Armbruster C, Dittrich K, et al (1998) Long-term outcome after open treatment of severe intra-abdominal infection and pancreatic necrosis. Arch Surg 133:140–144
   Open treatment was used for 147 patients with pancreatic necrosis, severe intra-abdominal infections due to benign diseases, and infections due to malignant neoplasm. All 92 surviving patients were followed up. The effective costs of treatment per surviving patient (including restorative surgery) were calculated, and postdischarge medical treatment, degree of - recovery, functional state, and employment status were assessed. The effective costs per survivor studied were $175,000 for patients with pancreatitis and $232,400 for the other patients. Most patients experienced good long-term results. Employment status was unchanged for 69 (75%) of the patients, the functional state was unchanged for 81 (88%) of the patients, and 75% described their quality of life as good. Open treatment of severe intra-abdominal infection and pancreatic necrosis is a cost-effective treatment with good long-term results for most patients.
5. Holley DT, McGrath PC, Sloan DA (1994) Necrotizing fasciitis as a complication of percutaneous catheter drainage of an intra-abdominal abscess. Am Surg 60:197–199
   The authors reported a case of necrotizing fasciitis complicating percutaneous drainage of a postoperative intra-abdominal abscess. This potentially fatal complication illustrates that successful percutaneous drainage of an abscess does not eliminate the need to closely monitor the patient's subsequent clinical course.
6. Thorell A, Nygren J, Ljungqvist O. Insulin resistance: a marker of surgical stress (1999) Curr Opin Clin Nutr Metab Care 2:69–78
   Surgery causes a marked, transient reduction in insulin sensitivity. The degree of the reduction is related to the magnitude of the operation. The type and duration of surgery performed, perioperative blood loss, and also the degree of postoperative insulin resistance have significant influences on the length of hospital stay. It is not clear which mediators are the most important for the development of insulin resistance after surgery. Nevertheless, marked insulin resistance can develop after elective surgery without concomitant elevations in cortisol, catecholamines, or glucagon. The main sites for insulin resistance seem to be extrahepatic tissues, probably skeletal muscle, where preliminary data suggest that the glucose transporting system is involved. A novel approach to minimize insulin resistance after surgery is presented. The authors suggest that simply pretreating the elective surgical patient with sufficient amounts of carbohydrates instead of fasting can significantly reduce postoperative insulin resistance.
7. Stone HH, Mullins RJ, Dunlop WE, Strom PR (1984) Extraperitoneal versus transperitoneal drainage of the intra-abdominal abscess. Surg Gynecol Obstet 159:549–552
   Controversy as to whether intra-abdominal abscesses should be drained extraperitoneally or through formal laparotomy was raging at the time of publication of this classic article, as percutaneous drainage was not yet accepted widely. A prospective study of each method enrolled 60 patients. With the transperitoneal approach, five patients had hollow viscus injury, whereas seven eventually had an intestinal fistula develop. Seven patients drained transperitoneally had additional abscesses discovered, and another operation was required to drain at least one subsequent abscess in seven patients. With the extraperitoneal route, only two patients needed reoperation to drain another abscess. Best results were noted with abscess identification through computerized tomography followed by an extraperitoneal drainage procedure.
8. Shapiro MB, Jenkins DH, Schwab CW, Rotondo MF (2000) Damage control: collective review J Trauma 49:969–978
   These authors, among the first to popularize the concept of limited abdominal surgery in the unstable patient, followed by a return to the operating room to complete the procedure once the patient has been stabilized, have provided a clear description of the techniques they employ and the pitfalls that must be avoided.
9. Sugerman HJ, Bloomfield GL, Saggi BW (1999) Multisystem organ failure secondary to increased intra-abdominal pressure. Infection 27:61–66

Acutely increased intra-abdominal pressure can lead to multisystem organ dysfunction. The diagnosis is made clinically in a patient with high peak inspiratory pressures, oliguria and an apparently tight abdomen, although urinary bladder pressure $\geq$ 20 cm H_2O is suggestive. Once the diagnosis is made, the patient's abdomen should be opened and the tension relieved. The intestinal contents need to be protected and evaporative water loss minimized by either closing the skin and not the fascia or, if this is not possible, using an impermeable protective dressing. If the abdomen is difficult to close at the primary operation, it is best to prevent the development of an acute abdominal compartment syndrome by closing only the skin or leaving it open and using an impermeable dressing.

10. Bertram P, Treutner KH, Stumpf M, Schumpelick V (2000) Postoperative necrotizing soft-tissue infections of the abdominal wall. Langenbecks Arch Surg 385:39–41
    The authors evaluated an aggressive surgical regimen for treatment of postoperative necrotizing soft tissue infection. Three of eight patients presented with generalized peritonitis. Cultures revealed polymicrobial infections in all eight patients. The mean interval between the primary operation and clinical symptoms of NSTI was 63 h. Three to six reoperations were required for in each patient. Temporary closure of the abdominal wall by absorbable mesh was used in six cases. Six patients survived, but the mean hospital stay was more than 110 days.)

11. McHenry CR, Piotrowski JJ, Petrinic D, Malangoni MA (1995) Determinants of mortality for necrotizing soft-tissue infections. Ann Surg 221:558–563
    The authors determined the risk factors for mortality in 65 patients with necrotizing soft tissue infections. Necrotizing soft tissue infections were polymicrobial in 45 patients (69%). *S. pyogenes* was isolated in only 17% of the NSTIs, but accounted for 53% of monomicrobial infections. Eight of ten idiopathic infections were caused by a single bacterium ($p = 0.0005$), whereas 82% of postoperative infections were polymicrobial. An average of 3.3 operative debridements per patient and amputation in 12 patients were necessary to control infection. The overall mortality was 29%. Early debridement of NSTI was associated with a significant decrease in mortality.

12. Leung FW, Serota AI, Mulligan ME, et al (1981) Nontraumatic clostridial myonecrosis: an infectious disease emergency. Ann Emerg Med 10:312–314
    Nontraumatic clostridial myonecrosis is a fulminant, usually fatal disease that is most often the result of bacteremia from an occult gastrointestinal lesion. Ulceration of the colon or terminal ileum is the most common predisposing condition, and is usually due to gastrointestinal or hematologic malignant tumor. Patients often present with nonspecific complaints, including fever and pain. The disease progresses rapidly to include bronze discoloration, edema, and hemorrhagic bullous lesions of the skin, subcutaneous emphysema, and myonecrosis. Favorable outcome depends on prompt institution of appropriate antimicrobial therapy and surgical debridement of involved soft tissues, as well as correction of the underlying disorder.

13. Talmor M, Hydo L, Barie PS (1999) Relationship of systemic inflammatory response syndrome to organ dysfunction, length of stay, and mortality in critical surgical illness: effect of intensive care unit resuscitation. Arch Surg 134:81–87
    A systemic proinflammatory response has been implicated in the pathogenesis of organ dysfunction. The effects of surgery, surgical stress, anesthesia, and subsequent intensive care unit resuscitation may affect the components of the systemic inflammatory response syndrome. Twenty-four hours of ICU resuscitation results in a decline in the SIRS score. The magnitude of the proinflammatory response on the second ICU day may be a useful predictor of outcome in critical surgical illness

14. Wittmann DH, Schein M (1996) Let us shorten antibiotic prophylaxis and therapy in surgery. Am J Surg 172(6A):26S–32S
    Excessive duration of antibiotics for prophylaxis and treatment of surgical infection appears to be the principal area of inappropriate administration in current surgical practice. The main factors to blame are the inability of the clinician to distinguish between contamination, infection, and inflammation. Failure to distinguish between contamination and infection is the reason that prophylaxis is unnecessarily carried through into the postoperative phase for prolonged periods. Failure to distinguish between infection and inflammation misguides surgeons to continue antibiotics for unnecessarily long treatment periods. Shortened courses of antibiotic administration should be utilized by tailoring the duration of administration to the intraoperative findings to shorten treatment courses.

15. Bone RC (1996) Sir Isaac Newton, sepsis, SIRS, and CARS. Crit Care Med 24:1125–1128
    In this article, the concept of a counter-regulatory anti-inflammatory response is espoused.
    But is it adequate to the task of counterbalancing inflammation, or immunosuppressive at a
    time when the patient is vulnerable to nosocomial infections?

16. Flowers F, Zimmerman JJ (1998) Reactive oxygen species in the cellular pathophysiology of
    shock. New Horiz 6:169–180
    Reactive oxygen species (ROS) mediate the fine balance between cellular physiology and patho-
    physiology. Accordingly it is not surprising that cellular redox homeostasis is disrupted by shock
    events related to ischemia-reperfusion and inflammation. ROS may initiate as well as amplify
    the shock cellular insult in a number of ways which include important contributions to inflam-
    mation as well as lytic and apoptotic cell death. In addition, ROS in the setting of shock represent
    important antecedents to cellular proliferation, differentiation, and adaptation by virtue of altered
    transcription and translation of antioxidant enzymes, stress proteins, and a variety of cytokines.
    It is likely that an eventual important biochemical therapeutic goal in the setting of shock will
    involve reestablishing cellular redox homeostasis not only to ensure cellular structural integri-
    ty, but also to reestablish normal secondary cellular signal transduction mechanisms.

17. Barie PS (2000) Importance, morbidity, and mortality of pneumonia in the surgical intensive
    care unit. Am J Surg 179[2A Suppl]:2S–7S
    Surgical patients are at high risk to develop nosocomial pneumonia, although an accurate
    diagnosis is difficult to make. *Staphylococcus aureus* and *Pseudomonas aeruginosa* are the
    most common pathogens, but *Acinetobacter* is emerging as an important pathogen. Because
    affected patients are often critically ill with multisystem pathology, it can be difficult to ascribe
    morbidity or mortality directly to the infection.

18. Malangoni MA (2000) Evaluation and management of tertiary peritonitis. Am Surg
    66:157–161
    Tertiary or recurrent peritonitis can occur after any operation for secondary bacterial
    peritonitis. The major risk factors for the development of tertiary peritonitis include mal-
    nutrition, a high APACHE II score, the presence of organisms resistant to antimicrobial
    therapy, and organ system failure. Most patients with tertiary peritonitis will have fever and
    leukocytosis, even though other signs of infection may be absent. The management of tertiary
    peritonitis should include the provision of appropriate physiologic support, the administra-
    tion of antimicrobial therapy, and operation or intervention to control the source of conta-
    mination and to decrease the bacterial load. Antibiotic-resistant organisms and bacteremia
    are present more commonly and mortality is greater in patients with tertiary peritonitis.
    Early recognition and effective intervention are critical to achieving a successful outcome.)

19. Wittmann DH (1998) Operative and nonoperative therapy of intra-abdominal infections.
    Infection 26:335–341
    The basic principles for treating intra-abdominal infections are to obliterate the infectious
    source, to purge bacteria and toxins, to maintain organ system function, and to suppress the
    inflammatory process. Operative and nonoperative treatment options are reviewed. The author
    is a major proponent of abdominostomy (leaving the abdomen open).

20. Donskey CJ, Chowdhry TK, Hecker MT, et al (2000) Effect of antibiotic therapy on the density
    of vancomycin-resistant enterococci in the stool of colonized patients. N Engl J Med
    2000;343:1925–1932
    For patients colonized with vancomycin-resistant enterococci in their stool, treatment with
    anti-anaerobic antibiotics promotes high-density colonization. Limiting the use of such
    agents in these patients may help decrease the spread of vancomycin-resistant enterococci.

21. Fry DE, Schermer CR (2000) The consequences of suppression of anaerobic bacteria. Surg
    Infect 1:49–56
    In this review, the authors argue that unnecessary suppression of anaerobic bacteria as a con-
    sequence of broad-spectrum antibiotic therapy may have several deleterious consequences
    for the patient.

22. Rice LB, Eckstein EC, deVente J, et al (1996) Ceftazidime-resistant *Klebsiella pneumoniae*
    isolates recovered at the Cleveland Veterans Affairs Medical Center. Clin Infect Dis 23:118–124
    The rate of ceftazidime resistance among *Klebsiella pneumoniae* isolates recovered from
    patients at the Cleveland Department of Veterans Affairs Medical Center increased markedly.

The outbreak was hospitalwide, with the highest rates of resistance occurring on wards where ceftazidime was administered most frequently. The addition of piperacillin/tazobactam to the hospital formulary and educational efforts focused on minimizing the administration of ceftazidime were associated with a marked decrease in the drug's use and a concomitant decrease in the percentage of ceftazidime-resistant isolates.

23. Fukatsu K, Saito H, Matsuda T, et al (1997) Influences of type and duration of antimicrobial prophylaxis on an outbreak of methicillin-resistant Staphylococcus aureus and on the incidence of wound infection. Arch Surg 132:1320–1325
    Overuse of third-generation cephalosporins for long periods caused an MRSA outbreak. Long-term prophylaxis did not lower infection rates. The briefest possible prophylaxis with first- or second-generation cephalosporins should be used in general surgery.

24. Dahms RA, Johnson EM, Statz CL, et al (1998) Third-generation cephalosporins and vancomycin as risk factors for postoperative vancomycin-resistant enterococcus infection. Arch Surg 133:1343–1346
    This matched control study showed that use of third-generation cephalosporins, alone or concurrently with vancomycin, was a risk factor for vancomycin-resistant enterococcal infection in surgical patients. Judicious administration of third-generation cephalosporins is warranted in surgical patients with other risk factors for vancomycin-resistant enterococcal infection.

25. Maier RV (2000) Pathogenesis of multiple organ dysfunction syndrome-endotoxin, inflammatory cells, and their mediators: Cytokines and reactive oxygen species. Surg Infect 1:197–206
    This is a succinct review of the evidence relating endotoxin, systemic activation of the inflammatory response, and organ dysfunction.

26. Cobb JP, Buchman TG, Karl IE, Hotchkiss RS (2000) Molecular biology of multiple organ dysfunction syndrome: injury, adaptation, and apoptosis. Surg Infect 1:207–216
    The authors describe succinctly their well-respected work on the regulation of programmed cell death and the consequences for inflammation and the survival of the host.

27. Barie PS, Hydo LJ (2000) Epidemiology of multiple organ dysfunction syndrome in critical surgical illness. Surg Infect 1:173–186
    The authors review their extensive experience with nearly 1,000 patients who developed multiple organ dysfunction syndrome.

28. Goris RJ, te Boekhorst TP, Nuytinck JK, Gimbrere JS (1985) Multiple-organ failure – generalized autodestructive inflammation? Arch Surg 120:1109–1115
    In this landmark study, the importance of bacterial sepsis was evaluated retrospectively in 55 trauma and 37 intra-abdominal-sepsis patients with multiple organ failure. The severity of organ failure was graded, and an analysis was made of day of onset, incidence, severity, sequence, and mortality of organ failures. No difference was found between groups in sequence, severity, or mortality of organ failures. It was concluded that sepsis is probably not the essential cause of organ failure. Instead, an alternative hypothesis is presented involving massive activation of inflammatory mediators by severe tissue trauma or intra-abdominal sepsis, resulting in systemic damage to vascular endothelia, permeability edema, and impaired oxygen availability to the mitochondria despite adequate arterial oxygen transport.

Invited Commentary

Arthur E. Baue

This book on source control in surgical infection has brought together all the movers and shakers in the Surgical Infection Society and the international surgical infection community. Barie and Eachempati use their extensive experience to fulfill very completely their assignment on the consequences of failed source control. They describe general approaches to failed source control, the abdominal complications with persistent peritonitis, the nonspecific consequences of failed source control, the development of SIRS, MODS, hypovolemia, ischemia, reperfusion injury and nutritional, metabolic complications. They provide an excellent review of the current problems in antibiotic use, resistant organisms and appropriate use of antibiotics. Then they discuss nosocomial infections, ventilator-associated pneumonia (VAP), vascular catheter infections, and other problems that are not specific to failed source control. Prolonged ICU stays, antibiotic usage and nosocomial infections have become real problems in ICUs everywhere.

What Do We Learn from All of This?

Certainly we learn about the problems of persistent infections in surgical patients. We also learn the jargon of the day. Surgeons over the age of 55 will learn the new terminology [1]. Younger surgeons will have grown up with it. It is different – but is it better? I am told that this new terminology and the associated acronyms are part of the standard nomenclature at the Centers for Disease Control and Prevention (CDCP) in their National Nosocomial Infection Surveillance (NNIS) system. The government has always been the leader in acronyms, beginning with SNAFU. There is failed source control and its acronym (FSC). We used to call it persistent infection (PI) but that could also be principal investigator or present illness. That won't do. I have tried to find the coiner of the expression "source control." The first reference to it I could find is an article in *Intensive Care Medicine* this year by Jimenez and Marshall entitled "Source Control in the Management of Sepsis" [2].

I am always amused by the use of the expression "toilet" or "peritoneal toilet" for cleaning things up in the wound or in the peritoneal cavity. Will irrigation and debridement not do the job? Incidentally, how do you treat FSC? The answer is you cannot unless you know the site, the source, the specific problem and the patient. So how does the concept of FSC help us? It does define a severe problem in surgical patients with persistent infections. Is that enough?

A wound infection is now called a surgical site infection, an SSI, no doubt. Is that an advance? Not for me. Necrotizing soft tissue infections are NSTIs. The authors describe damage control laparotomy (DCL). They cite and reference the excellent review on "Damage Control: Collective Review" by Shapiro et al. These authors refer to Harlan Stone and his group who, in 1983, developed the concept for this approach that proved to be life-saving in situations that were previously nonsalvageable [3]. This approach did not catch on until the 1990s.

The authors trace the concept of the sepsis syndrome on to SIRS and MODS but not to MOF [4, 5]. For one problem they describe, the evidence is a single-case report, hardly an epidemic. Has it happened again?

The compensatory anti-inflammatory response syndrome (CARS) is described but the authors do not espouse it. The fact is that inflammatory and anti-inflammatory mediators both begin together at the time of injury or operation and not one after another in sequence, as Roger Bone imagined it. There is no phase for CARS or MARS after an initial period of inflammation.

Finally, how do you treat sepsis syndrome, SIRS, MODS, or MOP? The answer again is you cannot. SIRS is sick, MODS is sicker, MOF is sickest, which may lead to death. I agree with the authors that prevention is the answer – prevention of FSC by better initial treatment.

References

1. Baue AE (1993) What's in a name? An acronym or a response? Am J Surg 165:299–301
2. Jimenez MF, Marshall JC (2001) Source control in the management of sepsis. Int Care Med 27:549–562
3. Stone H, Strom P, Mullins R (1983) Management of the major coagulopathy with onset during laparotomy. Ann Surg 197:532–535
4. Baue AE, Faise E, Fry D (eds) (2000) Multiple organ failure. Springer-Verlag, New York
5. Baue AE (1975) Multiple, progressive or sequential systems failure – a syndrome of the 70s. Arch Surg 110:779–781

Editorial Comment

In their exhaustive chapter, Drs. Barie and Eachempati describe everything that can go wrong after an operation, and the list is horrendously long and sadly well known to most of us.

In most instances source control can be achieved during the first operation – if it is not achieved, it is usually a result of poor technique or faulty judgment. On those rare occasions when source control cannot be immediately and effectively achieved, the surgeon should reattempt source control as soon as possible. Surgeons should realize that at least during the first postoperative week, the problem usually lies at the operative site: the cause of fever or "septic state" in the surgical patient is usually at the primary site of operation unless proven otherwise. The phenomenon of the "surgical ostrich" – treating the patient for "pneumonia" while he/she is slowly sinking into multiple organ failure from poorly controlled, or redeveloping, source of infection – still provides us with a constant source of SICU patients and experience.

Dr. Baue, a father of MOF and a prophet of MODS, aptly concluded that prevention is the key to treatment. Strive to achieve proper source control as early as possible; if impossible, drain, divert, leave open, and then come back – as discussed in other chapters in this book.

Part II: Source Control in Specific Locations

10 Diffuse Peritonitis

Beat Gloor, Mathias Worni, Markus W. Büchler

Key Principles

- Surgical intervention without delay
- Aggressive initial surgical source control including extensive intraoperative lavage, sufficient in the vast majority of cases (~ 90%)
- Continuous lavage, laparostomy and/or planned reexploration only if source control is not possible at initial operation
- Supportive therapy with adequate antibiotics and intensive care

Abdominal sepsis is one of the leading causes of death in surgical intensive care patients, and the treatment of choice continues to be controversial. With progress in supportive care, the mortality rate in referral hospitals has fallen to 20% or less

Table 1. Causes of diffuse peritonitis

Primary peritonitis (< 5% of all cases in a surgical institution)
Usually a single pathogen involved
Hematogenous spread of bacteria (e.g., remote infectious focus; following dental procedures)
Liver cirrhosis with ascites
Nephrotic syndrome
Metastatic malignant disease
Chronic ambulatory peritoneal dialysis
Secondary peritonitis > 90% of all cases in a surgical institution) Perforation of gastro-intestinal or genitourinary tracts
Necrosis of the gastrointestinal tract (e.g., strangulation, bowel obstruction, mesenteric vascular obstruction)
Bacterial translocation, abscess formation
Penetrating/blunt abdominal trauma
Intestinal neoplasm
Operative contamination of the peritoneum
Postoperative leakage of anastomoses or sutures
Tertiary or persistent peritonitis (< 10% of all cases in a surgical institution)
No recovery from secondary peritonitis despite timely surgical intervention and appropriate antibiotics
Occult infection
Impaired host defense or overwhelming infection

[1]. Peritonitis may be classified as primary, secondary, or tertiary (Table 1). This chapter deals only with secondary peritonitis, which represents 90% of all patients with peritonitis in surgical practice, and usually occurs as a result of gastrointestinal perforation or leakage.

General Approach

The hallmark of diffuse peritonitis is severe abdominal pain. Abdominal tenderness is always present, sometimes more intense over the area where the process started. Fever, tachypnea, tachycardia, hypotension, anorexia, nausea, vomiting, and hypoactive bowel sounds may also be noted. Laboratory tests should include a complete blood count, a chemistry profile, and a urinalysis. With the Mannheim peritonitis index (MPI), a peritonitis score that has been validated prospectively [2], or the APACHE II score, the severity of the disease can be determined and outcomes compared. If the plain abdominal radiograph shows free air in a patient with a clinical picture of diffuse peritonitis, rapid resuscitation and transfer to the operating room should be the next step in order to start source control without further delay.

Midline celiotomy allows access to all quadrants of the abdomen, regardless of the anatomic origin of the peritonitis. The treatment strategy depends on the cause and source of the peritonitis. In most cases, source control includes closure, resection or excision of the diseased segment. If the peritonitis is of colonic origin, the preferred approach is either a colostomy without anastomosis or an anastomosis with a protective diverting ileostomy. Source control is followed by an extensive intraoperative lavage to remove fibrin (which traps bacteria), blood, bacteria, toxins, and debris. Twenty to 30 l or more of (antibiotic-free) warm (37°C) saline solution is used. Irrigation is continued until the aspiration fluid from every compartment of the abdomen is clear, from the diaphragm to the pelvis, including every single loop of the bowel, indicating that there is no further intra-abdominal release of noxious chemical and/or bacterial material [3].

If the source of infection (focus) cannot be controlled (e.g., by closure, resection, or excision) during the initial operation, the strategy must be changed in order to allow continued removal of substances maintaining the inflammatory response. Continuous postoperative lavage, staged relaparotomy, or treatment by an open abdomen are therapeutic modalities aimed at preventing secondary and/or recurrent infection in such patients. We prefer postoperative continuous lavage, using two to four Salem Sump tube catheters. With this lavage system, the abdominal cavity is washed with 20 l of standard antibiotic-free peritoneal dialysis fluid. If closure of the abdominal wall is anatomically not possible, treatment with an open abdomen is indicated. However, it should be borne in mind that these techniques, especially "planned relaparotomy" and "open abdomen", are associated with considerable treatment-related morbidity. Therefore it is important to make every effort possible during the initial operation to control the source. A strategy of "conservative" surgical treatment of diffuse peritonitis, challenging the need for additional surgical treatment modalities, has been reported recently [4]. Of 258 patients with diffuse peritonitis, source control during the initial operation was possible in 230 (89%)

and not possible in 28 (11%). Twenty-one patients (9%) in whom source control was possible needed a second intervention. Only five patients were treated with staged reintervention or open abdomen. The overall morbidity rate was 41%; the rate of reoperation was 12%, and hospital mortality was 14% [4].

Controversies

For more than 100 years it has been well accepted that therapy in peritonitis must first aim for control of the source [5]. The key question is how best to perform source control. Do we need continuous postoperative lavage, or repeated, planned relaparotomy, or even treatment with an open abdomen? These aggressive techniques were established in order to prevent secondary and/or recurrent infection in patients with diffuse peritonitis [6]. However, it is our opinion that relaparotomy and treatment with an open abdomen were overused during the last decade, causing morbidity, which might have been prevented with a less aggressive approach. The best way to prevent secondary foci is a sufficient initial operation including extensive lavage. Provided that source control at the first intervention is adequate, fully 90% of patients with diffuse peritonitis will recover without additional surgical interventions [4]. The remaining patients with diffuse peritonitis present a challenge to the clinician; many are unsalvageable regardless of the therapeutic approach taken. In 52 patients with diffuse postoperative peritonitis, diffuse fecal peritonitis, or infected pancreatic necrosis, relaparotomy was associated with a mortality of 24% as compared to 58% in patients treated with an open abdomen [7]. The study's authors concluded that planned relaparotomy in patients with diffuse fecal peritonitis may be beneficial.

Critical Factors and Decision Making

Two factors are of paramount importance in the management of patients with diffuse peritonitis.

- The first is the timing of the intervention. The shorter the time after onset of disease or perforation, the earlier the inflammatory cascade can be interrupted, and its consequent morbidity prevented. Delayed intervention is reflected in high MPI and APACHE II scores. The higher these scores, the worse the outcome [8-11]. Early elimination of the focus – i.e., surgical treatment – is needed in all these patients.
- The second key factor in the management of patients with diffuse peritonitis is the effectiveness of the source control and the "price" of achieving it. Apart from the surgical strategy, which is primarily determined by the anatomy and the cause of peritonitis, extensive intraoperative lavage is the first choice for reducing intra-abdominal toxin levels [3]. In addition, this treatment is easy to perform, safe, inexpensive, and associated with almost no side effects.

If source control is not possible, other treatment modalities such as postoperative lavage, relaparotomy, or treatment with an open abdomen are necessary.

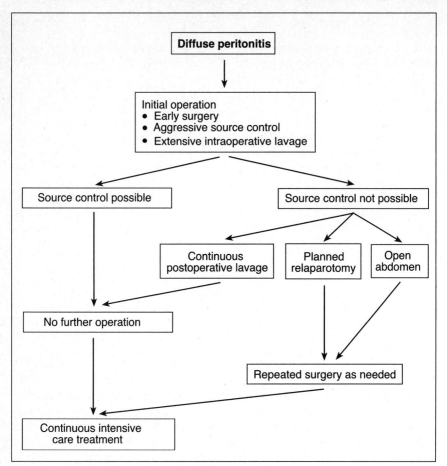

Diagram 1. Algorithm for management of diffuse peritonitis

References

1. Büchler MW, Baer HU, Brügger LE, Feodorovici MA, Uhl W, Seiler C (1997) Surgical therapy of diffuse peritonitis: debridement and intraoperative extensive lavage. Chirurg 68:811–815
2. Ohmann C, Wittmann DH, Wacha H (1993) Prospective evaluation of prognostic scoring systems in peritonitis. Peritonitis Study Group. Eur J Surg 159:267–274
3. Seiler CA, Balsiger BM, Feodorovici M, Baer HU, Buchler MW (1996) Extensive intraoperative lavage: the key maneuver in the treatment of severe peritonitis. Dig Surg 13:400–404
4. Seiler CA, Brugger L, Forssmann U, Baer HU, Buchler MW (2000) Conservative surgical treatment of diffuse peritonitis. Surgery 127:178–184
5. Mikulicz J (1889) Weitere Erfahrungen über die operative Behandlung der Perforationsperitonitis. Arch Klein Chir (Berl) 39:756–784
6. Hau T, Ohmann C, Wolmershauser A, Wacha H, Yang Q (1995) Planned relaparotomy vs relaparotomy on demand in the treatment of intra-abdominal infections. The Peritonitis Study Group of the Surgical Infection Society-Europe. Arch Surg 130:1193–1197

7. Schein M (1991) Planned reoperations and open management in critical intra-abdominal infections: prospective experience in 52 cases. World J Surg 15:537–545
8. Bosscha K, Reijnders K, Hulstaert PF, Algra A, van der Werken C (1997) Prognostic scoring systems to predict outcome in peritonitis and intra-abdominal sepsis. Br J Surg 84:1532–1534
9. Pacelli F, Doglietto GB, Alfieri S, Piccioni E, Sgadari A, Gui D, Crucitti F (1996) Prognosis in intra-abdominal infections. Multivariate analysis on 604 patients. Arch Surg 131:641–645
10. Ohmann C, Yang Q, Hau T, Wacha H (1997) Prognostic modeling in peritonitis. Peritonitis Study Group of the Surgical Infection Society Europe. Eur J Surg 163:53–60
11. Wickel DJ, Cheadle WG, Mercer-Jones MA, Garrison RN (1997) Poor outcome from peritonitis is caused by disease acuity and organ failure, not recurrent peritoneal infection. Ann Surg 225:744–756

Invited Commentary

WILLIAM G. CHEADLE

The chapter by Dr. Gloor and colleagues provides a succinct description of the management of diffuse peritonitis. The key principles of surgical intervention, aggressive source control, postoperative lavage, use of the open abdomen technique, planned reexploration if necessary, and antibiotics with intensive care support are certainly cornerstones of treatment. Secondary bacterial peritonitis cannot be considered as a single disease for its causes are legion and approaches to source control highly variable. Mortality from secondary and tertiary peritonitis is related to organ failure, and we found that recurrent infection responds well to repeat source control if not accompanied by organ failure [1]. I would argue whether 20-30 l of intraoperative lavage is necessary, particularly in light of the study by Fry and colleagues 20 years ago showing that radical peritoneal debridement did not confer benefit [2]. We have never used more than a few (3-4 l) liters of lavage and there are no prospective trials to justify a particular volume of lavage. Postoperative lavage is also controversial, but makes sense in certain patients. It too has yet to be proven effective in a prospective trial.

References

1. Wickel DJ, Cheadle WG, Mercer-Jones MA, Garrison RN (1997) Poor outcome from peritonitis is due to disease acuity and organ failure, not recurrent peritoneal infection. Ann Surg 225:744–756
2. Polk, HC, and Fry, DE (1980) Radical peritoneal debridement for established peritonitis: the results of a prospective randomized clinical trial. Ann Surg 192:350–355

Editorial Comment

Whether the 20-30 l of intraoperative peritoneal lavage so enthusiastically endorsed by Drs. Gloor, Worni, and Prof. Büchler are yet another gimmick is unknown in the absence of a properly conducted prospective trial.

One might also challenge the authors' recommendation that a midline celiotomy should be used regardless of the anatomic origin of the peritonitis. Common sense dictates that the most direct access to the specific intra-abdominal pathology is preferable. We should be pragmatic rather than dogmatic and tailor the incision to the individual patient and the disease process. The urgency of the situation, the site and nature of the condition, the confidence in the preoperative diagnosis, and the build of the patient should all be taken into consideration. Thus, the biliary system is often best approached through a transverse, right subcostal incision. Transverse incisions are easily extensible across, to offer additional exposure; a right subcostal incision can be extended into the left side (as a "chevron") offering an excellent view of the entire abdomen. When a normal appendix is uncovered through a limited incision like a McBurney's, one can extend across the midline to deal with any intestinal or pelvic condition. Alternatively, when an upper abdominal process is found, it is perfectly reasonable to close the small right iliac fossa incision and place a new, more appropriate, one. A preliminary diagnostic laparoscopy commonly allows the surgeon to place a limited, "minimally invasive" incision directly over the process, which can then be extended as necessary. The mandatory complications-prone, "maxi"-midline incision for any case of peritonitis belongs to the past.

The authors write that if the peritonitis is of colonic origin, the preferred approach is either a colostomy without anastomosis or an anastomosis with a protective diversion ileostomy. The third option, namely a selective use of primary "unprotected" anastomosis is discussed in Chap. 12.

11 Gastric and Proximal Small Bowel

DAREN DANIELSON, MICHAEL A. WEST

Key Principles

- Assess anatomic location
- Debride nonviable tissue
- Primary closure, usually

General Approach

Infections involving the stomach, duodenum, and proximal small intestine typically result from perforations of these structures, and management usually entails primary closure. The etiologic mechanism of perforation encompasses a wide range of surgical and medical problems and is beyond the scope of this discussion. In general, the surgical principles used to manage these perforations depend upon the anatomic location of the perforation (Fig. 1), in turn differentiated by the characteristics outlined in Table 1.

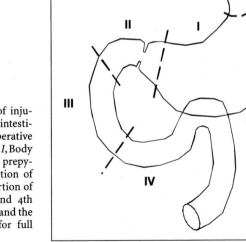

Fig. 1. Anatomic location of injuries in the proximal gastrointestinal tract determines the operative approach to source control. *I*, Body and fundus of stomach; *II*, prepyloric stomach and 1st portion of the duodenum; *III*, 2nd portion of the duodenum; *IV*, 3rd and 4th portions of the duodenum and the small intestine. See text for full discussion

Table 1. Characteristics affecting source control in the proximal gastrointestinal tract

	I	II	III	IV
Location	Gastric cardia and fundus	Prepyloric antrum and 1st portion duodenum	2nd Portion duodenum	3rd, 4th Portions duodenum and proximal small intestine
Blood supply	Excellent	Very good	Very good	Very good
Bacterial counts	$<10^2$ CFU/ml (10^5-10^6 if achlorhydric)	$\sim10^{3}$- 10^4 CFU/ml	$\sim10^{3}$- 10^4 CFU/ml	$\sim10^{3}$- 10^6 CFU/ml
Redundancy	Good	Little	None	Excellent
Mobility	Very good	Slight	Little	Excellent
Critical anatomic relationships	No	No	Yes	No
Serosa	Yes	Yes	No	Yes
Intra-peritoneal	Yes	Yes	No	Yes

I-IV, for description of location, refer to Fig. 1.
CFU, colony-forming units.

Under normal circumstances, the upper GI tract contains relatively few bacteria, in marked contrast to the abundant and varied flora associated with the lower GI tract. Gastric acid suppresses bacterial growth and kills ingested bacteria, resulting in a relatively sterile mucosal surface. Bacterial numbers are dramatically increased in the achlorhydric stomach, whether as a result of pharmacological therapy with H2-blockers or proton pump inhibitors, or pathologic conditions such as gastric carcinoma and pernicious anemia. As the gastric contents move into the duodenum and proximal small intestine, the bacterial numbers and diversity increase.

Surgical principles and techniques are discussed below for each of the four different anatomic locations shown:

I.   The gastric cardia and fundus
II.   The prepyloric antrum and 1st portion of the duodenum
III. The 2nd portion of the duodenum
IV.   The 3rd and 4th portions of the duodenum and small intestine

Injuries or perforations of the gastroesophageal junction are addressed elsewhere in this book (see Chap. 20).

The Gastric Cardia and Fundus

Repair of serosal injuries is usually not necessary. The management of full thickness injuries begins with the debridement of all nonviable tissue. When healthy tissue margins are obtained, and there is sufficient mobility of the edges, full thickness defects are repaired in either a one- or two-layer fashion (see "Controversies"). If a two-layer closure is used, the inner layer is constructed with a running absorbable (polyglycolic acid or polydioxane) 3-0 or 4-0 suture, followed by an outer interrupted layer of 3-0 suture placed in a Lembert fashion. A single layer of full thickness, Lembert 3-0 sutures, is also acceptable and can be performed more rapidly. The author prefers silk for such repairs, because it is inexpensive, readily available, and has excellent handling characteristics. Alternatively, absorbable synthetic sutures such as polyglycolic acid (Vicryl), polydioxane (PDS) and Maxon, or permanent monofilament sutures such as polypropylene can be used. These general issues of suture choice are applicable throughout this chapter. Catgut and chromic catgut should generally be avoided because they degrade rapidly and may compromise the repair. Extensive injury may require gastric resection. Billroth I reconstruction is preferred if the duodenum is not injured and mobile, otherwise Billroth II reconstruction can be performed. Descriptions of these procedures can be found elsewhere [1, 2].

Gastric resection is the preferred treatment for *perforated gastric ulcer* because of the high recurrence rate with patching alone. Gastric resections are usually performed with the aid of GIA or TA surgical stapling devices. Because of the thickness of the stomach wall, 4.2-mm staples should be used. The mucosal resection line should be carefully inspected for bleeding which may arise from the abundant submucosal vascular network. Hemodynamically unstable patients and poor surgical candidates should be treated with wedge resection, closure, and omental patching. If hemodynamic condition permits, patients with large or recurrent peptic ulcers should be considered for definitive ulcer surgery. Mucosal biopsies for *H. pylori* should be performed to assist with postoperative treatment. In addition, four quadrant biopsies should be performed to exclude gastric cancer.

Anastomotic leaks from Billroth I or II and Roux-en-Y gastroenterostomies require urgent definitive treatment. If possible, the anastomotic leak should be directly repaired and protected with an omental or jejunal serosal overlay. Internal NG drainage and external drainage should also be performed. Gastric pouch ischemia, which is the most common etiology of gastroenteric anastomotic leak, may be so severe as to require takedown of the anastomosis and creation of a gastrostomy and feeding jejunostomy with subsequent Roux-en-Y reconstruction.

Gastrocutaneous fistulas should be given a trial of conservative management with nasogastric drainage and supportive nutrition. If nonoperative treatment fails, operative excision with closure and omental patching, or gastric resection, is indicated.

Leaks after gastric bypasses deserve special mention. In many cases, these patients are too obese for US- or CT-guided drainage. A contained leak without signs of peritonitis or subphrenic abscess may be treated nonoperatively with antibiotics and nutritional support. If a nasogastric tube is still in place, it should be maintained, however, once removed, the NG tube should not be replaced for fear of further injury. With peritonitis or signs of clinical sepsis, immediate surgical exploration is indicated because of the high associated mortality, even if a leak cannot be proven radiographically. If the site of the leak can be located, it should be oversewn, patched with omentum, externally drained, and an NG placed under direct visualization. If the leak cannot be located, which is not uncommon, the same principles of anastomotic reinforcement, internal and external drainage apply. Consideration should also be given to feeding jejunostomy (see Chap. 15).

The Prepyloric Antrum and 1st Portion of the Duodenum

Most surgeons would advocate immediate definitive surgical management for perforations of the distal antrum or the 1st portion of the duodenum. Currently, the most common treatment is a one- or two-layer primary closure with an omental patch overlay, a modification of the technique originally described by Graham [3]. Performance of a definitive ulcer operation is controversial (see "Controversies"). Drain placement is neither safe nor effective and is mentioned here only to be condemned. A few authors have suggested selective management independent of the presence of peritonitis because upwards of 50% of perforations seal spontaneously within 12 h. Crofts et al. suggested that nonoperative management can therefore be considered, though it is not recommended in the elderly [4]. Mucosal biopsies for *H. pylori* should be sent and treatment begun if positive. If it is not possible to repair the first portion of the duodenum primarily and without fear of stenosis, resection with Billroth I reconstruction can be performed. If antral closure risks gastric outlet obstruction, a pyloroplasty should be performed. Extensive antral injuries may also necessitate resection with Billroth I reconstruction.

The 2nd Portion of the Duodenum

The 2nd portion of the duodenum enjoys the benefit of an excellent blood supply and minimal bacterial load, but suffers from its thin wall, lack of redundancy, and critical anatomic relationships. Despite these characteristics, the majority of duodenal defects can be repaired primarily. Larger defects and those with associated common bile duct (CBD) or pancreatic injuries require more complex surgical management.

Isolated duodenal injuries, those without CBD or pancreatic involvement and which involve less than 50% of the circumference, can be closed transversely in a one- or two-layer fashion. It is wise to buttress these repairs with omentum. Complete transection with minimal tissue loss may occasionally be repaired primarily after debridement of the wound edges. If the transection is near the ampulla, mobilization may risk CBD injury and primary repair may not be possible. A Roux-en-Y jejunal limb can be anastomosed to the proximal duodenum and the distal duodenum oversewn. Defects involving greater than 50% of the circumference of the lumen can be managed in the same fashion. External drainage with a silastic closed suction drain should be performed for all but the simplest of repairs, for the early detection and management of fistulas in the event of an anastomotic leak.

Duodenal diversion should be considered for large defects, when there has been a substantial interval between the timing of the injury and the repair, and in the presence of an associated pancreatic injury – risk factors for dehiscence and leak. Several methods of diversion have been described. Berne and Donovan advocated duodenal "diverticulization": antrectomy with truncal vagotomy, B-II reconstruction, oversewing the duodenal stump with an end duodenostomy, and common bile duct decompression with a T-tube [5]. Truncal vagotomy with T-tube placement are no longer routinely performed. Vaughan et al. described the less complex technique of "pyloric exclusion," which involves closing the pylorus with absorbable suture and constructing a gastrojejunostomy [6].

Some measure of "protection" of a primary repair may also be achieved with internal tube drainage. This may be accomplished via a gastrostomy combined with afferent and efferent jejunostomy, with or without tube duodenostomy. Alternatively, tube gastrostomy combined with transpyloric duodenostomy and efferent jejunostomy may be used selectively, according to Carrillo et al. [7].

A pancreaticoduodenectomy, or Whipple procedure, should be reserved for stable patients with the combination of *extensive* second portion tissue loss, ampullary or CBD disruption or *severe* injury of the pancreaticoduodenal complex. The complex nature of these injuries requires meticulous management. Excellent reviews of the intricacies of their management are provided by Carillo et al. and Jurkovich [7, 8] (see Chap. 32).

The 3rd and 4th Portions of the Duodenum and Proximal Small Intestine

The small bowel enjoys an excellent vascular supply (allowing primary repair or anastomosis), redundancy (allowing resection), and a lower bacterial load than the colon (minimizing the risk of contamination). Infections arising from perforations of the 3rd and 4th portions of the duodenum and of the proximal small intestine can all be handled in a similar manner. The principles of repair or resection, restoration of GI continuity, and decompression described above apply to injuries in this location. Extensive serosal injuries run the risk of delayed mucosal breakdown and leakage, and may be closed transversely. Small serosal defects do not require repair, and the risk of adhesion formation outweighs the risk of breakdown and leakage. Small full thickness defects can be closed directly using an interrupted Lembert suture. Larger, full thickness injuries involving less than 50% of the circumference of the lumen should be appropriately debrided and transversely closed using a one- or two-layer repair. Transverse closure minimizes the risk of luminal narrowing as illustrated by Bailey [9]. Small injuries in close proximity to one another should be connected and closed in the same fashion.

Extensive injuries, with more than 50% of circumferential tissue loss, are best managed by resection and primary anastomosis to avoid luminal narrowing and obstruction. Multiple small injuries within a short segment of bowel should also be treated with segmental resection and primary anastomosis. Resection may be liberal due to the redundancy of the small intestine, but in cases of massive small-bowel destruction where short-gut syndrome is risked, appropriate attempts at bowel preservation should be made. With resection, the type of anastomosis (hand sewn or stapled) is determined by surgeon choice and patient stability. Stapled anastomoses should be performed in a side-to-side, functional end-to-end fashion as described by Steichen and Ravitch [10] (see Chap. 32).

Aortoduodenal fistulas are rare but potentially lethal. Survival depends on early diagnosis and appropriate operative intervention. Throughout the literature, successful operative intervention has followed the same principles. First, the fistula is dissected free, next the duodenum is repaired in a two-layer fashion using polypropylene suture to minimize contamination, and finally the aortic pseudoaneurysm is repaired. Coverage of the duodenal repair should be performed, but interposed omentum is not necessarily required.

Controversies

Single- Versus Double-Layer Closure

Single-layer closures and anastomoses were met with resistance when first advocated. Multiple studies, including those in the review of Irwin et al. of single-layer anastomoses in the upper GI tract [11], have shown their complication rates to be similar to two-layer closures and anastomoses. Additionally, Burch showed in a randomized trial, that single-layer continuous anastomoses appear to be equivalent to interrupted techniques [12]. When there is a considerable risk of mucosal bleeding, a two-layer closure, with a running inner layer for hemostasis, may advantageous.

Operative Management of Perforated Ulcer in the Era of *H. pylori*

Traditional management of perforated ulcers in the stable patient included a definitive acid reducing operation to reduce recurrence rates. With recognition of the role of *H. pylori* as an etiologic agent, the proper operation for perforated ulcers has become controversial. Ng's recent study indicates that simple closure and omental patching with postoperative eradication of *H. pylori*, in the medically compliant patient, gives excellent results [13]. However, for those not infected with *H. pylori* or who have failed *H. pylori* treatment, as well as for chronic NSAID users, a definitive acid reducing operation should still be considered. It is often difficult to know these important aspects of a patient's medical history at the time of operation.

Critical Factors and Decision Making

Decision making for the repair of perforations involving the stomach, duodenum, and proximal small intestine depends on their location. Once adequate debridement of all nonviable tissue has been completed, primary closure can usually be performed if redundancy and mobility allow, as in the stomach and small intestine. In the 2nd portion of the duodenum, where mobility is limited, redundancy lacking, and critical anatomic relationships exist, more complex repairs are required to gain source control.

References

1. Siewert JR, Holscher AH (1997) Billroth I gastrectomy. In: Nyhus LM, Baker RJ, Fischer JE (eds) Mastery of surgery. Little, Brown, Boston, pp 848–857
   Excellent discussion and drawings illustrating the operative technique of gastrectomy and Billroth I reconstruction.
2. Branicky FJ, Nathanson LK (1997) Billroth II gastrectomy. In: Nyhus LM, Baker RJ, Fischer JE (eds) Mastery of surgery. Little, Brown, Boston, pp 858–872
   Excellent discussion and drawings illustrating the operative technique of gastrectomy and Billroth II reconstruction.
3. Graham RR (1937) The treatment of perforated duodenal ulcers. Surg Gynecol Obstet 64:235–238
   "Classic" description of patch repair of perforated duodenal ulcer.
4. Crofts TJ, Park KGM, Steele RJC (1989) A randomized trial of nonoperative treatment for perforated peptic ulcer. N Engl J Med 320:970–973
   Paper refuting the need for emergent operation in all patients with perforated peptic ulcer.
5. Berne C, Donovan A, White E, et al (1974) Duodenal "diverticulization" for duodenal and pancreatic injury. Am J Surg 127:503–507
   Original paper describing the operative technique and improved results for severe duodenal injuries with the use of duodenal diversion.
6. Vaughan G, Frazier O, Graham D, et al (1977) The use of pyloric exclusion in the management of severe duodenal injuries. Am J Surg 134:785–790
   First paper describing an alternative to the more extensive Berne duodenal diverticulization procedure. This is probably the current procedure of choice for extensive duodenal injuries.
7. Carrillo EH, Richardson JD, Miller FB (1996) Evolution in the management of duodenal injuries. J Trauma 40:1037–1045
   Recent review of experience with a wide range of duodenal injuries.
8. Jurkovich GJ (2000) Duodenum and pancreas. In: Mattox KL, Moore EE, Feliciano DV (eds) Trauma. McGraw-Hill, New York, pp 735–762
   Current trauma textbook chapter describing state of the art management of duodenal and pancreatic injuries.
9. Bailey H (1944) Intra-abdominal procedures, including wounds of the small intestine and mesentery. In: Bailey H (ed) Surgery of modern warfare, vol. 2, 3rd edn. Williams and Wilkins, Baltimore, pp 880–883
   "Classic" description of repair of small bowel injuries based upon experience in World War II.
10. Steichen FM, Ravitch MM (1983) Stapling in surgery. Year Book Medical Publishers, Chicago, p 277
    Original monograph describing the application of mechanical stapling devices to gastrointestinal surgery.
11. Irwin ST, Krukowski ZH, Matheson NA (1990) Single layer anastomosis in the upper gastrointestinal tract. Br J Surg 77:643–644
    Excellent discussion of technique and results with single layer GI anastomosis.
12. Burch JM, Franciose RJ, Moore EE, Biffl WL, Offner PJ (2000) Single-layer continuous versus interrupted intestinal anastomosis: a prospective randomized trial. Ann Surg 23:832–837
    Comparison of continuous versus interrupted single layer GI anastomosis – results of a prospective randomized study.
13. Ng EKW, Lam YH, Sung JJY, et al (2000) Eradication of *Helicobacter pylori* prevents recurrence of ulcer after simple closure of duodenal ulcer perforation: randomized controlled trial. Ann Surg 231:153–158
    Recent paper emphasizing the importance of eradication of *H. pylori* to minimize recurrence of peptic ulcer disease following perforation.

Invited Commentary

David Leaper

This chapter states that there is a small risk of infection from the stomach, duodenum, and upper small bowel with the implication that source control is not overly challenging. However, in disease, this situation is reversed and is well presented in Table 1. The influence and importance of various pathologies, which affect the upper gastrointestinal tract, cannot be overemphasized.

The stomach and duodenum have very low counts of intraluminal pathogens in health because of their active peristalsis and low pH. The gastric "mill" is able to break down large particles of swallowed food and this motility with an intact mucosa and low pH is bactericidal. Dysmotility from distal obstruction or infiltrative cancer changes this, as do disease processes that reduce gastric acid secretion, such as pernicious anemia or the presence of blood from acute gastritis or a bleeding ulcer. Patients taking proton pump inhibitors or histamine receptor antagonists are similarly at risk. Changes in gastric mucosal pH, measured by gastric tonometry reflect ischemia in septic or hemorrhagic shock that is associated with the development of gastritis. All these states, and in the absence of enteral nutrition (even prolonged preoperative starvation), favor early bacterial colonization, with aerobic Gram-negative bacilli in particular. In the absence of appropriate prophylaxis, the upper GI tract becomes the "undrained abdominal abscess," leading to translocation and progression or worsening of sepsis and organ failure, and the risk of nosocomial pneumonia and increased mortality. Prophylaxis, using selective antimicrobial decontamination or probiotic bacteria, has its adherents but early resumption of enteral feeding is probably the single most useful method to reduce the risk of upper gastrointestinal stasis, mucosal atrophy, and bacterial colonization. Small-bowel ischemia is a genuine emergency needing revascularization or more commonly excision.

The optimal management of a perforated gastric or duodenal ulcer is controversial. Conservative treatment of an early perforation with close surveillance is acceptable. Most duodenal ulcer perforations, which are the vast majority of upper GI perforations, usually seal quickly with minimum soiling of the peritoneum. Operation in this situation is unnecessary, provided postoperative follow-up includes antacid therapy (proton pump inhibitor) with endoscopy and eradication therapy for *H. pylori* if indicated. Older patients are perhaps more prone to perforated gastric ulcers and source control is less easy, requiring early surgical intervention, particularly when localization of signs is not rapid.

There are clear differences of opinion in surgical management of perforated upper gastrointestinal disease between the two sides of the Atlantic. Debridement is not considered necessary for duodenal perforations or clean incised injury, whereas a gastric perforation should always have a biopsy, or preferably excision biopsy of the whole ulcer prior to closure, to exclude cancer. In cases of dubious viable edges, debridement is advisable – in the small bowel this usually implies resection rather than direct repair. Duodenal injuries are often associated with other major injury and may be overlooked, leading to delayed intervention and dire consequences. All surgeons would agree that early recognition and intervention are crucial and that extensive surgery may be needed, with mobilization for assessment prior to resection or repair. Clearly, in appropriate circumstances a pancreaticoduodenectomy is indicated, but this option presupposes outstanding imaging for preoperative diagnosis and surgical expertise.

In general, gastrectomy is not advised for perforated benign duodenal or gastric ulcer, simple repair being complemented with antacid acid eradication therapy. We concur with the conservative approach to fistula; occasionally 3-6 months will be required, with attention to eradication of sepsis and nutritional support.

There is also widespread agreement on the east side of the Atlantic about the use of suture techniques. Although there here is little evidence-based proof, single-layer techniques appear to be as safe as two-layer techniques and are widely popular. However, catgut has been virtually discredited for use because of its unpredictability, and the modern absorbable polymers are tailor made. Silk is also increasingly unpopular despite its easy handling characteristics. A braided silk encourages bacterial colonization. It causes an appreciable inflammatory response and, anecdotally, may be the cause of postoperative adhesions.

Editorial Comment

MOSHE SCHEIN

Each of the conditions discussed in this chapter is complex enough to deserve a separate chapter. Spontaneous and traumatic sources in the UGI tract are relatively simple to control by simple closure, patch or, rarely, resection. Postoperative leaks after UGI procedures, on the other hand, are a surgical disaster, with a high mortality, and require complex and individualized approaches as discussed also in Chap. 30. Here are a few points which we would like to emphasize:

- The natural history of an uncontrolled source in the upper GI is unpredictable: in some patients it may seal spontaneously, in others present later as a lesser sac abscess, and in rare cases be rapidly lethal.
- We do not advocate primary treatment of a perforated ulcer with "onlay patch," as suggested by Drs. Danielson and West. We prefer the classic omentopexy as described by Graham: a few "through all layers" interrupted sutures are placed through both edges of the perforation and are left untied; a pedicle of the greater omentum is created and flipped over the perforation; the sutures are then gently tied over the omentum in order not to strangulate it. This obviates the approximation of the edematous, friable edges of the perforation, and indeed in many cases of postoperative duodenal fistula witnessed by us the simple suture-closure of perforated duodenal ulcer was the causative mechanism. Remember, you do not stitch the perforation but plug it with a viable omentum.
- *Nonoperative approach for perforated ulcers* – consisting of nil per mouth, nasogastric suction, systemic antibiotics, and acid secretion inhibitors – has

been proven effective by a few enthusiastic groups. The sine qua non for success is spontaneous sealing, radiologically proven, of the perforation by the omentum or other adjacent structures; if this occurs, nonoperative treatment will be successful in the majority of cases. This approach may be of particular value for two types of patients: the "late presenter" and the "extremely sick." The former presents a day or more after the perforation has occurred, with an already improving clinical picture and minimal abdominal findings. This, together with a radiographic evidence of free air, hints at a localized and spontaneously sealed perforation. Other candidates for conservative therapy are those in whom the risk of any operation could be prohibitive, such as the early post massive MI patient, the COPD grade IV or the patient with an APACHE II score over 25. Also in this group, however, conservative treatment may be successful only if the perforation is sealed and radiographically proven to be so. When sealing did not occur, in desperate situations we have successfully carried out omentopexy under local anesthesia.

• Definitive antiulcer procedures are today rarely indicated. The following table summarizes general guidelines in the selection of procedure.

	Text book options		We recommend	
Ulcer type	Good risk[a]	Poor risk	Good risk[a]	Poor risk
Duodenal	Omentopexy+/– TV+D or HSV or TV+A	Omentopexy	Omentopexy plus HSV	Omentopexy
Prepyloric	Omentopexy+/– TV+D or TV+A	Omentopexy	Omentopexy plus HSV+D	Omentopexy
Gastric	Omentopexy or wedge excision or partial gastrectomy	Omentopexy or partial gastrectomy	Omentopexy plus HSV+D or partial gastrectomy	Omentopexy or partial gastrectomy

[a] Recurrent ulcer, failed antiulcer therapy, noncompliant.
TV+D, truncal vagotomy and drainage procedure; HSV, highly selective vagotomy; TV+A, truncal vagotomy and antrectomy.
(Modified from *Schein's Common Sense Abdominal Surgery*, Springer Verlag, 2000)

JOHN MARSHALL

While I agree with the approach described by the authors for dealing with perforations secondary to ulcer disease (although I agree that plugging rather than suturing the ulcer is preferred; the ulcer is ischemic and will not heal), the approach to the duodenum and small bowel is more appropriate for trauma patients, without established inflammation. Extensive procedures, especially pancreaticoduodenectomy are dangerous if there is significant inflammation, or in a potentially unstable septic patient.

12 The Colon

Dietmar H. Wittmann

The Force Behind the Source: Colonic Bacteria

The large bowel contains up to 400 different bacterial species with concentrations of 10^{12-13}/ml of feces. All require an intact intracolonic environment to prosper and stay in balance for the benefit of the host [1, 2]. The colon wall has a mature host defense system to keep bacteria in check and prevent their transmural migration into the peritoneal cavity. Structural bowel wall changes such as diverticula, inflammatory bowel disease, and cancer interfere with the colonic wall's ability to contain bacteria and a perforation may result. Similarly, impaired blood supply may diminish oxygen and nutrient supply to cellular structures of the colonic wall, impair colon function in general and cellular defense in particular. Perfusion deficits may progress to frank ischemia when several factors add up. Such a scenario may be seen when edema increases intra-abdominal pressure and reduces venous and arterial blood flow, and when surgical sutures strangulate perianastomotic arterioles [3]. Rather than a barrier and defense against bacterial invasion, the ischemic colon wall now serves as nutrient for bacterial growth, fostering their access to the peritoneal cavity.

Few of these bacteria, however, can survive outside the colon following perforation or migration through a diseased colon wall. A comparison of bacteria from the healthy colon and the peritoneal cavity after colon perforation shows that only a small group of bacterial survivors adapt to the new environment (Fig. 1). Comparing their relative numbers may give a clue as to bacterial pathogenicity. *Escherichia coli* makes up less than 0.1% of the intracolonic flora, but following perforation it is the most commonly isolated bacterium, accounting for more than 50% of the isolates. Conditions outside the colon favor its growth, and it releases large amounts of endotoxin when attacked by powerful peritoneal and systemic defenses. *Bacteroides* species are more common intracolonic microorganisms and are often present in cultures taken from the peritoneal cavity after perforation – but this indicates mere survival and not special affinity for the host because they do not find living conditions optimized outside the colon as *E. coli* does. In peritonitis, *E. coli* is isolated at 300 times its intracolonic concentration.

The pathogenic potential of colonic bacteria that adapt well to the extracolonic environment, therefore, is the force that causes disease following perforation. The perforation itself is the source of this process, and must be closed or otherwise eliminated to save the patient. About 100 years ago when this was not possible virtually all patients with perforations died [4].

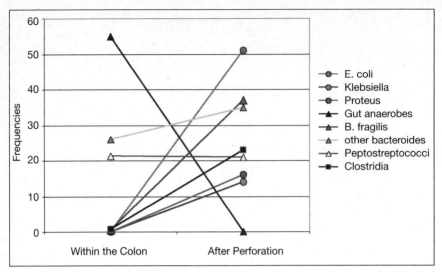

Fig. 1. Relative frequency of colonic bacteria within the normal colon and compared to bacterial frequencies within the peritoneal cavity following perforation

The Therapeutic Effect of Source Control

The therapeutic effect of source control may be best assessed by looking at situations where source control was the only available therapeutic option and other means of therapy such as antibiotics and fluid resuscitation were not developed.

Towards the end of the nineteenth century, surgeons learned to access the abdominal cavity to treat intra-abdominal infections [5]. Dramatic therapeutic successes were seen and gradually more abdominal procedures were introduced and performed. In 1902, Rehn recommended "radical elimination of the cause (source) of peritonitis" [6], and in 1909, W. Noetzel reported a dramatic improvement of mortality that was attributed to radical source control as mandated by his teacher Rehn [7]. His reports covered 449 operations for peritonitis from 1891 to March 1909 of which 178 were successful – a 38% mortality. All patients with diffuse suppurative peritonitis, including the most desperate cases, were treated without exception. Considering that no antibiotics were available, that fluid resuscitation was in its infancy, and that critical care therapy was not developed yet, one must conclude that source control, perhaps with the addition of purging of the abdominal cavity of pus (they used copious intraoperative irrigation with saline), was the most important factor responsible for a 62% mortality reduction. Other institutions gradually applied the source control philosophy. Their successful efforts to surgically close the source of infection were rewarded by decreasing mortality rates (Fig. 2). Kirschner in 1926 presented an impressive statistical analysis of 5,468 patients with peritonitis treated in seven major institutions from 1890 to 1924 [4]. The mortality curves indicate a parallel decline in all seven hospitals (Fig. 2).

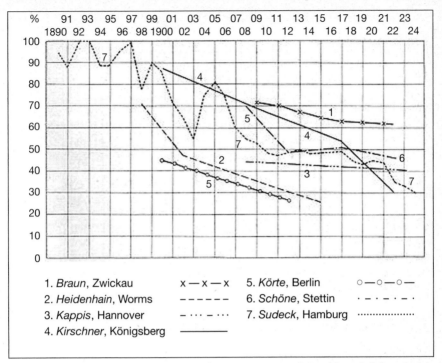

Fig. 2. Mortality of 5,468 cases of peritonitis from 1990 to 1924. During this period the principle of source control was introduced and applied clinically. (From [4])

When the Source of Peritonitis Is the Colon

During the period when the principle of source control was first introduced, peritonitis of colonic origin had a poorer outcome than peritonitis from other sources such as a perforated appendix or perforations of the upper GI tract. The mortality associated with peritonitis of colonic origin was 100% during the period from 1895 to 1914. It decreased to 68% and 50% from 1915 to 1924, while in the latter period the mortality of peritonitis from appendiceal and upper GI origins had decreased to 20% and 42.2%, respectively [4], emphasizing the importance of source control. While an appendectomy affords a safe source control, it is surgically more difficult to close or eliminate a perforation of the upper GI tract or the colon. The technique of exteriorizing a colon perforation had not yet been developed, and colostomies as a source control measure were introduced only during the Second World War. The higher concentration of bacteria entering the peritoneum after colon perforation in contrast to upper GI tract perforations may have contributed to the higher mortality.

Source Control: Refocus on a Solved Problem

Following the recognition of its importance and clinical application about 100 years ago, source control has become a fundamental feature of clinical practice. Recent developments in clinical research, however, have shown that the adequacy of source control has a significant impact on the interpretation of clinical trials. It has become evident that it is very difficult to evaluate outcomes in trials testing new antimicrobials [8] and new immunological strategies [9-11] without a precise definition of source control. This problem has prompted researchers to refocus on source control [12].

How Is a Source of Colonic Origin Controlled?

Colonic perforations leading to free bacterial flow into the peritoneal cavity can be classified into three distinct groups:
• Traumatic perforation following accidental and nonaccidental injury
• Perforation following localized necrosis from disease
• Transmural ischemic necrosis due to impaired vascular flow

The choice of therapy depends on the general condition of the patient, the inflammatory response of the peritoneum, the magnitude of increased intra-abdominal pressure, and the pathology itself. Treatment options include:
• Simple suture closure of the perforation
• Resection of the diseased colon segment with concomitant anastomosis
• Exteriorization of the colon segment that is perforated
• Resection of the perforated colon segment without anastomosis and formation of a terminal colostomy with or without a mucous fistula
• STAR (staged abdominal repair) to secure source control by daily inspection during abdominal reentries

The goal of each of these procedures is to prevent the perforation from permitting further bacterial entry into the peritoneal cavity. If increased intra-abdominal pressure prevents fascial closure at the initial operation, or if sepsis has created a situation of hemodynamic instability that allows for emergency measures only, a damage control procedure may be a meaningful initial step to control the source by simple resection and closing the transected colon openings temporarily – deferring definitive repair for 24 h or more so that the patient can be stabilized.

The STAR procedure, by using an artificial bur device as a temporary fascial prosthesis, permits fascial expansion and abdominal closure, at the same time allowing for planned abdominal reexploration to complete the repair and close fascia. The method offers the advantage of an ability to inspect the abdominal cavity and check that the source has been closed permanently. If necessary, defective closures can be rerepaired before bacteria regain access to the peritoneum (Fig. 3) [13-16].

Table 1 lists possible source control procedures for the three types of colon perforations. There are no prospective randomized trials to guide the surgeon's

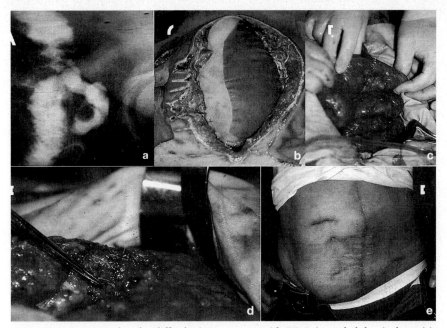

Fig. 3a-e. Source control under difficult circumstances with STAR (staged abdominal repair). This 62-year-old man with macronodular liver cirrhosis developed diffuse peritonitis from an anastomotic leak following sigmoid colon resection. A diverting colostomy was performed and the leak was sutured. The infection, however, continued because of continuous bacterial flow through a persistent anastomotic leak (*a*). The patient was transferred with multiple retention sutures cutting through the edges of a pararectal incision. Upon exploration we found multiple small bowel perforations (injuries from retention sutures), diffuse peritonitis, and a leaking colon anastomosis. We resected the small bowel and the leaking anastomosis, sutured two new anastomoses during STAR entry no. 1 (*d*), and closed with the artificial bur (Wittmann Patch) after debridement and copious irrigation with R/L. At STAR entry no. 3 on the 3rd day, the colostomy was taken down and anastomotic healing controlled (*c*). b The artificial bur in place neutralizing increased intra-abdominal pressure and also the previous colostomy site in the *upper left corner. e* The patient after recovery

choice for any particular procedure. In recent publications, however, the evolving consensus seems to favor abandoning operations to exteriorize the colon or to create a colostomy, because of the morbidity associated with surgery to reverse these procedures. It may be preferable to perform a primary anastomosis, and to evaluate the healing process at a subsequent abdominal operation, closing the abdomen only when source control is certain [4, 17].

For the conduct of clinical trials testing newer non-operative therapies, the source control criteria outlined in Table 1 may be useful to assess outcomes more effectively. It is not possible to favor one of the mentioned procedures over the other and further research is needed to clarify optimal operative management. Success, however, hinges on permanently controlling the source of infection within the colon wall. Postsurgical follow-up information must be included in the study design to document the safe closure of the source or a recurrent leak.

Table 1. Source control operations for colon perforations

Operation\Pathology	Traumatic perforation following accidental and non-accidental injury	Perforation following localized necrosis such as diverticulitis	Transmural ischemic necrosis due to impaired vascular flow
Simple suture closure of the perforation	Yes	Possible	No
Resection of the diseased colon segment with concomitant anastomosis	Yes	Yes	Yes
Resection of the diseased colon wall with delayed anastomosis	Yes	Yes	Yes
Exteriorization of the colon segment that is perforated	Possible	Possible	Difficult
Resection of the perforated colon segment without anastomosis and formation of a terminal colostomy	Possible	Possible	Possible
STAR procedure with multiple abdominal reentries and final fascial closure	Yes	Yes	Yes

References

1. Clarke JS, Bartlett JG, Finegold SM, et al (1874) Bacteriology of the gut and its clinical implications. Western J Med 121:390–403
2. Finegold SM (1982) Microflora of the gastrointestinal tract. In: Wilson SE, Finegold SM, Williams RA (eds) Intra-abdominal infection. McGraw-Hill, New York, pp 1–22
3. Wittmann DH, Iskander GA (2000) The compartment syndrome of the abdominal cavity: a state-of-the-art review. J Intensive Care Medicine 15:201–220
4. Kirschner M (1926) Die Behandlung der akuten eitrigen freien Bauchfellentzuendung. Langenb Arch Chir 142:53–267
5. Tait, L (1883) Laparotomy for septic peritonitis. Brit Med J 1155:1–15
6. Rehn L (1902) Behandlung infectiös eitriger Processe im Peritoneum. Arch Klin Chir 67:1–56
7. Noetzel W (1908) Die operativer Behandlung der diffusen eitrigen Peritonitis Die operativer Behandlung der diffusen eitrigen Peritonitis. Verhandlungen der Dtsch Gesellschaft für Chir 34:638–707
8. Solomkin JS, Dellinger EP, Christou NV, Mason AD (1987) Design and conduct of antibiotic trials: a report of the Scientific Studies Committee of the Surgical Infection Society. Arch Surg 122:158–164

9. Ziegler E, Fisher CF, Sprung CL, Straube RC, Sadoff JC, Foulke GE, Wortel CH, Fink MP, Dellinger RP, Teng NH, Allen IE, Berger HJ, Knatterud GL, LoBuglio AF, Smith CR (1991) HA-1A Sepsis Study Group. Treatment of gram-negative bacteremia and septic shock with HA-1A human monoclonial antibody against endotoxin. N Engl J Med 324:429–436
10. Greenman RL, Schein RM, Martin MA, Wenzel RP, MacIntyre NR, Emmanuel G, Chmel H, Kohler RB, McCarthy M, Plouffe J (1991) A controlled clinical trial of E5 murine monoclonal IgM antibody to endotoxin in the treatment of gram-negative sepsis. The XOMA Sepsis Study Group. JAMA 266:1097–1102
11. Fisher CJ, Dhainaut JFA, Opal SM, Pribble JP, Balk RA, Slotman GJ, Iberti TJ, Rackow EC, Shapiro MJ, Greenman RL, Reines HD, Shelly MP, Thompson BW, LaBrecque JF, Catalano MA, Knaus WA, Sadoff JC (1994) Phase III rhIL-Ira Sepsis Syndrome Study Group. Recombinant human interleukin 1 receptor antagonist in the treatment of patients with sepsis syndrome. JAMA 271:1836–1843
12. Marshall JC, Lowry SF (1995) Evaluation of adequacy of source control in clinical trials. In: Sibbald WJ, Vincent JL (eds) Clinical trials for the treatment of sepsis. Springer-Verlag, New York, pp 327–344
13. Wittmann DH, Aprahamian C, Bergstein JM (1990) Etappenlavage: advanced diffuse peritonitis managed by planned multiple laparotomies utilizing zippers, slide fastener, and velcro analogue for temporary abdominal closure. World J Surg 14:218–226
14. Wittmann DH (1996) Newer methods of operative therapy for peritonitis. In: Nyhus LM, Baker RJ, Fischer JE (eds) Mastery of surgery. Little, Brown, Boston, pp 146–152
15. Wittmann DH, Schein M, Condon RE (1996) Management of secondary peritonitis. Ann Surg 224:10–18
16. Wittmann DH (1998) Operative and nonoperative therapy of intraabdominal infections. Infection 26:335–341
17. Wittmann DH (1980) Chemotherapeutic principles in difficult-to-treat infections in surgery. I. Peritonitis. Infection 8:323–329

Invited Commentary

LEWIS FLINT

Dr. Wittmann's review of the pathophysiologic features and historical origins that form the intellectual foundation of modern surgical practice for the management of secondary bacterial peritonitis draws on his experience and longstanding interest in this area. There is no doubt that the massive bacterial inoculation of the peritoneum, which occurs at the time of colonic perforation, combines with medical co-morbidities and the nutritional and immunologic reserves of the patient, to determine the severity of the physiologic derangement and the clinical presentation. There is strong evidence that luminal bacterial content not only contributes to problems outside the bowel but also can contribute to the progression of ischemia of the colon to transmural necrosis. The mass of necrotic tissue and products of inflammation produce, within the peritoneal cavity, a hypoxic environment, which is hostile to immune and inflammatory cells. Moreover, this environment prevents the influx of immune defense cells as well as cytotoxic factors. It is a consistent observation that patients who localize infection and produce mature abscesses do well while patients whose peritoneal cavities are filled with thin murky fluid filled with necrotic debris and bowel content develop organ failure, anastomotic failure, and wound healing failure, with death the frequent final outcome.

As Dr. Wittmann points out, early operation in the face of adequate peritoneal defense mechanisms leaves the surgeon many options including simple closure, resection and colostomy, or resection and protected anastomosis (proximal colostomy or ileostomy). With the exception of patients with recent injuries to the colon, I have been unwilling to perform resection and primary anastomosis without protection and would not do so in the face of established peritonitis. In the severely compromised patient without adequate peritoneal defenses, edema and necrosis make any suture line hazardous. Dr. Wittmann points out the difficulty in mobilizing tissues and forming a colostomy in this setting. His suggestion that "damage control" measures could be combined with some form of open abdomen or planned reentry strategy makes good sense intuitively.

My only argument would be with the method of abdominal closure and the timing of reentry procedures. I have used the STAR device, or "Wittmann patch," in managing trauma patients at risk of abdominal compartment syndrome, and have found it easy to use and valuable for these patients. I do not have confidence in the planned reentry strategy since my view of the basic pathophysiology of severe peritonitis is that physical removal of exudate and fluid is as likely to be harmful as helpful. When the source control procedure is not completed at the primary operation, I would reenter the abdomen once the patient is stable, and complete the procedure with a minimal amount of manipulation and dissection. I would strive not to have anastomoses exposed and would not plan to expose them by reentering the abdomen except when directed to do this by clinical evidence of an anastomotic problem. In my view, it is essential to accomplish a definitive solution to the problem causing peritonitis within the first 7 days following the primary operation since, beyond this point, damage to the bowel is a common complication of any dissection.

We use systemic antibiotics, but antibiotic irrigation and forceful peritoneal irrigation are not used routinely. As Dr. Wittmann points out, prospective randomized controlled trials are not available, nor are they likely to be done, to answer all of these questions with convincing data. The trial of Fry and Polk [1] comes as close as any we have to providing an answer, and they found that physical debridement of the peritoneum was not associated with improved outcomes in their study. Notably, the study subjects were very similar to those referenced by Dr. Wittmann. The individual differences in patients presenting to surgeons, even those in large referral centers, confounds efforts to develop generalized strategies for these unfortunate individuals.

Reference

1. Polk HC, Fry DE (1980) Radical peritoneal debridement for established peritonitis: the results of a prospective randomized clinical trial. Ann Surg 192:350–355

Editorial Comment

That not all colonic sources need an operative source control has been mentioned already in Chap. 8. Pericolonic, diverticular abscesses do not necessarily require surgical therapy, or even percutaneous drainage (PCD). Ambresetti and Morrel's prospective experience included 61 diverticular abscesses diagnosed by CT [1]: 57 mesocolic and pelvic abscesses were treated conservatively, and PCD was only undertaken in the absence of clinical improvement within 48 h. The majority of mesocolic abscesses (82%) and pelvic abscesses (70%) settled without an invasive procedure. The size of the abscess was a predictor; most abscesses which were smaller than 5 cm responded to conservative treatment [2].

Dr. Wittmann provides a historical perspective on the management of colonic trauma. Over the years, there has been an evolution in the management of non-traumatic colonic origin peritonitis such as acute diverticulitis. Diverting colostomy was the procedure of choice in the early years of the twentieth century, and even until the 1980s. Laparotomy with an appropriate "peritoneal toilet" was performed, after which the inflamed or perforated sigmoid colon was drained and a proximal "diverting colostomy" was performed. Once the patient had "improved," the sigmoid colon was resected – the "second stage"; the colostomy was closed during yet another operation – the "third stage." The problem with this approach was that it left in situ a diseased, perforated organ, with a column of feces proximal to it (distal to the colostomy) that perpetuated the local and systemic infection. Gradually surgeons realized that the mortality and morbidity of an immediate resection of the sigmoid was lower than that of diverting colostomy [3], that each of the subsequent stages carried additional morbidity and mortality [4], and that only half of patients eventually had their colostomy closed [5]. The only randomized trial evaluating this "orthodox-conservative" approach [6] randomized 62 patients with diffuse peritonitis from perforated diverticulitis of the left colon to transverse colostomy, suture and omental covering of a visible perforation, or acute resection without primary anastomosis. For purulent peritonitis the postoperative mortality rate was significantly higher after acute resection (6 of 25) than after colostomy (0 of 21). Significantly, however, stomas became permanent in 4 of 25 patients with diverticulitis surviving acute colostomy and in 7 of 22 surviving acute resection.

A one-stage sigmoid resection plus an immediate anastomosis would be the ideal operation for perforated diverticulitis, but is it safe? Madden and Tan championed one-stage approach as early as 1961 [7] but remained its only advocates for many years; primary anastomosis in the face of an unprepared colon and adverse local circumstances was considered unsafe by mainstream American Surgery. Since the late 1980s the paradigm has begun to change and primary colorectal anastomosis is being gradually accepted.

The issue of unprepared colon is solved by some surgeons through the use of intraoperative, antegrade colonic lavage [8]. Others do not bother with bowel preparation at all [9]. Notably, the obsession of surgeons with the need to mechanically prepare the colon prior to an anastomosis is based more on dogma than on science. There is ample evidence to suggest that anastomosis can be safely performed in an unprepared colon [10-12]. Variables other than bowel preparation may be pertinent in the proper selection of patients in whom a primary anastomosis would be advisable. Common sense dictates that the additional time required for constructing an anastomosis should not be spent in unstable or critically ill patients. Poor nutritional status or steroid dependence are adverse prognostic factors that would deter most surgeons from the creation of an emergency primary anastomosis. Traditionally, an abscess or diffuse or localized peritonitis are contraindications to anastomosis. It appears, however, that an anastomosis may be safely attempted in selected patients suffering from localized peritonitis or suppuration, as opposed to those with diffuse forms of established peritonitis [13-15]. Recently, however, Schilling et al. [16] reported superb results with primary sigmoid resection and anastomosis in diffuse peritonitis (Hinchey Stage III and IV) of diverticular origin. In an audit, 500 U.S. gastrointestinal surgeons were asked: "What is your procedure of choice in a hemodynamically 'stable' 72-year-old patient suffering from diverticular perforation of sigmoid with localized purulent peritonitis?" One-third of the responders recommended a one-stage procedure in a "good-risk" patient with perforated diverticulitis associated with local peritonitis – most of these would perform this without an "on table" colonic lavage. In "high-risk" patients most surgeons (88%) would opt for a Hartmann's procedure [17]. It thus seems that the long-time obsession with a mandatory colostomy for any complicated colonic surgery is undergoing a paradigm shift [18].

Emerging, innovative methods of laparoscopic control of colonic sources are discussed in Chap. 36 while more opinions on Dr. Wittmann's STAR-planned relaparotomies approach are given in Chaps. 5, 7, 9, 10, 30, 35, 41, and 42.

References

1. Ambrosetti P, Morel P (1998) Acute left-sided colonic diverticulitis: diagnosis and surgical indications after successful conservative therapy of first time acute diverticulitis. Zentralbl Chir 123:1382–1385
2. Ambrosetti P (1999) Invited comment. Acute diverticulitis. In: Schein M, Wise L (eds) Crucial controversies in surgery, vol 3. Lippincott Williams & Wilkins, Philadelphia, pp 122–126
3. Krukowski ZH, Matheson NA (1984) Emergency surgery for diverticular disease complicated by generalized and faecal peritonitis: a review. Br J Surg 71:921–927
4. Classen JN, Bonardi R, O'Mara CS, Finney DC, Sterioff S (1976) Surgical treatment of acute diverticulitis by staged procedures. Ann Surg 184:582–586
5. Wara P, Sorensen K, Berg V, Amdrup E (1981) The outcome of staged management of complicated diverticular disease of the sigmoid colon. Acta Chir Scand 147:209–214
6. Kronborg O (1993) Treatment of perforated sigmoid diverticulitis: a prospective randomized trial. Br J Surg 80:505–507
7. Madden JL, Tan PY (1961) Primary resection and anastomosis in the treatment of perforated lesions of the colon with abscesses or diffuse peritonitis. Surg Gynecol Obstet 113:640–650
8. Lee EC, Murray JJ, Coller JA, Roberts PL, Schoetz DJ Jr (1997) Intraoperative colonic lavage in nonelective surgery for diverticular disease. Dis Colon Rectum 40:669–674
9. Trillo C, Paris MF, Brennan JT (1998) Primary anastomosis in the treatment of acute disease of the unprepared left colon. Am Surg 64:821–824
10. Burke P, Mealy K, Gillen P, Joyce W, Traynor O, Hyland J (1994) Requirement for bowel preparation in colorectal surgery. Br J Surg 81:907–910

11. Schein M, Assalia A, Eldar S, Wittmann DH (1995) Is mechanical bowel preparation necessary before primary colonic anastomosis? An experimental study. Dis Colon Rectum 38:749–752

12. Platell C, Hall J (1998) What is the role of mechanical bowel preparation in patients undergoing colorectal surgery? Dis Colon Rectum 41:875–82 (discussion 882–883)

13. Seiler CA, Brugger L, Maurer CA, Renzulli P, Buchler MW (1998) Peritonitis in diverticulitis: the Bern concept. Zentralbl Chir 123:1394–1399

14. Wedell J, Banzhaf G, Chaoui R, Fischer R, Reichmann J (1997) Surgical management of complicated colonic diverticulitis. Br J Surg 84:380–383

15. Hoemke M, Treckmann J, Schmitz R, Shah S (1999) Complicated diverticulitis of the sigmoid: a prospective study concerning primary resection with secure primary anastomosis. Dig Surg 16:420–424

16. Schilling MK, Maurer CA, Kollmar O, Buchler MW (2001) Primary vs. secondary anastomosis after sigmoid colon resection for perforated diverticulitis (Hinchey Stage III and IV): a prospective outcome and cost analysis. Dis Colon Rectum 44:699–703

17. Goyal AJ, Schein M (2001) Current practices in left-sided colonic emergencies. Dig Surg 18:399–402

18. Jimenez MF, Marshall JC (2001) Source control in the management of sepsis. Intensive Care Med 27[Suppl 1]:S49–S62

13 Infection and Trauma of the Rectum and Anus

Per-Olof Nyström

Key Principles

Perianal Abscess and Infected Fistulae

- Perform incision and curettage for drainage of abscess.
- Lay open associated low fistula.
- Insert seton in high fistula.
- Do not insert drains or pack wounds.
- Antibiotics are of uncertain value.

Fournier's Gangrene

- Emergency surgery is required.
- Broad-spectrum antibiotics should be used.
- Wide excision of necrotic tissue is necessary.
- Leave wounds open and plan for revision.
- Diverting stoma is usually not necessary.

Anal and Perineal Trauma

- Debride devitalized tissue.
- Suture external sphincter if possible.
- Leave wounds open.
- Diverting stoma is usually not necessary.

Rectal Trauma

- Perform a defunctioning sigmoidostomy.
- Suture rectal wounds.
- Drain the presacral space.
- Perform a rectal washout.

Perianal Infection

Perianal abscesses are common in emergency departments. Patients complain of increasing anal pain and tenderness caused by the inflammation and increasing pressure of the abscess. Eventually there will be fever if the abscess is large enough to cause systemic inflammation. If it is not surgically drained the abscess will usually drain spontaneously through the skin, often with some skin necrosis, or drain into the anal canal if there is a fistula associated with the abscess. Both after spontaneous drainage and after an incision it is not uncommon that the abscess recurs or that the patient returns with a history of cyclic complaints of pain and secretions. This is the typical chronic anocutaneous fistula, but occasionally the internal orifice is hard to demonstrate or absent, in which case the situation may be called a chronic sinus.

Any patient with acute signs of perianal abscess should be examined and treated under general anesthesia as an emergency case. The condition is too painful to allow proper examination in the conscious patient. The abscess may be deep within the ischiorectal fat, peripheral to the sphincter but below the levator muscles, and may not produce an obvious swelling. The basic rule is that patients with acute localized pain of the anus have an abscess until proven otherwise at surgery. Surgeons should not fool themselves that the abscess is not "mature" yet and therefore not ready for surgical drainage.

Surgical Drainage

If the prominence of the abscess is readily identified a direct incision into the abscess is made. If the abscess is covered by necrotic skin associated with spontaneous perforation, the affected skin is excised. Otherwise a straight skin incision of about the same length as the abscess should be made. It does not matter if the incision is radial or follows the anal circumference, but the surgeon should choose what is optimal for drainage. The abscess cavity should be curetted and irrigated with normal saline to remove residual blood from the cavity. There is no need to insert a drain or packing as long as the incision itself is adequate. There is no reason to do a cruciate incision, which delays healing and causes bad scarring.

With simple perianal abscesses, a fistula tract is identified in varying rates depending on how carefully the surgeon searches for it. If there is pus in the anal canal at examination, the fistula is obvious. The tract may be laid open at the time of the abscess drainage if the surgeon is confident that it is a low fistula. Several studies have shown that the subsequent problem of recurrent fistula is avoided, but many of the associated fistulae appear to heal anyway [1-4]. Surgeons who are less experienced with unroofing a fistula-in-ano can insert a loose draining seton until subsequent definitive surgery of the fistula can be accomplished.

Perianal abscesses can be incised, curetted, and suture closed under antibiotic cover, as shown in several studies [5-7]. I have personally been unconvinced of the usefulness of this procedure because an open incision heals as quickly and causes less discomfort to the patient than do sutures. Antibiotics are not needed if the incision is left open.

The need for antibiotic treatment has not been sufficiently researched. If the patient has pyrexia, I believe that a preoperative dose of an adequate antibiotic is sufficient, and that there is no need for postoperative treatment if the abscess has been adequately drained. Postoperatively the patient should be relieved of the pain, but tenderness may persist for a few days. If pain relief is insufficient, it is advisable to return the patient to the operating room to ascertain that the abscess has been completely drained.

Anocutaneous Fistulae with Abscess

Both high and low anocutaneous fistulae, in their initial presentation, have identical internal and external orifices because the tracts follow muscle planes. The internal orifice is in the glandular crypts of the dentate line of the anal canal. The external opening is at the peripheral margin of the subcutaneous muscle about 4 cm from the anal verge (lower margin of the internal sphincter). From the dentate line the tract passes between the internal and external sphincters downwards (in low fistula) and turns at the lower margin of the external sphincter to continue deep to the subcutaneous muscle until it breaks through the skin. The tract of a high fistula passes upwards between the sphincters to the upper margin of the external sphincter and curves around it downwards to follow outside the external sphincter and then deep to the subcutaneous muscle until it breaks through the skin. Any previous surgery may change the position of the external orifice, e.g., after incision of an associated abscess.

Low fistula is much more common than high. Because the tract is low the associated abscess is superficial in the ischiorectal compartment and therefore readily identified on examination. The abscess may be intersphincteric but more commonly extends lateral to the subcutaneous muscle. It is unusual that the low fistula produces extensive perianal infection; rather it usually presents as a simple perianal abscess. The abscess is incised with fistulotomy, or a seton may be inserted for resolution of the inflammation in anticipation of elective surgery of the fistula.

High Anocutaneous Fistula with Abscess

Because the tract of the high fistula is deep into the ischiorectal compartment, right below the levator, it is always associated with an abscess cavity that extends to the levator and may push the levator cranially to give the false impression that the abscess extends above the levator. Such penetration of the levator is rare or iatrogenic. Most often the internal orifice of the high fistula is in the posterior midline associated with a retroanal abscess cavity formed by cranial and caudal fascial septa from the coccyx to the sphincter. The septa prevent an external opening in the midline behind the anus, but the abscess and tract must extend laterally, peripheral to the external sphincter, to penetrate the skin lateral on one or both sides of the anus (Goodsall's rule) as a horseshoe abscess.

If neglected, a high fistula can present with extensive deep infection of the posterior and lateral infralevator compartment with multiple necrotic external orifices. The operation for source control is rather straightforward following the rules stated previously, but the incisions need to be extended to lay open the tracts and abscess. It is nearly always evident that there is an internal opening because it drains pus into the posterior anal canal. It is usually best to begin at the external opening. Excise necrotic skin if present. It is often advisable to gain better access by circumcising the external orifice and follow the tract as it extends posteriorly and upwards to the retroanal abscess. Multiple openings on either side are joined by laying open the common tract. Both sides of the anus are treated

similarly as needed. The retroanal abscess cavity is accessed by extending the incision to the midline behind the anus or through a separate incision behind the
anus. The cavity is curetted and a seton is inserted. The wounds are left open.
Small incisions with plastic drains (e.g., Penrose) are painful and unreliable for
source control so I prefer the more extensive incisions through which the tracts
can be partially cored out or laid open. The seton will be loose but short as its external exit will now be in the midline right behind the anus. The wounds to the
sides of the anus will heal well if the tract has been adequately cored out or laid
open. The clinical harbinger of good source control is the rapid disappearance of
pain. If pain persists it is advisable to return the patient to the theatre for revision. The wounds should not be packed because changing the dressings can be very
painful. The wounds are better left open for the patient to manage with showers
or sitz baths. These patients probably benefit from antibiotic therapy until the
acute pain subsides after a few days but there are no studies addressing this question.

Controversies of Anocutaneous Fistulae

The simple classification of anocutaneous fistulae into high and low depending
on whether the tract goes above or below the external sphincter is not accepted
by all. Indeed, most surgeons writing on the subject favor a classification that in
addition incorporates transsphincteric fistulae (through the external sphincter)
and supralevator fistulae (above the puborectalis muscle) in following the classification given by Parks [8]. The supralevator fistula with an associated supralevator abscess, i.e., an abscess in the perirectal compartment above the levator, is
very rare. Whatever classification is favored, the abscess needs to be properly
drained [9]. The low, intersphincteric, fistula associated with an abscess can always be laid open without risk of incontinence but any fistula affecting the external sphincter must not be incised [4]. A draining seton is better until elective
definitive surgery can be performed.

Traditional management of wounds after incision of an abscess with or without fistula includes the insertion of plastic drains and packing of wounds created by cross-formed incisions [10]. All of these cause unnecessary pain and scarring. The resolution of pain immediately after drainage is the best clinical sign of
source control. A few prospective studies have specifically prescribed straight
incision without drainage [4].

Synergistic Infection of the Anus and Perineum (Fournier's Gangrene)

The perineum is the most common site for synergistic infection [11], and in this location the infection is usually called Fournier's gangrene (although it is essentially
the same infectious process that is called necrotizing fasciitis in other parts of the
body). Synergistic infection is a polymicrobial infection that spreads along the subcutaneous fascia or muscle fascia planes so rapidly that body defenses are unable

to contain the infection. As a consequence, the vascular bed of the subcutaneous fat is destroyed with foul-smelling necrosis of fat and secondary skin necrosis. The infection usually respects muscle boundaries and hence will not invade the levator ani or the anal sphincter, although it may appear to do so because the muscle fascia is involved. Because of the necrotic separation of the planes, emphysema of the tissues is characteristically observed on plain X-ray films or CT scan.

The infection may be seen as a special case of a triad of infections involving the skin (erysipelas), the subcutaneous fat compartment (fasciitis), or the muscle compartment (myositis). Group A and B streptococci are sufficiently virulent to attack the skin and muscle, while less virulent streptococci in combination with other bacteria cause fasciitis. The distinction of infected compartments may be not so clear in later stages of the infection when the patient is toxic and the infection overwhelms all defenses. Because the subcutaneous defenses are unable to contain the infection it spreads quickly from the anal region to the perineum, external genitals, and beyond.

Fournier's gangrene may appear spontaneously, may be associated with anal pathology, or may develop as a complication after anal or perineal surgery. Patients with insulin-dependent diabetes, or who are severely immunocompromised as in AIDS or after bone marrow transplantation are at increased risk of perineal infection [11-14].

The surgical treatment is urgent wide debridement of all necrosis. Necrotic skin is excised but the fat necrosis extends much further and must be exposed through skin incisions to the margin of viable fat. All necrotic fat and remnants of the subcutaneous fascia are excised with scissors. The muscle fascia can be left unless there is obvious necrosis of the muscle. The wounds are left open with light packing with gauze. It is advisable to take the patient back to theatre for revision of the wounds within 24 h to make sure that the infection has been arrested. The subsequent course may require further minor revision of necrosis. If the patient's condition permits, a preoperative CT scan will assist in determining the extent of the infection and any supra-levator extension.

Antibiotic treatment should be instituted immediately on diagnosis. The antibiotic regimen must cover both aerobic and anaerobic bacteria, and both the Gram-positive flora (streptococci) and the Gram-negative flora (enteric bacteria). High-dose penicillin with clindamycin and a cephalosporin, or imipenem combined with clindamycin are two options. These patients can be severely toxic and may require support of vital functions in the intensive care unit preoperatively and postoperatively. The operation must not be delayed because only surgery can reverse the infection.

Traumatic Injury of the Anus and Rectum

The spectrum and incidence of anorectal trauma varies from one society to another. Penetrating trauma due to missile wounds is uncommon in Europe [15]. Accidental impalement injury and assault rectal injuries are occasionally encountered. Pelvic fractures may be complicated by tears of the anorectum. Thermometer injury, especially in small children, has largely disappeared as a cause. Laceration of the anus may be seen in accidental injury, sexual abuse, and more commonly as obstetric tears.

Surgical Treatment of the Injured Anus

Accidental lacerations of the anus are debrided, sparing as much as possible of the sphincter ani. The wounds are left open and the patient may be referred to a colorectal surgeon for immediate (within days) or delayed reconstruction of the sphincters. A sigmoid colostomy should be created if the sphincters and perineal tissue are severely torn, but can be avoided in minor injury.

Rectal Injury

Penetrating injury of the abdominal (intraperitoneal) rectum is treated as any other colonic injury. Penetrating trauma of the extra-abdominal rectum was a fatal injury in wartime until the basic principles of treatment were developed, including diverting sigmoidostomy and presacral drainage behind the anorectum. Suture of the rectal wound and rectal washout were added.

There is now considerable controversy about the optimal management of the rectal injury. Several retrospective studies show that the management had often omitted one or several of the four cornerstones of the treatment [16-20]. Most of the larger injuries were diverted but many patients had not had the rectal hole repaired, nor was the presacral space always drained or the rectum emptied of feces with washouts. It appears that surgeons had taken a practical view of the management by grading the rectal injury, the number and severity of associated injuries, the patient's general condition, and the time delay of treatment [19]. The more severe the injury the more the comprehensive principles were adhered to. One prospective randomized study showed that when the rectal injury was diverted, presacral drainage did not influence the local infection rate [21]. Prospective studies that challenge the various components of the management are difficult because such injuries are rare and represent a wide spectrum of severity.

Most civilian missile injuries are operated within 1 or 2 h, when contamination is present but infection has not yet developed. In nonmissile injury the diagnosis may be delayed until infection is present. In such instances, diversion should be undertaken and the infected pocket drained. Whether rectal washout is required is debatable, and solid feces are perhaps better left since their removal is not a requisite for healing of the rectal wound.

Summary

Infection and injury of the perineum and anorectum require the same treatment principles as infections in other anatomic locations. Contained infection (abscess) is drained by incision. Soft tissue necrotizing infection must be debrided of all necrosis and laid open. Traumatic injuries represent such a wide spectrum of severity that treatment must be adapted to the circumstances, but any large injury should be diverted and the perforation resected, closed, or drained. Because of the important function of the anorectum, the surgeon needs to be familiar with the anatomy to preserve future function without compromising source control.

References

1. Hebjorn M, Olsen O, Haakansson T, Andersen B (1987) A randomized trial of fistulotomy in perianal abscess. Scand J Gastroenterol 22:174–176
2. Schouten W, vanVroonhoven T (1991) Treatment of anorectal abscess with or without primary fistulectomy: results of a prospective randomized trial. Dis Colon Rectum 34:60–63
3. Tang C-H, Chew S-P, Seow-Choen F (1996) Prospective randomized trial of drainage alone vs. drainage and fistulotomy for acute perianal abscess with proven internal opening. Dis Colon Rectum 39:1415–1417
4. Ho YH, Tan M, Chui CH, Leong A, Eu KW, Seow-Choen F (1997) Randomized controlled trial of primary fistulotomy with drainage alone for perianal abscesses. Dis Colon Rectum 40:1435–1438
5. Leaper D, Page R, Rosenber I, Wilson D, Goligher J (1976) A controlled study comparing the conventional treatment of idiopathic anorectal abscess with that of incision, curettage and primary suture under systemic antibiotic cover. Dis Colon Rectum 19:46–50
6. Kronborg O, Olsen H (1984) Incision and drainage v. incision, curettage and suture under antibiotic cover in anorectal abscess. Acta Chir Scand 150:689–692
7. Mortensen J, Kraglund K, Klaerke M, Jaeger G, Svane S, Bone J (1995) Primary suture of anorectal abscess: a randomized study comparing treatment with clindamycin vs. clindamycin and Gentacoll. Dis Colon Rectum 38:398–401
8. Parks AG, Gordon PH, Hardcastle JD (1976) A classification of fistula-in-ano. Br J Surg 63:1–12
9. Onaca N, Hirshberg A, Adar R (2001) Early reoperation for perirectal abscess: a preventable complication. Dis Colon Rectum 44:1469–1473
10. Cox SW, Senagore AJ, Luchtefeld MA, Mazier WP (1997) Outcome after incision and drainage with fistulotomy for ischiorectal abscess. Am Surg 63:686–689
11. Elliott D, Kufer J, Meyers R (1996) Necrotizing soft tissue infections: risk factors for mortality and strategies for management. Ann Surg 224:672–683
12. Cohen JS, Paz IB, O'Donnell MR, Ellenhorn JD (1996) Treatment of perianal infection following bone marrow transplantation. Dis Colon Rectum 39:981–985
13. Barrett WL, Callahan TD, Orkin BA (1998) Perianal manifestations of human immunodeficiency virus infection: experience with 260 patients. Dis Colon Rectum 41:606–612
14. Buyukasik Y, Ozcebe OI, Sayinalp N, et al (1998) Perianal infections in patients with leukemia: importance of the course of neutrophil count. Dis Colon Rectum 41:81–85
15. Marti MC, Morel P, Rohner A (1986) Traumatic lesions of the rectum. Int J Colorectal Dis 1:152–154
16. Shannon F, Moore E, Moore F, McCroskey B (1988) Value of distal colon washout in civilian rectal trauma: reducing gut bacterial translocation. J Trauma 28:989–994
17. Burch JM, Feliciano DV, Mattox KL (1989) Colostomy and drainage for civilian rectal injuries: is that all? Ann Surg 209:600–611
18. Levy RD, Strauss P, Aladgem D, Degiannis E, Boffard KD, Saadia R (1995) Extraperitoneal rectal gunshot injuries. J Trauma 38:273–277
19. Morken JJ, Kraatz JJ, Balcos EG, et al (1999) Civilian rectal trauma: a changing perspective. Surgery 126:693–698
20. Renz BM, Feliciano DV, Sherman R (1993) Same admission colostomy closure (SACC). A new approach to rectal wounds: a prospective study. Ann Surg 218:279–292
21. Gonzalez RP, Falimirski ME, Holevar MR (1998) The role of presacral drainage in the management of penetrating rectal injuries. J Trauma 45:656–661

Invited Commentary

Luis A. Carriquiry

There are very few randomized studies concerning emergency anorectal surgery, so there is scant level I or II evidence to justify most of our common management strategies. Thus, Dr. Nyström cannot count upon many compelling certainties, but only upon his outstanding capacity of judgment applied to his vast experience.

Perianal Infection

I strongly endorse his preference for examination (and drainage) of patients with acute signs of perianal abscess under general anesthesia. Contrary to the widely held opinion of cost-conscious surgeons, I think exploration and drainage are too painful to be done in the awake patient and local anesthesia does not work well in these circumstances. Most patients subjected to drainage in the emergency ward have sad memories of their suffering. Furthermore, I prefer to perform a gentle debridement of the abscess cavity with the finger (if it is done gently, there is no risk of creating additional tissue damage) and this procedure is extremely painful in the conscious patient.

If examination is performed by a surgeon-in-training – as is quite usual – incision and drainage of the abscess is appropriate and leads to satisfactory healing, although a fistula will develop in subsequent months in 40% of patients. But if the attendant were a well-trained surgeon, with experience in anorectal surgery, I would recommend to search the primary fistula track and to manage it adequately to prevent further recurrence of the fistula. In this case it is of paramount importance to locate the internal opening, looking for the appearance of pus in the anal canal when compressing the abscess before drainage or for the appearance of bubbles when injecting hydrogen peroxide into the drained cavity. Even exploration of the cavity with Lockhart Mummery probes can be useful if done gently. If the fistula track is subcutaneous or intersphincteric, it may be safely laid open; if it is transsphincteric, or if there is any doubt about the anatomy concerning the external sphincter, a draining seton is a better choice. As Dr. Nyström points out, four randomized studies have shown that primary fistulotomy leads to a substantial decrease in recurrence of abscesses or fistulas. Of course, this is another argument favoring examination and treatment under general anesthesia.

I share Dr. Nyström's approach to the surgical treatment of horseshoe abscess, but I prefer to use separate lateral and posterior incisions with drainage of the tracts with rubber Penrose drains for the first few days. They do not cause pain and healing is quicker. In this situation I also use antibiotics for 3 or 4 days, although there is no evidence that this is necessary.

Necrotizing Perineal Infections

Wide debridement of all necrotic tissue is the mainstay of treatment. Skin incisions should be extended as far as necessary to achieve full excision of necrotic tissue till reaching healthy bleeding fat. Careful revisions should not be spared. Concerns about reconstruction should be left to the plastic surgeon, but it is always convenient to wrap the testicles in healthy tissues if the incision extends to the scrotum. Dr. Nyström dismisses the diverting stoma. I am not convinced of that position, at least in cases of necrotizing infection originating in the anal canal, and especially if after treatment a floating anus results. Some authors [1] have strongly recommended the use of hyperbaric oxygen chambers. However, this is a cumbersome practice which has not been demonstrated to be useful [2].

Traumatic Injury of the Anus and Rectum

I share Dr. Nyström's views on intraperitoneal rectal injuries, where primary repair should be the rule and on anal canal injuries: they should be repaired by a well trained colorectal surgeon without proximal sigmoidostomy, as has been shown to be appropriate for sphincteroplasties [3]. The problem arises with injuries of the extraperitoneal rectum. The four basic principles of surgical treatment: diverting sigmoidostomy, presacral drainage, repair of the wound, and rectal washout were developed for war injuries and demonstrated as very effective in reducing mortality and morbidity. But their dogmatic application in all cases of civil injury has been increasingly challenged in recent years. Suture repair of the wound is the weakest principle: doing it through a transanal approach is not easy, and everybody agrees that opening the pelvic peritoneum during abdominal exploration is only indicated in case of extensive bony and soft tissue damage. In most civilian rectal injuries, suture has been omitted without affecting morbidity and mortality, as similarly happens in the case of full-thickness local excision of rectal tumors without suture of the rectal hole. Rectal washout has been the second victim of iconoclasts. Most recent series have omitted it and results have not been worse. Presacral drainage has also been debated. Even a prospective randomized trial showed that it did not affect the final result, although the study included very few patients and a beta-type error could not be ruled out. Only proximal fecal diversion seems to remain firm, although recent debates about its protective role in very low rectal anastomosis, and about the necessity of mechanical preparation in colon and rectal surgery – an ongoing Swedish trial is addressing the issue – seem to challenge its status. I look at these developments with an open mind: probably colostomy may be omitted in low-velocity missile wounds, but I am inclined to keep it in the management of most injuries. The colostomy should be created as distal as possible and a properly constructed loop sigmoidostomy, with an adequate spur, has been demonstrated to be completely diverting, with no need for a terminal or loop-end colostomy. The only recent development to consider is use of a laparoscopic approach [4] to look for associated intraperitoneal injuries and to exteriorize the sigmoid, without a formal laparotomy. Although not an unconditional fan of laparoscopic approaches, I think it is a good suggestion and probably one of the best indications for laparoscopic colon surgery.

References

1. Lucca M, Unger H, Devenny A (1990) Treatment of Fournier's gangrene with adjunctive hyperbaric oxygen therapy. Am J Emerg Med 8:385–387
2. Iorianni P, Oliver G (1992) Synergistic soft tissue infections of the perineum. Dis Colon Rectum 35:640–644
3. Hasegawa R, Yoshioka K, Keighley MR (2000) Randomized trial of fecal diversion for sphincter repair. Dis Colon Rectum 43:961–964
4. Navsaria PH, Graham R, Nicol A (2001) A new approach to extraperitoneal rectal injuries: laparoscopy and diverting loop sigmoid colostomy. J Trauma 51:532–535

14 Acute Appendicitis

James M. Watters

Key Principles

- Early appendectomy, open or laparoscopic, is standard therapy for acute appendicitis.
- Appendiceal phlegmon commonly resolves with antibiotic therapy alone.
- Appendiceal abscess may also respond to antibiotic therapy but will require percutaneous (or surgical) drainage in many instances.
- Appendicitis occasionally manifests as a more severe, potentially life-threatening problem which may include generalized peritonitis, bacteremia, pylephlebitis, and/or liver abscesses, and requires appropriate surgical, antibiotic, and supportive therapy.

General Approach

The source control problem in appendicitis ranges from a localized inflammatory process, requiring only appendectomy, to generalized purulent peritonitis, for which formal laparotomy and peritoneal toilet are required.

Uncomplicated, Gangrenous, or Locally Perforated Appendicitis

Open or laparoscopic appendectomy conducted in a timely manner is by far the most common approach to appendicitis which is uncomplicated, gangrenous, or perforated, but without phlegmon or abscess. Such patients typically present within the first few days of their illness, and outcomes are generally excellent, with postoperative intra-abdominal abscess uncommon and the incidence of wound infection relatively low. Early appendectomy provides a definitive diagnosis, avoids possible progression to perforation, prevents recurrent appendicitis, and minimizes the need for antibiotic therapy. Most appendectomies continue to be open procedures although a laparoscopic approach is attractive when diagnostic uncertainty is high (see Chap. 37).

The likelihood of perforated appendicitis is greater when the appendix is retrocecal, as well as in children and the elderly. In these circumstances, symptoms may be less prominent or atypical, leading to a delay in presentation or diagnosis. The duration of symptoms is more than twice as long on average in patients with perforated compared with nonperforated appendicitis [1]. This association is usually interpreted as indicating that nonperforated appendicitis will normally progress to perforated appendicitis, and is the rationale for a policy of early appendectomy. It is argued that immediate surgery should be undertaken in order to avoid progression to perforation, accepting an increased likelihood that the appendix will be normal. If this concept is correct, one would expect the rate of normal appendectomies to increase as the rate of perforated appendectomies decreased. Such an inverse relationship between perforated and normal appendectomy rates has been described in a report compiling data from a number of published series [2]. However, the range of duration of symptoms in patients with perforation is very wide, and other observations suggest that perforating and nonperforating appendicitis are different entities [1, 3]. For example, the greater likelihood of perforation in the elderly arises because of a progressive, age-associated decrease in the incidence of nonperforated appendicitis while the incidence of perforated appendicitis remains constant [3]. Further, other population-based studies show that diagnostic accuracy decreases as the rate of appendectomy increases, but the rate of perforation does not change [4]. The strong association between duration of symptoms and risk of perforation may also arise from a selection bias. Specifically, nonperforated appendicitis will resolve spontaneously in some patients who are likely to have short-lived symptoms and may not be identified as having appendicitis, whereas perforated appendicitis is presumed invariably to worsen [3]. Much of the difference in time to therapy between nonperforated and perforated appendicitis occurs before presentation to hospital [1]. Thus, from the perspective of effective surgical source control, a limited period of observation in hospital does not expose patients with an equivocal presentation to an increased rate of perforation, and will allow the diagnosis and need for surgical intervention to be established [1, 5, 6].

Antibiotic therapy has been demonstrated to be effective for appendicitis in a small randomized trial comparing it with appendectomy, as well as in larger case series [7-9]. However, recurrence of appendicitis occurs in 35% of patients by 12 months [7]. In addition, the role of nonoperative management in pediatric and elderly patients, and in patients with significant co-morbidity, has not been established. Antibiotic therapy may be a useful strategy for presumed appendicitis in selected circumstances, for example, when facilities for surgery and anesthesia are not available.

Appendiceal Phlegmon and Abscess

Some patients present with a palpable mass and have a significant phlegmon or abscess on diagnostic imaging. They have typically had symptoms for longer than 3 or 4 days. Antibiotic therapy is often effective in resolving the acute process, especially phlegmon, and avoids a surgical procedure, which is usually more complex than routine appendectomy [10-12]. The possibility of alternative or additional diagnoses (e.g., cecal cancer, Crohn's disease) must be kept in mind when a nonoperative approach is selected. Nonoperative measures will not be successful in some patients, as judged by persistence or worsening of pain, abdominal findings, and systemic manifestations of acute inflammation. Surgical exploration and, if feasible, appendectomy should be carried out when there is failure to improve by 48 h, and sooner if there is concern about adequate localization of the inflammatory process, uncertainty about the diagnosis, or clinical deterioration. Appendicitis may recur following resolution, and interval appendectomy (open or laparoscopic) should be considered. However, reported recurrence rates are quite variable, published recommendations about interval appendectomy conflicting, and compelling data few.

Antibiotic therapy may also be effective in resolving appendiceal abscesses, particularly smaller abscesses, but a substantial proportion will fail to improve and will require drainage [12]. Antibiotic therapy and percutaneous drainage may be chosen from the outset if the abscess is large or systemic signs and symptoms prominent [11]. Surgical drainage of a well-defined abscess does not offer any particular advantage over percutaneous drainage. Limited cecal or ileocecal resection has been used infrequently when the viability and integrity of the appendiceal stump and adjacent cecum are questionable, or if the diagnosis remains uncertain even at laparotomy [13]. The role of surgical drains is uncertain, but their use is probably best confined to those cases in which an established abscess cavity is present.

Generalized Peritonitis

Occasionally, when peritoneal defenses are inadequate to contain the infective process, appendicitis presents as generalized purulent peritonitis. Laparotomy is the conventional approach when there are clinical findings of generalized peritonitis. If appendicitis is suspected, then laparoscopy may be a useful alternative. Confirming the diagnosis of appendicitis laparoscopically allows optimal placement of an incision for laparotomy. Whether appendectomy and measures appropriate for generalized purulent peritonitis (e.g., irrigation of the abdomen and pelvis) can be accomplished effectively by laparoscopy will depend on the judgment and experience of the surgeon. There is little information about laparoscopic management of generalized peritonitis.

Management of the Appendiceal Stump

Pericecal abscess can arise if closure of the stump of the appendix is insecure, and may result in a fecal fistula. When the appendiceal stump is wide, a more formal closure by oversewing or stapling is preferable to simple ligation or suture ligature. If the appendiceal stump is of questionable integrity or necrotic, then it may be prudent to invert the stump or excise a margin of cecal wall so that the closure is of healthy tissue. Routine inversion of the stump offers no advantage over ligation or suture ligature and is potentially hazardous if the wall of the cecum is indurated, inflamed, or noncompliant. Appendectomy may be difficult or even unsafe when there is an appendiceal phlegmon or abscess, since inflamed and necrotic tissues and adherent tissue planes make dissection hazardous. In such circumstances, necrotic tissue and any fecalith which might serve to perpetuate local infection should be removed. Recent case reports have drawn attention to the problem of recurrent appendicitis arising in a long appendiceal stump following laparoscopic appendectomy. Whether this problem is more common than following open appendectomy is unknown, but the principle of careful and complete visualization, leaving only a very short stump applies equally to open and laparoscopic surgery.

Controversies and Changing Practices

The Timing of Surgery for Appendicitis

Our understanding of the natural history of appendicitis is evolving. The concept that immediate surgery is necessary to prevent the progression from simple to perforated appendicitis is probably not warranted. A limited period of observation in hospital is safe when the clinical presentation is equivocal, in order to establish the diagnosis of appendicitis with greater confidence, and to ascertain the need for surgical source control.

The Choice of Open or Laparoscopic Approaches to Appendicitis

Laparoscopic appendectomy, combining diagnostic laparoscopy and "minimally invasive" appendectomy, offers an attractive alternative when there is diagnostic uncertainty. It remains unclear, however, whether routine laparoscopic appendectomy is superior to conventional open appendectomy. At present, the choice of surgical approach varies with patient, surgeon, and institutional factors. Laparoscopic appendectomy for uncomplicated and locally perforated appendicitis is well supported, as is a laparoscopic approach to interval appendectomy. Favorable experience with perforated appendicitis and small abscesses has been reported, but the role of laparoscopic techniques in more complicated appendicitis remains to be defined. Wound infection rates may be reduced and postoperative recovery accelerated with a laparoscopic approach [14, 15]. However, analyses of the impact of laparoscopic appendectomy on health-related quality of life or costs are lacking [15].

Wound Management Following Perforated Appendectomy

Delayed wound closure has traditionally been advocated following open appendectomy for gangrenous or perforated appendicitis to improve wound infection rates ranging in some reports as high as 32% with immediate closure [16]. Recent analyses suggest that immediate closure is preferable when appropriate antibiotics are employed [16, 17]. A meta-analysis identified similar wound infection rates, between 4% and 5%, for both primary and delayed wound closure [17]. A cost-utility analysis, incorporating patient preference and economic factors, concluded that immediate closure is the favored option as long as wound infection rates are not excessive [16].

Interval Appendectomy

Interval appendectomy following resolution of appendicitis prevents recurrence. Whether the potential for recurrence is great enough to warrant routine interval appendectomy is controversial. If appendectomy is not carried out, the possibility that other appendiceal or ileocecal pathology is present needs to be considered and addressed by appropriate radiologic and/or endoscopic assessment.

Critical Factors and Decision Making

Appendectomy should be carried out in patients with uncomplicated, gangrenous, or perforated appendicitis who present within the first few days of their

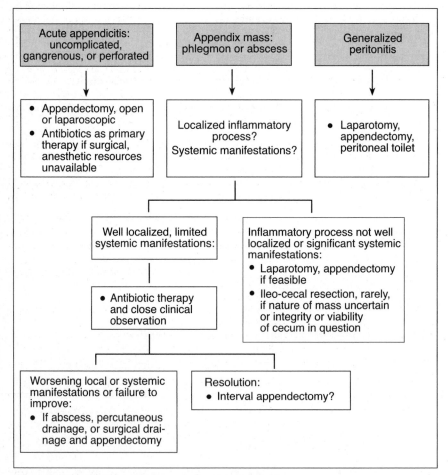

Diagram 1. Algorithm for management of acute appendicitis

illness. The procedure may be open or laparoscopic. Patients with phlegmon or abscess typically present later in their course. Antibiotic therapy alone is often effective for a localized abscess or phlegmon, although percutaneous drainage may be required for some abscesses. Generalized peritonitis is an indication for laparotomy.

References

1. Temple CL, Huchcroft SA, Temple WJ (1995) The natural history of appendicitis in adults: a prospective study. Ann Surg 221:278–281
   A prospective observational study of 95 consecutive adult patients undergoing appendectomy with the purpose of relating pre-hospital and in-hospital delays to the incidence of perforation.
2. Velanovich V, Satava R (1992) Balancing the normal appendectomy rate with the perforated appendicitis rate: implications for quality assurance. Am Surg 58:264–269
   A decision analysis using data for 10,023 appendectomies compiled from publications of the previous 15 years with the aim of quantifying and exploring the inverse relationship between the perforated appendicitis rate and the normal appendectomy rate.
3. Luckmann R (1989) Incidence and case fatality rates for acute appendicitis in California: a population-based study of the effects of age. Am J Epidemiol 129:905–918
   An analysis of hospital discharge abstracts for 24,794 patients who had appendectomy or abscess drainage for appendicitis in California in 1984 to determine age- and sex-specific incidence and case fatality rates for perforating and nonperforating appendicitis.
4. Andersson RE, Hugander A, Thulin AJG (1992) Diagnostic accuracy and perforation rate in appendicitis: association with age and sex of the patient and with appendectomy rate. Eur J Surg 158:37–41
   A retrospective study of consecutive patients operated on for suspected appendicitis in a defined population (Jonkoping County, Sweden, 1984–1989), and an analysis of diagnostic accuracy, perforation rate, and appendectomy rate in other published reports.
5. Walker SJ, West CR, Colmer MR (1995) Acute appendicitis: does removal of a normal appendix matter, what is the value of diagnostic accuracy and is surgical delay important? Ann R Coll Surg Engl 77:358–363
   A single-center, prospective, observational study of 248 patients who had emergency appendectomy during a 1-year period, with follow-up up to 8 years.
6. Dolgin SE, Beck AR, Tartter PI (1992) The risk of perforation when children with possible appendicitis are observed in the hospital. Surg Gynecol Obstet 175:320–324
   A prospective, observational study of 150 consecutive children referred for possible appendicitis, managed with appendectomy when clinically clear (74 patients) and admitted for observation when initially unconvincing (76 patients).
7. Eriksson S, Granstrom L (1995) Randomized controlled trial of appendicectomy versus antibiotic therapy for acute appendicitis. Br J Surg 82:166–169
   A prospective, randomized trial of a 10-day course of antibiotics or appendectomy for appendicitis of less than 72 h duration in patients (n=20 per group) aged 18–75 years.
8. Coldrey E (1959) Five years of conservative treatment of acute appendicitis. J Int Coll Surg 32:255–261
   A single-center, retrospective review of 471 patients with appendicitis during 1953–1957, including 334 managed nonoperatively initially (including antibiotics) as a routine in the last 2 years.
9. Adams ML (1990) The medical management of acute appendicitis in a nonsurgical environment: a retrospective case review. Military Med 155:345–347
   A case series of nine young males with appendicitis on submarines managed with antibiotics.
10. McPherson AG, Kinmonth JB (1945) Acute appendicitis and the appendix mass. Br J Surg 32:365–370
    A retrospective, single-center analysis of 730 patients with simple appendicitis, appendicitis with diffuse peritonitis, and appendicitis with mass treated from 1937–1942.

11. Bagi P, Dueholm S (1987) Nonoperative management of the ultrasonically evaluated appendiceal mass. Surgery 101:602–605
    A single-center, retrospective study to evaluate the routine nonoperative management of 40 consecutive patients with an appendiceal mass (abscess in 31 patients and phlegmon in 9) evaluated by ultrasonography 1976–1985.
12. Yamini D, Vargas H, Bongard F, Klein S, Stamos MJ (1998) Perforated appendicitis: is it truly a surgical urgency? Am Surg 64:970–975
    A single-center, retrospective study of 66 patients with appendicitis and phlegmon or abscess (54 with abscess, 10 with phlegmon, 2 not imaged) from 1992–1997 whose initial management was nonoperative.
13. Sarkar R, Bennion RS, Schmit PJ, Thompson JE (1997) Emergent ileocectomy for infection and inflammation. Am Surg 63:874–877
    A single-center review of 83 patients over a 7-year period who underwent emergency ileocecal resection to control intra-abdominal inflammation and sepsis, among whom 32 had appendicitis.
14. Sauerland S, Lefering R, Holthausen U, Neugebauer EAM (1998) Laparoscopic vs conventional appendectomy – a meta-analysis of randomised controlled trials. Langenbeck's Arch Surg 383:289–295
    A recent meta-analysis of randomized clinical trials (to March 1998) comparing open and laparoscopic appendectomy.
15. Temple LKF, Litwin DE, McLeod RS (1999) A meta-analysis of laparoscopic versus open appendectomy in patients suspected of having acute appendicitis. Can J Surg 42:377–383
    A recent meta-analysis of randomized clinical trials (to March 1997) comparing open and laparoscopic appendectomy.
16. Brasel KJ, Borgstrom DC, Weigelt JA (1997) Cost-utility analysis of contaminated appendectomy wounds. J Am Coll Surg 184:23–30
    A decision and cost-utility analysis of primary closure, delayed primary closure and secondary closure of right lower quadrant wounds following appendectomy for perforated or gangrenous appendicitis.
17. Rucinski J, Fabian T, Panagopoulos G, Schein M, Wise L (2000) Gangrenous and perforated appendicitis: a meta-analytic study of 2532 patients indicates that the incision should be closed primarily. Surgery 127:136–141
    A meta-analysis of clinical trials and prospective studies published 1981–1997, examining the hypothesis that advances in the use of antibiotic prophylaxis for wound infection and surgical techniques obviate the need for delayed wound closure.

Invited Commentary

Roland E.B. Andersson

The most important issue concerning source control in appendicitis is how to identify the small proportion of patients that need surgical treatment among the patients with suspected appendicitis. The traditional principles for the management of patients with suspected appendicitis were formulated at a time when perforated appendicitis with generalized peritonitis was an important cause of death. The development of new diagnostic tools and nonsurgical treatment with potent antibiotics, the low mortality due to improvements in anesthetic and intensive care methods, and new knowledge about the natural course of the disease calls for a reformulation of these principles.

The management of patients with suspected appendicitis has traditionally focused on the prevention of perforation by early operation, but at the expense of a high proportion of unnecessary operations. New diagnostic techniques have been introduced, but despite promising initial results, experience in everyday practice is disappointing. An emphasis on the need for early exploration associated with a liberal use of ultrasound, CT, and diagnostic laparoscopy has had a limited impact on the number of unnecessary explorations, but the costs have increased enormously.

As proposed by Dr. Watters, the principle of early appendectomy to prevent perforation must be questioned. Most perforations have likely already occurred before the patient arrives at the hospital [1-3]. Studies have not shown a decreased risk of perforation with a liberal attitude toward early exploration [4, 5]. An apparently lower rate of perforation appears to be a consequence of increased treatment of cases of uncomplicated appendicitis that would otherwise have resolved without treatment, since the absolute number of perforations has not decreased. Resolution of appendicitis with nonoperative management appears to be quite common.

The existence of *resolving appendicitis* is further supported by histopathological evidence, and by reports of cases of resolving appendicitis where the clinical diagnosis has been supported by typical findings on ultrasound [6, 7]. Up to 6.5% of patients operated for appendicitis have had previous symptoms, indicating that *recurrent appendicitis* may occur [8]. There is also historical evidence; at the time when expectant treatment was still practiced, it was generally accepted that in most instances appendicitis would resolve spontaneously [9]. Epidemiological studies suggest that perforated and nonperforated appendicitis are different entities [4, 10, 11]. Obstruction is frequently found in gangrenous and perforated appendicitis but is rare in nonperforated appendicitis, suggesting a different pathogenesis [12].

As discussed by Dr. Watters, an evolving knowledge of the natural history of appendicitis has important implications. The management of patients with suspected appendicitis should focus on the early identification and surgical management of the more advanced cases. Patients with an equivocal diagnosis can safely be observed, reserving surgery for patients in whom clear signs of the disease develop or symptoms do not resolve. Signs of spontaneous resolution should also be actively sought, and support an approach of ongoing expectant management.

A restrained attitude to exploration will not only decrease the number of negative appendectomies but also allow cases with self-limiting appendicitis to resolve without surgery. As a consequence, the proportion of perforations will be high due to the reduction in the detection of simple appendicitis. *A high proportion of perforations is therefore not necessarily a sign of bad management.*

In-hospital observation, based on repeated examinations for the signs of local peritonitis and systemic inflammatory response that is associated with appendicitis [13], should be sufficient for the majority of patients. Diagnostic techniques such as CT and ultrasound may be used selectively in patients in whom the risks of a negative exploration are higher [14].

When the likelihood of appendicitis is high, laparoscopy offers very limited benefit compared with open appendectomy but is more expensive. Laparoscopy should therefore be reserved for the situation when an exploration is thought to be needed although a surgical condition is less likely.

I agree with the approach of nonsurgical treatment of appendiceal phlegmon and appendicitis with localized abscess as advocated by Dr. Watters. The efficacy of antibiotic treatment and percutaneous drainage of abscesses is well documented, whereas surgical exploration is traumatic and may result in an unnecessary right-sided colectomy. After resolution of the phlegmon, a workup for colonic cancer is indicated in older patients. The patient should be informed about the risk of recurrent appendicitis, but the low risk does not necessitate an interval appendectomy.

A short trial of nonoperative antibiotic management of patients with suspected appendicitis has been shown to be safe, and is a reasonable option, particularly in patients whose anesthetic risk is increased [14]. In acute appendicitis as in many other diseases the pendulum is swinging back towards medical treatment after 100 years of surgical treatment.

References

1. Hale DA, Jaques DP, Molloy M, Pearl RH, Schutt DC, d'Avis JC (1997) Appendectomy: improving care through quality improvement. Arch Surg 132:153–157
2. Temple CL, Huchcroft SA, Temple WJ. The natural history of appendicitis in adults: a prospective study. Ann Surg 221:278–281
3. Koepsell TD, Inui TS, Farewell VT (1981) Factors affecting perforation in acute appendicitis. Surg Gynecol Obstet 153:508–510
4. Andersson R, Hugander A, Thulin A, Nyström PO, Olaison G (1994) Indications for operation in suspected appendicitis and incidence of perforation. BMJ 608:107–110
5. Howie JGR (1964) Too few appendectomies? Lancet i:1240–1242
6. Ciani S, Chuaqui B (2000) Histological features of resolving acute, non-complicated phlegmonous appendicitis. Pathol Res Pract 196:89–93
7. Cobben LP, de Van Otterloo AM, Puylaert JB (2000) Spontaneously resolving appendicitis: frequency and natural history in 60 patients. Radiol 215:349–352
8. Barber MD, McLaren J, Rainey JB (1997) Recurrent appendicitis. Br J Surg 84:110–112
9. Stengel A (1908) Appendicitis. In: Osler W, McCrae T (eds) Modern medicine, vol 5. Diseases of the alimentary tract. Lea & Febiger, Philadelphia, p 428
10. Andersson R (1999) "Can perforating appendicitis be considered a separate disease entity"? Eur J Surg 165:481–482
11. Luckman R (1989) Incidence and case fatality rates for acute appendicitis in California. Am J Epidemiol 129:905–918
12. Arnbjörnsson E, Bengmark S (1984) Role of obstruction in the pathogenesis of acute appendicitis. Am J Surg 147:390–392
13. Andersson RE, Hugander A, Ravn H, Offenbartl K, Ghazi SH, Nystrom PO, Olaison G (2000) Repeated clinical and laboratory examinations in patients with an equivocal diagnosis of appendicitis. World J Surg 24:479–485
14. Blomqvist R, Andersson RE, Granath F, Lambe MP, Ekbom AR (2002) Mortality after appendectomy in Sweden, 1987–1996. Ann Surg 233:455–460

Editorial Comment

The following scenario is not uncommon: you admit for observation a patient with right lower quadrant pain and ambiguous clinical findings. Meanwhile the ER doctor orders a CT, which is reported by the radiologist the following morning. At this stage the patient feels much better, his abdomen is benign, and he wants to go home, but the radiologist claims that the appendix is grossly inflamed. You choose not to treat the radiological image, and send the patient home. The HMO, however, denies any payment for the "unnecessary hospitalization for observation." Of course they would pay for the CT and the appendectomy – if performed.

This leads us to the myths concerning acute appendicitis, a few of which are exposed above by Drs. Watters and Andersson.

- Myth 1: The rate of perforation reflects on the quality of care provided by the surgical team.
- Myth 2: Clinical observation may lead to an increased rate of perforation.
- Myth 3: Unattended simple appendicitis, if untreated, progresses to perforation.
- Myth 4: Early use of imaging improves results.
- Myth 5: Nonlocalized abdominal findings call for a "formal" laparotomy.
- Myth 6: The appendiceal stump has to be cauterized, touched with an antiseptic, and/or inverted.
- Myth 7: The wound has to be left open following appendectomy for complicated appendicitis (gangrenous/perforated).
- Myth 8: A prolonged course of IV antibiotics should be given following the operation for complicated appendicitis.
- Myth 9: Drains should be used whenever periappendicular pus is encountered.
- Myth 10: An interval appendectomy is necessary following successful conservative management of appendiceal mass/abscess.

Amazingly, more than 100 years after it was recognized as a treatable surgical entity, acute appendicitis still fascinates surgeons and is surrounded by a growing list of controversies and uncertainties. Like other surgical conditions, acute appendicitis represents a spectrum of disease. To reach the diagnosis, historical, physical, laboratory, and imaging variables should be considered together. No isolated variable can confirm or exclude the diagnosis, while the more "typical" variables are present, the higher is the chance that this is appendicitis. Whether one operates immediately or tomorrow, whether one observes or obtains additional tests is determined selectively, based on the individual patient.

15 Bariatric Operations

Robert E. Brolin

Key Principles

- Gastrointestinal (GI) leaks after bariatric operations can kill.
- Aggressive treatment of wound infection after open bariatric operations rarely includes opening the entire incision.
- Atelectasis after bariatric operations is a surprisingly uncommon cause of delayed discharge and is almost never the cause of florid sepsis.

Introduction

Table 1 shows the relative incidence of septic complications following various bariatric operations. The incidence of wound infection after gastroplasty and gastric banding is lower than that following operations such as jejunoileal bypass (JIB), Roux-en-Y gastric bypass (RYGB), and biliopancreatic diversion (BPD) that involve open intestinal anastomoses. The incidence of septic pulmonary complications and urinary complications is not included in many large clinical reports, probably because these problems rarely result in disability or increased length of hospitalization. The incidence of gastrointestinal (GI) leaks is in the range of 1%-2% in most large series, and does not appear to have decreased during the past three decades. However, it is the author's belief that the mortality rate following leaks may have decreased during this interval.

Pulmonary Complications

Atelectasis is the most common cause of fever in the first 24-48 h following open bariatric operations; most large series do not list it as a "complication" of bariatric surgery. Hess estimates that about 20% of his duodenal switch patients develop atelectasis during postoperative convalescence [1].

Mechanical breathing treatments are the mainstay of treatment of atelectasis; antibiotics are never used as first-line treatment. With conservative treatment, atelectasis typically resolves after 1 or 2 days. In rare cases where pneumonia develops, appropriate antibiotics should be given after obtaining reliable sputum cultures.

Adult respiratory distress syndrome (ARDS) almost never develops from postoperative atelectasis alone. ARDS is typically associated with major sepsis arising from some other organ system, usually the GI tract. The most common

Table 1. Relative incidence of septic complications[a]

Series/Year	Operation	Leaks	Pulmonary	Wound	UTI	Other
Starkloff (1975) [2]	JIB	4 (1%)	–	17 (5%)	–	0
Scott (1977) [7]	JIB	0	15 (8%)	5 (3%)	0	
Yale (1989) [3]	RYGB	3 (1%)	19 (8%)	15 (6%)	5 (2%)	0
Brolin (2000) 4]	RYGB	5 (1%)	1 (0.2%)	4 (1%)	–	2 (0.5%)
Wittgrove (1999) [5]	L-RYGB	11 (2%)	7 (1%)	28 (6%)	–	–
Schauer (2000) [6]	L-RYGB	13 (5%)	15 (6%)	13 (5%)	7 (3%)	–
Yale (1989) [3]	VBG	0	5 (5%)	2 (2%)	–	
Scopinaro (1996) [10]	BPD	2 (0.3%)	–	9 (1%)	1 (0.1%)	
Hess (1998) [1]	BPD-DS	17 (4%)	"20%"	–	–	
Belachew (1998) [9]	SAGB	1 (0.3%)	–	0	0	
Hauri (1999) [11]	SAGB	1 (0.5%)	–	9 (4.3%)	–	

UTI, urinary tract infection; JIB, jejunoileal bypass; RYGB, Roux-en-Y gastric bypass; L-RYGB, laparoscopic RYGB; VBG, vertical banded gastroplasty; BPD, biliopancreatic diversion; BPD-DS, BPD with the duodenal switch; SAGB, silicone adjustable gastric banding.
[a] The number (n) and percentage of complications in each series are given. Blanks indicate that no data were reported for a given complication.

cause of ARDS in bariatric patients is intra-abdominal sepsis resulting from a GI leak or perforation, and ARDS is often the cause of death in cases of overwhelming abdominal sepsis after bariatric operations.

Leaks

The incidence of GI leaks after primary gastric bariatric operations is reported to be in the range of 1%-2% [2-4]. Leaks can be difficult to recognize in bariatric surgical patients because fever and abdominal tenderness are frequently absent during the first 48 h after a leak has occurred. Other symptoms in patients who have leaks include left shoulder and/or suprapubic pain and occasionally a feeling of impending doom. Persistent tachycardia and progressive tachypnea are the most common early signs. Urine output is often decreased.

The leukocyte count is usually elevated but may be within normal limits. An isolated left-sided pleural effusion is a common finding on the plain chest radiograph. Because tachypnea and tachycardia are the typical presenting signs, pulmonary embolism is often suspected initially in a patient with a gastric leak.

Most surgeons attempt to identify leaks using radiographic GI contrast studies. However, a normal contrast study does not exclude a leak, since extravasation from the gastric staple line is usually not identified by upper GI contrast studies. Because failure to recognize a leak can result in death, exploratory laparotomy should be considered in patients with progressive tachypnea and tachycardia in whom pulmonary embolism has been ruled out, and for patients who are rapidly deteriorating, exploratory surgery without GI radiographs may be indicated.

At laparotomy the left upper quadrant should be liberally drained using large suction catheters. Suture repair of leaks at the gastrojejunostomy is rarely successful in the face of florid infection. Conversely, leaks in the gastric staple line usually can be suture closed. If the leak involves the distal bypassed stomach, a tube gastrostomy should be performed. Leaks from enteroenterostomies are extraordinarily rare after bariatric operations.

Laparoscopic Leak Syndrome

With the growing popularity of minimally invasive bariatric surgery, it has become apparent that leaks following laparoscopic procedures are often not as serious as those that follow open bariatric operations. The clinical presentation of laparoscopic leaks is similar but of a lesser magnitude to those that follow open procedures. Although most patients typically have fever and tachycardia, they tend not to develop a precipitous downhill course with progressive signs of overwhelming sepsis and organ system failure. Occasionally these leaks are virtually asymptomatic and are recognized when the patient sees a liquid diet come out through the drain tubing. Wittgrove, Schauer and others have shown that the great majority of leaks following minimally invasive operations can be treated by drainage alone rather than by a second surgical procedure [5, 6]. Moreover, many of these laparoscopic leaks are managed successfully using the indwelling drain placed at the original procedure.

The incidence of leaks following minimally invasive operations appears to be somewhat higher than following open procedures [4, 6, 7]. Much of this difference has been attributed to the so-called learning curve. After a surgeon has performed more than 100 cases it appears that the leak rate after laparoscopic procedures is in the range of 1%-2%, similar to that following open operations.

The usual nonoperative treatment regimen consists of drainage of the leak in conjunction with nutritional support. Parental antibiotics directed against Gram-positive organisms are given. Fungal superinfections are occasionally problematic after prolonged use of broad-spectrum intravenous antibacterial agents. Occasionally, these leaks will close after only 2-3 weeks of drainage. If a patient's clinical condition deteriorates with nonoperative management laparotomy should be performed. Follow-up evaluation of leaks consists of performing radiographic contrast studies at 2-3 week intervals until the leak is shown to be closed. A minimum of two different radiological contrast studies, including a contrast swallow and a sinogram through the drain, should be performed before pulling the drain out and restarting a patient on an oral diet. The author has found CT to be less useful than contrast studies in following bariatric leaks.

The incidence of leaks following revision procedures is 5-10 times higher than after primary bariatric operations, presumably as a result of ischemic damage to the stomach [4, 8]. Although the published mortality rate of leaks after open operations is in the range of 10%-20%, it may well be higher in the hands of less experienced surgeons. Delayed recognition and treatment of GI leaks is the most common cause of preventable death after bariatric operations, and the most common reason for litigation.

Wound Infection

Primary infection of the subcutaneous wound is surprisingly uncommon after bariatric operations. The incidence in most large series ranges between 1% and 5% [4, 7, 9]. In the author's experience the majority of wound infections arise from inadequately drained seromas. Seromas are common following open bariatric operations with an incidence approaching 50%, and wound infection in the absence of a preexisting seroma is rare.

Both seromas and subcutaneous wound infections can usually be treated conservatively. Most seromas drain spontaneously, however, evacuation of additional fluid by the surgeon is occasionally required, using a sterile cotton tip applicator. It is rarely necessary to open the wound more than 5-10 cm to evacuate a seroma.

Most primary wound infections involve *Staphylococcus aureus* species with *Streptococcus* species a distant second in terms of frequency. Gram-negative infections are less common.

The principles of treatment of infected incisions following bariatric operations differ somewhat from the surgical principles employed for other wound infections. Incision and drainage is used to treat the infection, and the wound must be opened sufficiently to achieve adequate drainage. However, opening the entire length of a large incision condemns the patient to months of wound care prior to secondary closure. Even a more limited approach for drainage can result in several months of wound care for patients with an extremely deep fat layer. Certainly, vigilant and aggressive wound care is imperative in order to adequately treat these infections. Use of antibiotics is generally of secondary importance. The choice of antibiotics should be guided by the culture results.

Urinary Infection

Urinary tract infection is relatively uncommon after bariatric operations, occurring in 2%-3% of patients, and directly related to the length of time indwelling urinary catheters remain in place [3, 6]. Occasionally bariatric patients are so immobilized by their obesity that they are unable to use a bed pan or walk to the bathroom, with the result that they require urinary catheters for several days postoperatively.

Rare Causes of Sepsis

Septic Phlebitis

Septic phlebitis is a rare cause of sepsis in postoperative bariatric patients. Peripheral deep venous thrombosis (DVT) in the absence of pulmonary embolism is also remarkably uncommon in bariatric surgical patients, occurring in approximately 0.4% of patients in our series [4]. However, catheter sepsis in patients with long standing central venous access is relatively common.

Fournier's Gangrene

Fournier's gangrene, a mixed bacterial infection that produces massive necrosis of the skin and subcutaneous fat, is a rare but recognized complication of severe obesity. Many cases are associated with type II diabetes. Presentation may be subtle, and pain or fever are not evident until extensive infection has set in. The treatment is radical debridement of dead and ischemic tissue in conjunction with broad spectrum parenteral antibiotics. The mortality of Fournier's gangrene in severely obese patients exceeds 50%.

References

1. Hess DS, Hess DW (1998) Biliopancreatic diversion with duodenal switch. Obesity Surg 8:267–282
2. Starkloff GB, Donovan JF, Ramach R, Wolfe BM (1975) Metabolic intestinal surgery: its complications and management. Arch Surg 110:652–657
3. Yale CE (1989) Gastric surgery for morbid obesity: Complications and long term weight control. Arch Surg 124:941–947
4. Brolin RE (2000) Complications of surgery for severe obesity. Prob in Gen Surg 17:55–61
5. Wittgrove AC, Clark GW, Schubert KR (2000) Laparoscopic gastric bypass, Roux-en-Y: the results in 500 patients with 5 year followup. Obes Surg 10:233–239
6. Schauer PR, Ikramuddin S, Gourash W, et al (2000) Outcomes after laparoscopic Roux-en-Y gastric bypass for obesity. Ann Surg 232:515–529
7. Scott HW Jr, Dean RH, Schull HJ, Gluck R (1977) Results of jejunoileal bypass in two hundred patients with morbid obesity. Surg Gynecol Obstet 145:661–670
8. Schwartz RW, Strodel WE, Simpson WS, Griffen WO Jr (1988) Gastric bypass revision: lessons learned from 920 cases. Surgery 104:806–812
9. Belachew M, Legrand M, Vincent V, et al (1998) Laparoscopic adjustable gastric banding. World J Surg 22:955–963
10. Scopinaro N, Gianetta E, Adami FG, et al (1996) Biliopancreatic diversion for obesity at eighteen years. Surgery 119:261–268
11. Hauri P, Steffen R, Richlin T, et al (2000) Treatment of morbid obesity with the Swedish adjustable gastric band (SAGB): complication rate during a 12 month follow up period. Surgery 127:484–488

Invited Commentary

Nicolas V. Christou

The chapter on source control in bariatric surgery is written by a very experienced bariatric surgeon and offers a unique perspective in the management of infectious insults in this specialized patient population.

The section on *pulmonary complications* highlights the need to mobilize these patients *early*. All our patients are urged to walk to their commode the evening of their surgery in the step down unit of the intensive care area. Since sleep apnea can be undiagnosed in as many as 40% of morbidly obese patients, monitoring of oxygen saturation in the first 24 h helps to identify those patients who may need support. Starting their pulmonary toilet and mobilization early diminishes the risk of pulmonary complications in this high-risk patient population.

There is no doubt among experienced bariatric surgeons that *anastomotic leaks* are the "Achilles' heal" of this procedure as far as mortality is concerned. Leaks can kill. In our institution we have a standing order that a pulse rate of >120 bpm along with fever (>38°) and white cell count of >12,000 cells per milliliter indicates an anastomotic leak until proven otherwise. To date, this clinical triad has alerted us to investigate and diagnose an anastomotic leak in 100% of suspected patients. With the use of subcutaneous heparin prophylaxis and early mobilization, tachypnea and tachycardia more commonly presages an anastomotic leak than a pulmonary embolus. If a patient can be accommodated in the CT scan (even with a heavy duty CT scanner, in our practice where the mean BMI is 59, over 50% of our patient population cannot fit because of size and weight) we will proceed to abdominal CT scan with oral contrast, followed by a spiral CT scan of the chest. If the CT scan does not indicate a leak we proceed to gastrografin swallow. At times a chest radiograph will demonstrate increased subdiaphragmatic air from a leak. It should be stressed, as Dr. Brolin has done, that failure to demonstrate a leak radiologically in a patient with sign of a systemic inflammatory response, especially if progressive, should be followed by exploratory laparotomy. The cost of missing a leak could be the patient's life. The management of anastomotic leaks should be limited. Although an attempt at repair can be made, repair is usually unsuccessful because of inflammation. Adequate drainage must be provided, including the placement of a gastrostomy tube.

We have no experience with laparoscopic bariatric procedures. Dr. Brolin suggests that leaks following laparoscopic procedures are often not as serious as those that follow open procedures and that patients do not develop a precipitous downhill course. The theoretical explanation might be that laparoscopic bariatric surgery results in less damage to host tissue (e.g., no large incision) and therefore less "priming" of the host for a second-hit – the anastomotic leak. I stress that this is a theoretical explanation and that this hypothesis has not been tested in a well-controlled clinical trial.

Dr. Brolin states that *infections of the primary wound* are "surprisingly uncommon" after bariatric operations. Perhaps we are treating different patient populations, but our wound infection rate is 10%-20%. I agree that these are always preceded by wound seromas, usually in the dependent area of the wound above the umbilicus. Perhaps the difference in wound infection is a semantic one. By strict definition, any wound that opens and drains spontaneously, or is opened intentionally by the surgeon for that purpose, should be considered infected. The presence of purulent drainage is based on interpretation, and considerable inter-observer variability has been documented. Platt et al. describe the difficulties of obtaining adequate data, such as those reported by NISS [1]. The management of these seromas/wound infections should be tailored to the patient. I agree that they need not be opened completely, as long as adequate drainage is provided. In our experience, incisional hernias often follow these wound infections.

Avoiding placing a urinary catheter in these patients can minimize *urinary tract infections*. Hence, we do not insert them perioperatively. We also have an 18-h Foley catheter rule: one is not to be placed unless the patient has not voided 18 h after their surgery, or unless the patient is physiologically unstable. We find that this rule achieves two objectives. First, it encourages early patient mobilization by having the patient get out of bed and use the commode. Second, it avoids the higher incidence of urinary tract infection associated with placement of the Foley catheter. Even patients with BMI of 70 tolerate this approach quite well. Actually, if properly instructed prior to surgery they are proud to show "what they can do" on the evening of their operation.

I agree with all concepts outlined in the "Rare Causes of Sepsis" section. Like Dr. Brolin, we have not seen a case of Fournier's gangrene at our institution.

Reference

1. Platt, R. Yokoe DS, Sands KE, CDC Eastern Massachusetts Prevention Epicenter Investigators (2001) Emerging Inf Dis 7:212-216

Editorial Comment

While agreeing with Dr. Brolin that "a normal contrast study by no means excludes a leak," we are not enthusiastic about his contention that "extravasation from the gastric staple line is usually not identified by upper GI contrast studies.". True, one should never say "never" or "always" but the leaking foregut in the morbidly obese patient should not differ from that of the nonobese patient following major upper gastrointestinal surgery. A leak is a leak, and if it is significant, contrast will leak through as well. Routine water-soluble contrast UGI study following bariatric operations in 413 patients identified all clinical leaks. The authors admit, however, that the "as the interpretation of these radiographs is often difficult, involving different projections or patient's positions, or other technical managements, surgeons and radiologists must interact" [1].

Similarly, we would take issue with the contention that exploratory laparotomy is indicated in the absence of a documented leak. The objective of surgery in the patient with a gastrointestinal leak, is to convert an abscess to a controlled fistula; if no collection is evident, then there is no evidence of an abscess, and no potential benefit to surgery. Empiric laparotomy may be indicated, as suggested by Dr. Christou, in the patient whose size precludes the performance of satisfactory radiographic contrast studies.

Like Dr. Christou, we are skeptical about the notion that leaks following laparoscopic bariatric procedures are less lethal than those developing after open procedures. Results of laparoscopic bariatric procedures are currently reported only by experienced, high-volume laparoscopic bariatric surgeons from large centers. Open bariatric surgery, on the other hand, is widely practiced in the community. One can draw a parallel to pancreatic leaks following the Whipple procedure: in modern studies from centers of excellence it is rarely fatal – when occurring, however, in the community such leaks remain a significant complication. The parallel is self-explanatory.

The message of this chapter is clear: early out of bed, early removal of lines and catheters, and early identification and treatment of leaks. Septic fatalities are usually associated with some sort of delay.

Reference

1. Toppino M, Cesarani F, Comba A, Denegri F, Mistrangelo M, Gandini G, Morino F (2001) The role of early radiological studies after gastric bariatric surgery. Obes Surg 11:447–454

16 The Gallbladder and Biliary Tree

Peter Götzinger, Reinhold Függer

Key Principles

- Early cholecystectomy is the treatment of choice in acute cholecystitis.
- Endoscopic sphincterotomy is the treatment of choice in ascending cholangitis.

Acute Cholecystitis

Acute Calculous Cholecystitis (ACC)

Approximately 90% of cases of acute cholecystitis are associated with cholelithiasis. The clinical findings of acute cholecystitis may include symptoms of local inflammation – such as right upper quadrant tenderness or mass, peritoneal signs, hypoactive bowel sounds, positive Murphy's sign – and systemic toxicity (fever, leukocytosis). Jaundice is noted in approximately 15% of patients even in the absence of associated choledocholithiasis [1]. Hyperbilirubinemia may result from local edema and inflammation secondary to a stone impacted in the cystic duct, or from compression of the common hepatic duct or common bile duct (Mirizzi's syndrome). In the event of prolonged cystic duct obstruction, the gallbladder may become distended with clear mucoid fluid, resulting in a hydrops.

Acute Acalculous Cholecystitis (AAC)

Acalculous cholecystitis is a consequence of a disturbed microcirculation, causing mucosal injury and secondary bacterial invasion of gallbladder wall. AAC is a life-threatening condition that may develop in postoperative patients, after severe injury or burns, and in patients receiving prolonged total parenteral nutrition.

Diagnostic Steps

- *Laboratory tests.* Leukocytosis with a left shift is commonly observed in patients with acute cholecystitis, although a normal white blood cell count does not exclude the diagnosis. Serum bilirubin and serum alkaline phosphatase may be elevated.
- *Ultrasonography* (US). US provides more than 95% sensitivity and specificity for the diagnosis of gallstones greater than 2 mm in diameter [2]. Criteria for acute

cholecystitis include gallstones with associated focal gallbladder tenderness, dilatation of the gallbladder, sludge, generalized wall thickening, gallbladder wall echoes indicating necrosis, and a pericholecystic fluid collection or abscess.

- *Hepatobiliary scintigraphy* (HS). Nonvisualization of the gallbladder in symptomatic patients at 1 h – with visualization of the liver, bile ducts and the duodenum – is diagnostic of acute cholecystitis. *A normal scan virtually rules out the diagnosis of acute cholecystitis in patients who present with abdominal pain.* HS has a better diagnostic accuracy for acute cholecystitis than US (sensitivity 88% vs. 50%, specificity 93% vs. 88%) [3]. We believe that HS should be used in the confirmation or exclusion of acute cholecystitis.
- *Computed tomography* (CT) *and magnetic resonance imaging* (MRI). The role of these imaging modalities is controversial. Although CT is over 90% specific and sensitive, it offers no advantages to the simpler and less costly diagnostic tests described above [4].

Therapeutic Steps

Initial therapy of acute cholecystitis is directed towards general support of the patient, including fluid and electrolyte replacement, correction of metabolic imbalances, and antibacterial therapy.

Antibacterial Therapy

Gram-negative bacteria are the most commonly involved organisms [5]. Although anaerobes have been detected in more than 15% of patients, they are seldom proven as the sole isolates [6]. Selection of antibacterial treatment is based on the severity of the disease process, the probable biliary pathogens, and the in vitro activity of the antibacterial agents. A broad-spectrum therapeutic regimen against both Gram-negative and Gram-positive organisms is the preferred treatment. The literature recommends ureidopenicillins, which exhibit a broad-spectrum activity that includes many anaerobes, the Gram-positive streptococci and Gram-negative bacilli [7]. Anaerobic coverage (for example, with metronidazole) is warranted in the initial management of biliary tract infections [5].

Surgical Treatment

- The cornerstone of treatment of acute cholecystitis (calculous/acalculous) is removal of the inflamed gallbladder. Laparoscopic cholecystectomy is increasingly employed as the initial surgical approach, offering the advantage of shorter length of stay, quicker recovery, and a faster return to full activity with less postoperative pain compared with the open approach [8–10]. Overall morbidity and mortality rates for laparoscopic cholecystectomy in acute cholecystitis range between 10% to 13% and 0.4%, respectively [11]. Duration of surgery is not significantly prolonged and outcome reflected in admission to the intensive care unit and hospital stay is significantly better in patients in whom laparoscopic cholecystectomy is successful [12].

- Laparoscopic operation should be undertaken within 48 h of onset of the disease. Recent reports cite conversion rates (from laparoscopic to open surgery) of 11% to 32% in laparoscopic cholecystectomy for acute cholecystitis, which may be reduced to 1.8% by performing this procedure within 48 h after onset of the disease [11, 13-15]. Nonetheless, in cases of severe inflammation of the gallbladder, or when it is difficult to identify ductal anatomy clearly, the threshold to convert to an open procedure should be low. The laparoscopic experience of the surgeon has a significant influence on the conversion rate [16].
- In the laparoscopic approach to the difficult gallbladder, conversion rates may be further lowered by performing the technique of laparoscopic subtotal cholecystectomy. By leaving the posterior wall of the gallbladder intact to avoid excessive bleeding or damage to bile ducts, the conversion to open procedure may be avoided [17, 18].
- The management of ACC is dictated by the overall condition of the patient. Because AAC is often aggravated by local complications such as gangrene and perforation, the diagnosis should mandate prompt operative approach [19]. In patients in whom operation is considered, prompt cholecystectomy is indicated, either laparoscopically or open.
- Percutaneous cholecystostomy has been proposed as an alternative measure for critically ill patients at extreme risk for general anesthesia. Resolution of the inflammation usually follows decompression of the gallbladder. Once sepsis and acute infection resolved and the underlying critical illness is dealt with, interval laparoscopic cholecystectomy may be safely performed in up to 91% of the patients [20].
- The indication for intraoperative cholangiography does not differ from that used in the elective setting. There is no evidence that routine cholangiography is necessary. However, cholangiography is indicated when the anatomy is uncertain, in order to avoid or diagnose bile duct injury, and when ductal stones are suspected [21]. It appears that routine drainage of the gallbladder bed is unnecessary [22, 23].

Acute Cholangitis

Acute cholangitis is an infection of the biliary tree caused by biliary stasis leading to ascending bacterial infection. Its causes include ductal stones, strictures, or tumors, as well as endoscopic manipulation. Increased intrabiliary pressure may cause retrograde spread to the perihepatic lymphatics and portal system, in turn causing bacteremia [24].

Clinical Signs

The classic presentation of acute cholangitis is Charcot's Triad (pain, chills, and jaundice), rarely accompanied by shock and mental confusion (Reynold's Pentate), although one or more of these features may be absent.

Laboratory findings show leukocytosis, elevated C-reactive protein, and elevation of the bilirubin and alkaline phosphatase.

Diagnosis

Ultrasonography

Ultrasonography may show dilated bile ducts, but the technique is insensitive in diagnosing common bile duct stones or establishing the exact cause of cholangitis. The presence of cholelithiasis suggests, but does not prove, that ductal stones are the underlying cause.

Endoscopic Retrograde Cholangiopancreatography

Endoscopic retrograde cholangiopancreatography (ERCP) is particularly useful in the management of the jaundiced patient suspected of having biliary obstruction, causing acute cholangitis. Endoscopic cholangiography should be achievable in 85%-90% of patients and will detect extrahepatic biliary obstruction if it is present. A completely normal study excludes extrahepatic obstruction. Acute cholangitis is not a contraindication to cholangiography provided that prompt endoscopic, radiographic, or surgical decompression is available.

Magnetic Resonance Cholangiopancreatography

Magnetic resonance cholangiopancreatography (MRCP) can be a useful tool to complete the diagnostic steps in patients with acute cholangitis if ductal cannulation by ERCP is unsuccessful or incomplete. As a diagnostic tool MRCP, unlike ERCP, is noninvasive.

Treatment

Initial management includes supportive care and intravenous antibiotics; the majority of patients (70%-85%) will respond to these measures. However approximately 15% of patients will not respond, and require immediate ductal decompression. In severe suppurative cholangitis biliary drainage is life-saving. Endoscopic biliary decompression with a nasobiliary drain or stent placement is generally considered the treatment method of choice [25]. Sphincterotomy and ductal clearance is possible when stones are small and few in number.

Another therapeutic option is ultrasound-guided percutaneous transhepatic biliary drainage of the obstructed ductal system [26]. If endoscopic or transhepatic biliary drainage fails in the presence of severe suppurative cholangitis, emergency surgical decompression is indicated. Surgical decompression consists of ductal clearance when ductal stones are present, accompanied by placing a transcystic tube or T-tube.

If cholangitis is secondary to a tumor, the initial step is endoscopic/transhepatic decompression. After resolution of inflammatory signs, the tumor is evaluated for resectability and further treatment planned electively.

Controversies

- *Optimal timing for surgical treatment in acute cholecystitis*: Until recently, this has been a subject of debate. The literature shows mortality rates for early and delayed surgical procedures to be comparable, with no significant difference in the frequency or severity of postoperative complications [11]. The primary benefit of early (within 48 h of admission) laparoscopic cholecystectomy is that laparoscopic management is more likely to be successful [27].
- *Open or laparoscopic cholecystectomy*: Although conversion rates are higher in acute cholecystitis then when operation is undertaken electively, randomized studies show that laparoscopic cholecystectomy is safe, and patients benefit from the known advantages of the minimal invasive approach [28].

Algorithm

Acute Cholecystitis (Calculous/Acalculous)

a) Prompt diagnosis (clinical findings, US, laboratory findings]
b) General fluid replacement, organ monitoring, antibiotic therapy
c) Surgical treatment

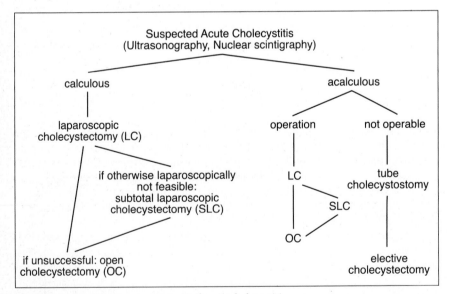

Diagram 1. Algorithm for management of acute cholecystitis

Cholangitis

a) Prompt diagnosis (clinical findings, US, laboratory findings, ERCP, MRCP)
b) General fluid replacement, organ monitoring, antibiotic therapy
c) Therapy (see Diagram 1)

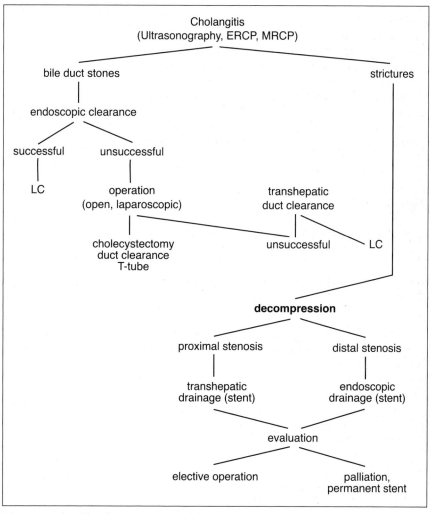

Diagram 2. Algorithm for management of cholangitis

References

1. Voyles CR, Sanders DL, Hogan R (1994) Common bile duct evaluation in the era of laparoscopic cholecystectomy: 1050 cases later. Ann Surg 219:744–750
2. Bortoff GA, Chen MY, Ott DJ, Wolfman NT, Routh WD (2000) Gallbladder stones: imaging and intervention. Radiographics 20:751–766
3. Chatziioannou SN, Moore WH, Ford PV, Dhekne RD (2000) Hepatobiliary scintigraphy is superior to abdominal ultrasonography in suspected acute cholecystitis. Surgery 127:609–613
4. Mirvis SE, Vainright JR, Nelson AW, et al (1986) The diagnosis of acute acalculous cholecystitis: A comparison of sonography, scintigraphy and CT. AJR 147:1171–1175
5. Westphal JF, Brogard JM (1999) Biliary tract infections: a guide to drug treatment. Drugs 57:81–91
6. Brook I (1989) Aerobic and anaerobic microbiology of biliary tract disease. J Clin Microbiol 27:2373–2375
7. Eliopoulos GM, Moellering RC (1982) Azlocillin, mezlocillin, and piperacillin: new broad spectrum penicillins. Ann Intern Med 97:755–760
8. Schwesinger WH, Sirinek KR, Srodel WE 3rd (1999) Laparoscopic cholecystectomy for biliary tract emergencies: state of the art. World J Surg 23:334–342
9. Cuschieri A (1993) Approach to the treatment of acute cholecystitis: open surgical, laparoscopic or endoscopic? Endoscopy 25:397–398
10. Garber SM, Korman J, Cosgrove JM, Cohen JR (1997) Early laparoscopic cholecystectomy for acute cholecystitis. Surg Endosc 11:347–350
11. Lillemoe KD (2000) Surgical treatment of biliary tract infections. Am Surg 66:138–144
12. Habib FA, Kolachalam RB, Khilnani R, Preventza O, Mittal VK (2001) Role of laparoscopic cholecystectomy in the management of gangrenous cholecystitis. Am J Surg 181:71–75
13. Chandler CF, Lane JS, Ferguson P, Thompson JE, Ashley SW (2000) Prospective evaluation of early versus delayed laparoscopic cholecystectomy for treatment of acute cholecystitis. Am Surg 66:896–900
14. Lo CM, Lai EC, Fan ST, Liu CL, Wong J (1996) Laparoscopic cholecystectomy for acute cholecystitis in the elderly. World J Surg 20:983–986
15. Willsher PC, Sanabria JR, Gallinger S, Rossi L, Strasberg S, Litwin DE (1999) Early laparoscopic cholecystectomy for acute cholecystitis: a safe procedure. J Gastrointest Surg 3:50–53
16. Liu CL, Fan ST, Lai EC, Lo CM, Chu KM (1996) Factors affecting conversion of laparoscopic cholecystectomy to open surgery. Arch Surg 131:98–101
17. Ransom KJ (1998) Laparoscopic management of acute cholecystitis with subtotal cholecystectomy. Am Surg 64:955–957
18. Michalowski K, Bornman PC, Krige JE, Gallagher PJ, Terblanche J (1998) Laparoscopic subtotal cholecystectomy in patients with complicated acute cholecystitis or fibrosis. Br J Surg 85:904–906
19. Traverso LW (1993) Clinical manifestations and impact of gallstone disease. Am J Surg 165:405–409
20. Berber E, Engle KL, String A, Garland AM, Chang G, Macho J, Pearl JM, Siperstein AE (2000) Selective use of tube cholecystostomy with interval laparoscopic cholecystectomy in acute cholecystitis. Arch Surg 135:341–346
21. Snow LL, Weinstein LS, Hannon JK, Lane DR (2001) Evaluation of operative cholangiography in 2043 patients undergoing laparoscopic cholecystectomy. Surg Endosc 15:14–20
22. Monson JRT, Guillon PJ, Keane FBV, Tanner WA, Brennan TG (1991) Cholecystectomy is safer without drainage: the result of a prospective, randomized clinical trial. Surgery 109:740–746
23. Fritsch A, Függer R (1993) Drainage in hepatobiliary surgery. Chirurg 64:85–89
24. Raraty MG, Finch M, Neoptolemos JP (1998) Acute cholangitis and pancreatitis secondary to common duct stones: management update. World J Surg 22:1155–1161
25. Lai EC (1990) Management of severe acute cholangitis. Br J Surg 77:604–6055
26. Huang MH, Ker CG (1988) Ultrasonic guided percutaneous transhepatic bile drainage for cholangitis due to intrahepatic stones. Arch Surg 123:106–109

27. Rattner DW, Ferguson C, Warshaw AL (1993) Factors associated with successful laparoscopic cholecystectomy. Ann Surg 218:129–137
28. Kiviluoto T, Siren J, Luukkonen P, Kivilaakso E (1998) Randomized trial of laparoscopic versus open cholecystectomy for acute and gangrenous cholecystitis. Lancet 351:321–325

Invited Commentary

JACK PICKLEMAN

In general, I find much to agree with in the authors' approach to the management of patients with acute cholecystitis and ascending cholangitis. Their chapter is concise, up to date, and displays mature clinical judgment throughout.

The authors outline the standard ultrasonographic criteria for acute cholecystitis and this diagnosis can be presumed in patients with a compatible clinical history and any of these radiologic signs. The real utility of ultrasonography rests in the fact that it is quickly obtainable, inexpensive, and, when coupled with a clinical history suggestive of acute cholecystitis, very reliable. Hepatobiliary scintigraphy, although favored by the authors, is used far less frequently than ultrasonography in the United States. An additional disadvantage of this test is that it may yield a false-positive result (e.g., nonvisualization of the gallbladder) in a sick or fasting patient, as the gallbladder is already distended with bile and may not take up the radioisotope. With respect to antibacterial therapy in acute cholecystitis, this author would favor a single preoperative dose of a second-generation cephalosporin, without specific anaerobic coverage. Importantly, no postoperative antibiotic therapy is necessary.

This reviewer strongly agrees with the authors' recommendation for laparoscopic cholecystectomy early in the course of acute cholecystitis. Delaying operation invites problems associated with uncontrolled sepsis and a higher conversion on rate to open cholecystectomy secondary to an increased inflammatory reaction. Additionally, patients who are thought to harbor gallbladder perforation, or those in whom a large tender mass is palpable preoperatively indicating a walled off inflammatory process, may be better and more cost effectively served by proceeding initially with open cholecystectomy. The authors stress the importance of a low threshold for conversion to open cholecystectomy if technical difficulties are encountered or if delineation of biliary anatomy is impaired. I could not agree more with them on this point. However, I would personally discourage the performance of subtotal laparoscopic cholecystectomy if technical difficulties are encountered. If the operation is that difficult, conversion to an open procedure represents sound surgical judgment.

Percutaneous ultrasonographic or CT-guided cholecystostomy will surely improve most critically ill patients with acute cholecystitis and concomitant morbidity. Although large series of such successfully treated patients have been published, it is difficult to determine how many such patients would have responded to antibiotic therapy alone and in whom the cholecystostomy was an unnecessary adjunct. However, in the occasional ICU patient with multiple organ system failure secondary to occult sepsis or suspected acute cholecystitis, this procedure may have merit. I agree with the authors' recommendation against routine operative cholangiography, unless there is a strong suspicion of the presence of common duct stones or if biliary ductal anatomy is unclear.

Regarding the management of ascending cholangitis, the authors' diagnostic and therapeutic steps are optimal. It should, however, be stressed that, in patients with ascending cholangitis, there is no role for either percutaneous or operative tube cholecystostomy, as this procedure will not reliably decompress the common bile duct.

Editorial Comment

We wish to add a few practical points to the otherwise solid advice given by the contributors and the commentator.

- *The high-risk patient.* It is today rare to encounter a patient who cannot be subjected to an emergency procedure under general anesthesia. But what to do with the occasional extremely sick patient who is even "not fit for a haircut under local"? The options are a tube cholecystostomy under local anesthesia; either ultrasound guided, percutaneous-transhepatic, by the radiologist, or an operative cholecystostomy. Failure of the patient to improve within 24 h, particularly after the percutaneous procedure, should suggest the presence of undrained pus or necrotic gallbladder wall, and the need to operate. Laparoscopic procedures are contraindicated in critically ill patients because the laparoscopic CO_2 pneumoperitoneum causes intra-abdominal hypertension The latter, with its adverse cardiorespiratory and renal physiological effects, further compromises the condition of the already compromised patient [1]. Furthermore, experimental studies suggest that laparoscopic CO_2 pneumoperitoneum increases the infective-septic complications and mortality rate in "late peritonitis" [2]. As a general rule, during laparoscopic cholecystectomy the lowest possible intra-abdominal pressure should be used. This together with gradual insufflation and limiting the head-up degree to minimum, avoids cardiovascular instability in high-risk patients [3] (see Chap. 36).
- *The cirrhotic patient.* An emergency cholecystectomy in cirrhotics with portal hypertension may quickly degenerate into a *bloody disaster* due to an intra- or postoperative hemorrhage from the congested gallbladder's hepatic bed, or from large venous collaterals at the duodenohepatic ligament. Although conventional laparoscopic cholecystectomy has been judged as safe in selected "Child A" or even B patients [4], the secret is to stay away from trouble – not to dissect near the engorged and rigid hepatic parenchyma and the excessively vascular triangle of Callot. For us, a subtotal or partial cholecystectomy is the procedure of choice in this situation – as discussed below.

- *Choledocholithiasis associated with acute cholecystitis.* About a tenth of patients who suffer from AC have associated common bile duct stones. As Drs. Götzinger and Függer stressed, AC may produce jaundice and liver enzyme disturbances in the absence of any ductal pathology. AC is very rarely associated with active complications of choledocholithiasis. Thus, the combinations of AC with acute pancreatitis, ascending cholangitis, or obstructive jaundice is uncommon. The emphasis, therefore, should be on the treatment of AC, which represents the life-threatening condition; ductal stones, if present, are of secondary importance.
- *Acalculous cholecystitis.* Acalculous cholecystitis is another common sequel of the disturbed micro-circulation in the critically ill patient. Clinical diagnosis is extremely difficult in the critically ill or traumatized patient. Abdominal complaints and the background disease mask signs. Fever, jaundice, leukocytosis, and disturbed liver function tests are commonly present but are entirely nonspecific. The early diagnosis requires a high index of suspicion: *suspect and exclude cholecystitis as the cause of an otherwise unexplained septic state or SIRS.* Ultrasonography performed at the bedside is the diagnostic modality of choice. Gallbladder wall thickness (>3.0-3.5 mm), intramural gas, the "halo" sign, and pericholecystic fluid are very suggestive. Similar findings on CT examination confirm the diagnosis. False-positive and negative studies have been reported with both imaging modalities. Hepatobiliary radioisotope scanning is associated with a high incidence of false-positive studies. However, filling of the gallbladder with the radioisotope (morphine assisted, if necessary) excludes cholecystitis. A highly suggestive clinical scenario and diagnostic uncertainty is an invitation to treat, as indicated by the contributors. However, acalculous cholecystitis is an uncommon entity in critical illness, whereas nonspecific distention – the equivalent of gall bladder ileus – is quite common.
- We agree with Dr. Pickleman that routine anti-anaerobic coverage is unnecessary in acute cholecystitis and that postoperative antibiotics are not needed in the absence of established purulent or biliary peritonitis. Acute cholecystitis represents a resectable type of infection, necessitating only perioperative antibiotics [6].

A Few Additional Technical Points

- As Dr. Pickleman stressed, very difficult gallbladders should be removed through an open approach. In addition, most converted cases will be difficult. In this situation it is wise to *go fundus down and stay near the gallbladder.* After needle decompression (connect a wide bore needle to the suction) of the distended gallbladder, hold the fundus up with an instrument and dissect down towards the cystic duct and artery, which are the last attachments to be secured and divided. Observing this rule, it is virtually impossible to damage the bile duct.
- Subtotal (partial) cholecystectomy is an excellent solution in problematic situations such as a difficult-to-dissect triangle of Calot, portal hypertension, or coagulopathy. The gallbladder is resected starting at the fundus; the posterior

wall (or what is left of it when a necrotizing attack has occurred) is left attached to the hepatic bed and its rim is oversewn for hemostasis with a running
suture. At the level of the Hartmann pouch, the cystic duct opening is identified from within. The accurate placement of a purse-string suture around this
opening as described by others is not satisfactory, as the suture tends to tear
out in the inflamed and friable tissues. Best is to leave a 1 cm rim of the Hartmann pouch tissue and suture-buttress it over the opening of the cystic duct.
When no healthy gallbladder wall remains for closing the cystic duct, it is absolutely safe just to leave a suction drain and bail out. In the absence of distal
common bile duct obstruction the drain will remain dry because the cystic
duct is obstructed by the inflammatory process. The exposed and often necrotic mucosa of the posterior gallbladder wall is destroyed with diathermy and
the omentum is brought into the area. In this operation the structures in the
Calot's triangle are not dissected out, and bleeding from the hepatic bed is
avoided; it is a fast and safe procedure having the advantages of both cholecystectomy and cholecystostomy [5].

* *Cholecystostomy.* This procedure may be indicated in the very rare patient who
  must be done under local anesthesia and when percutaneous cholecystostomy
  is not available or successful. After the infiltration of local anesthesia place a
  "mini" incision over the point of maximum tenderness or the palpable GB
  mass. You can mark the position of the fundus on the skin during preoperative ultrasound – as it is embarrassing to enter the abdomen, under local
  anesthesia, and find that the gallbladder is far away. The visualization of gallbladder wall necrosis at this stage mandates a subtotal cholecystectomy; otherwise, open the fundus and remove all stones from the gallbladder and Hartmann's pouch. For improved inspection of the gallbladder lumen, and
  complete extraction of stones and sludge, a sterile proctoscope may be useful.
  Thereafter, insert into the fundus a tube of your choice (we prefer a large
  Foley), securing it in place with a purse-string suture. Fix the fundus to the
  cholecystostomy site at the abdominal wall, as you would do with a gastrostomy. A tube cholangiogram performed 1 week after the operation will tell you
  whether the cystic duct and bile ducts are patent; if so, the tube can be safely
  removed. Whether an interval cholecystectomy is subsequently indicated is
  controversial.

References

1. Safran DB, Orlando R 3rd (1994) Physiologic effects of pneumoperitoneum. Am J Surg 167:281–286
2. Bloechle C, Emmermann A, Strate T, Scheurlen UJ, Schneider C et al (1998) Laparoscopic vs. open repair of gastric perforation and abdominal lavage of associated peritonitis in pigs. Surg Endosc 12:212–218
3. Dhoste K, Lacoste L, Karayan J, Lehuede MS, Thomas D, Fusciardi J (1996) Haemodynamic and ventilatory changes during laparoscopic cholecystectomy in elderly ASA III patients. Can J Anaesth 43:783–788
4. Poggio JL, Rowland CM, Gores GJ, Nagorney DM, Donohue JH (2000) A comparison of la-paroscopic and open cholecystectomy in patients with compensated cirrhosis and sympto-matic gallstone disease Surgery 127:405–411

5. Schein M (1991) Partial cholecystectomy in the emergency treatment of acute cholecystitis in the compromised patient. J Roy Coll Surg Edinb 36:295–297
6. Wittmann DH, Schein M (1996) Let us shorten antibiotic prophylaxis and therapy in surgery. Am J Surg 172[Supp 6A]:26S–32S

17 Pancreatic Infection

PATCHEN DELLINGER

Key Principles

- Timely diagnosis of infection
- Prompt debridement when infection is diagnosed
- Easier and safer late debridement, when possible
- Debridement of sterile necrosis, late in the course of the disease, if needed at all
- Removal of necrotic and/or infected tissue
- Avoidance of acute morbidity associated with necrotic tissue debridement (bleeding, fistula, devascularization of viscera, splenic injury)
- Preservation of functional tissue – pancreas, endocrine and exocrine
- Avoidance of late morbidity (prolonged open wounds, fistulas, hernias)

General Approach

Necrotizing pancreatitis [1] presents a number of challenges to the treating physician (Table 1), including diagnosis of pancreatitis, early treatment decisions, timely recognition of infection, timing of intervention for source control, and best techniques of source control. Patients with infected necrotizing pancreatitis have a high morbidity and mortality. The disease is common enough that most practicing surgeons will see several cases in a career, but uncommon enough that most do not accumulate an extensive experience. Even referral centers that publish series of cases see only from 6 to 22 cases per year on average [2-6]. Thus, controlled trials of different approaches to treatment are not common and frequently are not decisive. Older trials that have been conducted in pancreatitis often include all degrees of severity and are not relevant to the management of

Table 1. General approach

Diagnosis of necrotizing pancreatitis

Stabilization of cardiorespiratory status

Support of organ failure

Diagnosis of infection

Debridement of necrotic and infected tissue

Re-debridement and/or drainage as needed – scheduled or unscheduled

Wound closure

patients with severe necrotizing pancreatitis. Prospective trials of treatment for pancreatitis have failed to demonstrate consistent benefit for nasogastric suction, H_2 blockers, atropine, glucagon, somatostatin, calcitonin, indomethacin, aprotinin, gabexate, lexipafant, fresh frozen plasma, parenteral nutrition, peritoneal lavage, sump drainage, or pancreatic resection [7]. Regarding timing and technique for operative source control, almost no controlled trials have been conducted. One trial evaluating the timing of operative intervention was stopped prematurely with small numbers and no definitive conclusion [4]. This trial entered all patients with necrotizing pancreatitis with or without infection, and showed a trend that favored operation *after* 12 days. The information that is available to us comes from institutional series, either compared with their own prior experience as their techniques and procedures evolved, compared with other published series, or not compared.

Initial Presentation

The issues in diagnosing and caring for a patient with severe pancreatitis begin with the initial presentation, since even sterile pancreatitis in the absence of infection typically presents with fever, leukocytosis, tachycardia, and abdominal pain and tenderness, all signs consistent with abdominal infection [8]. The initial process is chemical rather than infectious; severe cases produce necrosis of pancreatic parenchymal tissues and surrounding peripancreatic, retroperitoneal adipose tissues. Patients with greater degrees of retroperitoneal necrosis and/or a more severe physiologic disturbance (measured by APACHE II or Ranson scores, or an organ failure score) have a higher incidence of infection [8-10]. The route of infection in individual cases is not usually known, but it can occur through bacteremia, biliary organisms entering the pancreatic duct, especially in cases of biliary pancreatitis, and through translocation. Animal models support all routes of contamination. Operative intervention in cases of sterile necrosis also introduces nosocomial contamination and infection in up to 30 % of cases [11, 12]. The time of onset of infection can be very difficult to determine; the clinical course of the patient is rarely helpful since infected patients cannot be distinguished from uninfected patients on the basis of white blood cell count, temperature, or abdominal exam [8]. Documented infection may occur during the first week of disease, or as late as 8-10 weeks later, but is more commonly diagnosed in the third and fourth week [10].

The role of ERCP in patients with severe biliary pancreatitis has been debated. Current data support its use primarily for patients with evidence of biliary obstruction and cholangitis [7].

Diagnosis and Antibiotics

Infection can be confirmed by culture of retroperitoneal tissues obtained at operation, but operation on clinical grounds alone results in intervention in sterile necrosis as often as 60 % of the time, and carries the risk of secondary infection following operation [11]. A preoperative CT scan demonstrating extensive gas collections in an area of necrosis almost always indicates infection, but occurs in a minority of cases. The only reliable preoperative diagnostic test for infection is CT or ultrasound-guided percutaneous aspiration of necrotic retroperitoneal tissues. This technique is approximately 90 % accurate and can be repeated as necessary in prolonged cases. Ninety percent of errors with this technique occur during the first week of the disease, a time when aspiration can usually be avoided [11]. Needle aspiration appears to be reliable even in patients receiving antibiotics at the time of the aspiration, probably because the antibiotics do not penetrate into the necrotic, unperfused areas where infection occurs.

Whether or not to begin systemic antibiotics in patients with retroperitoneal necrosis but no diagnosis of infection is controversial. Many experienced surgeons favor the early use of systemic antibiotics, but the trials that have been performed in this area have a number of shortcomings, and tend show a reduction in infections without a corresponding reduction in the number of operations required, morbidity, or mortality [8].

Operation in Sterile Necrosis?

There is also controversy regarding the role of operative intervention in patients with necrosis visible on CT scan and no documented infection, but a progressive course with organ failure despite aggressive ICU support. There are no comparative studies available to answer this question. Individual series reporting the results of operative debridement of sterile necrosis have suggested benefit [13], however, other series have reported patients with sterile necrosis who survived without operative intervention [12]. It is clear that a significant number of patients with pancreatic and peripancreatic necrosis but without infection will improve without operative intervention, the published figures showing a survival of 261/287 (90.9 %, 95 % confidence interval = 87.6 %-94.2 %) [12]. Whether patients with sterile necrosis who do not respond to nonoperative management might benefit from intervention and debridement cannot be determined from available published data. Recent publications, even from centers previously favoring debridement of sterile necrosis, acknowledge that many patients do not benefit, and recommend it only for patients who remain symptomatic weeks after the onset of disease [11, 14].

The Operation

When the diagnosis of retroperitoneal infection is made, all agree that intervention is required, and no studies regarding management of these patients without source control exist. The controversies relate to the method of operative intervention or source control. All agree that most necrotic tissue must be removed, and there are no reports of deliberately incomplete debridement. However, complete debridement at the first operation is impossible in the majority of patients. Most of the infected necrotic tissue is in the retroperitoneum of the lesser sac, often

Table 2. Controversies

Should systemic (preventive) antibiotics be started for patients with necrotizing pancreatitis before the diagnosis of infection is established?

What is the role of ERCP?

Should sterile necrosis be debrided?

What is the best time for operative debridement?

What is the best operative approach when debridement is done?

Percutaneous drains?
   Temporizing
   Definitive
   To provide guidance/access for a videoendoscopic approach

Videoendoscope?
   As the sole approach
   As an adjunct to an open procedure

Open operation?
   Incision
     Midline
     Subcostal
     Posterior approach
   Follow-up care
     Reoperate when indicated
       Open
       Percutaneous
     Close with scheduled reoperation (+ "zipper")
     Close with postoperative lavage
       Leave open

extending to the retrocolic gutters on the left and right and sometimes into the perirenal spaces. The process commonly extends into the transverse mesocolon and into the base of the small bowel mesentery, and on occasion, can extend as far as the mediastinum or the groin. The involved tissues surround the pancreas and the major visceral vessels, and injury to splenic vessels, spleen, pancreas, and mesentery with secondary injury to bowel can easily occur during debridement – or after as a result of pressure from drains or trauma from dressing changes. The response to these challenges has generated a number of published approaches to source control in these patients (Table 2).

Which Procedure?

The most widely described methods involve open laparotomy with exposure of the lesser sac and blunt debridement of the involved tissues. Viable tissues should be left both to avoid bleeding and to minimize late endocrine and exocrine dysfunction [15]. It is important to have a high-quality recent CT scan available in the operating room. During the operation the scan should be consulted to ensure that the debridement has been carried to all involved areas. Different authors champion a midline incision or a bilateral subcostal incision. The subcostal incision may provide slightly better access to the upper abdomen but makes debridement of caudal areas and management of submesocolic intra-abdominal complications more difficult. The choice of specific incision is better left to the experience and preference of the operating surgeon. Some prefer a posterior, 12th rib approach to the retroperitoneum to avoid complications of open laparotomy that will be discussed below. This approach is more difficult for many surgeons and gives a more limited access to the retroperitoneum but can be used to good effect if the surgeon has the experience, and if the CT scan demonstrates that all areas needing debridement will be accessible by this approach.

When the initial debridement is completed the abdomen can be closed primarily, closed over drains of various types with or without irrigating catheters, or left open with or without gauze packing and/or drains. Following surgery, the patient can be managed in the ICU and reexplored only if clinical indications for reoperation arise, or alternatively scheduled for mandatory reoperation at defined intervals until specific criteria regarding the state of the wound and the retroperitoneum are achieved. Mandatory reoperation often requires some type of prosthetic temporary closure of the abdomen, which can be accomplished with or without a zipper, bur, or similar fastening device. The choice of prosthetic material and use of fastening device are personal preferences of the operating surgeon and have never been demonstrated to affect outcome. Series reporting the outcome of each possible strategy listed above have been published, usually claiming superiority for the approach being published; no comparative series are available.

The concept of mandatory reexploration arose because first operations for necrotizing pancreatitis are typically incomplete, and reflected an attempt to return the patient to the operating room prior to clinical deterioration caused by persistent infection in the remaining areas of infected necrosis. An aggressive program of scheduled relaparotomy is very labor intensive and is most successful when performed by the same surgeon each time. It exposes the patient to an increased risk of wound complications and hernias, and to the repeated risk of bowel injury and fistula formation that increases as granulation tissue covers the viscera and exploration becomes more difficult. Leaving the abdomen open with gauze packing achieves earlier complete debridement, but exposes the patient to an almost inevitable giant incisional hernia and a very high risk of fistula from the gauze packing.

Centers that close the abdomen primarily and place large numbers of drains, with or without irrigation catheters, report that remaining areas of necrosis will ultimately separate from viable tissues and be removed by the drains. For this strategy to work, large drains must be used, and there is a significant risk of bowel or blood vessel injury by pressure and erosion from the drains. For this reason, I favor soft drains such as Penrose drains exiting through large flank incisions. When the abdomen is closed over drains following initial debridement, the treating surgeon must always be prepared to intervene if the patient's condition demonstrates a recurrent or persistent infection. In my experience, this second intervention can often be achieved successfully by *percutaneous techniques* obviating the need for a second open operation. A report of this technique from the Massachusetts General Hospital showed that 44 of 69 patients could be managed by a single surgical procedure, and that another 9 could be managed with a subsequent percutaneous drainage alone [6]. Thus, 83 % had only one trip to the operating room for an open surgical procedure. Retrospective analysis of this experience suggested that the patients benefited when the interval between onset of pancreatitis and operation increased up to 4 weeks. The consensus among pancreatic surgeons is that with time the necrotic tissues separate from surrounding vascularized, viable tissue, and debridement can be more complete. What remains has a better chance of being evacuated by drains.

Percutaneous Treatment

Following reports of successful treatment of intra-abdominal abscesses by percutaneous catheters placed in the radiology department in the early 1980s, this new technique was attempted in patients with infectious complications of pancreatitis. Early reports indicated a high failure rate due to the tenacious nature of the infected necrotic tissue that quickly clogged the catheters, and thus percutaneous drainage for pancreatic infection developed a bad reputation. Other reports indicated that placing catheters into sterile collections that included necrotic elements frequently converted these into infected collections. However, there has recently been a renewed interest in the use of percutaneous catheters, and published series have demonstrated successful management of patients with infected pancreatitis when catheters have been carefully managed by the use of frequent studies, changing and upsizing catheters, vigorous irrigation, and even percutaneous debridement with stone baskets and other such devices via percutaneous access [16-18]. Even when not ultimately successful as the definitive management technique for infected necrotizing pancreatitis, percutaneous catheter drainage can function as a temporizing maneuver, allowing a patient to stabilize and providing some additional time to allow subsequent open surgical drainage to be more complete when it is undertaken.

Videoendoscopic Techniques

Reports of videoendoscopic techniques applied to debridement of infected pancreatic necrosis have recently been published. Videoendoscopic instruments have been used to provide better visualization in areas of the retroperitoneum as part of an open operative procedure [19]. In other reports, the treating surgeon has dilated an existing percutaneous catheter tract and used that to introduce either an operating nephroscope [20] or other videoendoscopic instruments directly into the affected area for debridement under direct video observation. Others have reported small series of patients debrided by a traditional transabdominal laparoscopic approach analogous to laparotomy [21], or by a blunt retroperitoneal approach guided by CT scans [21, 22]. All of these "less invasive" approaches to debridement of infected necrotizing pancreatitis have the potential advantages of minimizing the physiological disturbance of an ill patient and reducing the risk of subsequent incisional hernia, which is common with all of the open approaches.

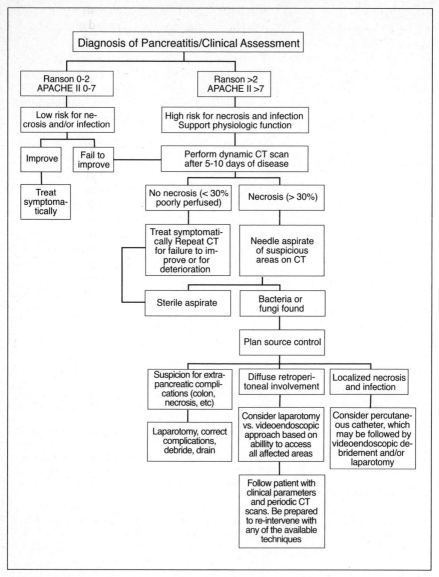

Diagram 1. Algorithm for necrotizing pancreatitis (modified from [8])

Summary

The principles presented above are components of successful source control for the patient with infected necrotizing pancreatitis. The presence of infection of retroperitoneal tissues must be recognized, and is most commonly accomplished with cultures and Gram stains of percutaneous aspirates guided by CT scan.

Whether to operate and debride patients with sterile necrosis who are not responding to nonoperative management remains an unresolved question, however, if operative intervention is contemplated, it should be done late in the course of the disease. Debridement of infected necrotic peripancreatic and pancreatic tissues is more likely to be nearly complete, thus avoiding the need for subsequent debridements, if at least 2 weeks have passed since the onset of acute pancreatitis. There may be a role for percutaneous drains as temporizing procedures in combination with antibiotics for patients who are diagnosed with infected peripancreatic tissue during the first 2 weeks. When debridement is performed it should be as complete as possible, accessing all affected areas and removing as much necrotic tissue as possible. On the other hand, debridement carries a significant risk of bleeding or bowel injury. These complications can be very serious and should be avoided if possible. The aggressiveness of debridement depends on the operative experience of the surgeon. The published literature does not support one technical approach over another with respect to choice of incision, use of drains, closure of the abdomen, mandatory reexploration, or other such options. It is likely that an increasing experience will be available with less invasive percutaneous and videoendoscopic approaches. Whatever approach and schedule are employed, the surgeon must be prepared for additional interventions, the details of which will depend on the circumstances of the individual patient. Most of the controversies listed in Table 2 are amenable to prospective multicenter trials.

References

1. Bradley EL (1993) A clinically based classification system for acute pancreatitis. Summary of the International Symposium on Acute Pancreatitis, Atlanta, Ga, September 1992. Arch Surg 128:586–590
2. Beger HG, Isenmann R (1999) Surgical management of necrotizing pancreatitis. Surg Clin North Am 79:783–800
3. Tsiotos GG, Luque-de Leon E, Soreide JA, et al (1998) Management of necrotizing pancreatitis by repeated operative necrosectomy using a zipper technique. Am J Surg 175:91–98
4. Mier J, Leon EL, Castillo A, Robledo F, Blanco R (1997) Early versus late necrosectomy in severe necrotizing pancreatitis. Am J Surg 173:71–75
5. Pederzoli P, Bassi C, Vesentini S, et al (1990) Necrosectomy by lavage in the surgical treatment of severe necrotizing pancreatitis: results in 263 patients. Acta Chir Scand 156:775–780
6. Fernandez-del Castillo C, Rattner DW, Makary MA, Mostafavi A, McGrath D, Warshaw AL (1998) Debridement and closed packing for the treatment of necrotizing pancreatitis [see comments]. Ann Surg 228:676–684
7. Steinberg W, Tenner S (1994) Acute pancreatitis N Engl J Med 330:1198–1210
8. Dellinger EP (1999) Infectious complications of pancreatitis. In: Root RK, Waldvogel F, Corey L, Stamm WE (eds) Clinical infectious diseases: a practical approach. Oxford University Press, New York, pp 605–611
9. Rau B, Pralle U, Uhl W, Schoenberg MH, Beger HG (1995) Management of sterile necrosis in instances of severe acute pancreatitis [see comments]. J Am Coll Surg 181:279–288
10. Beger H, Bittner R, Block S (1986) Bacterial contamination of pancreatitis necrosis. Gastroenterology 91:433–438
11. Schoenberg MH, Rau B, Beger HG (1999) New approaches in surgical management of severe acute pancreatitis. Digestion 60:22–26
12. Bradley EL (1996) Indications for debridement of necrotizing pancreatitis. Pancreas 13:220–223

13. Rattner DW, Legermate DA, Lee MJ, Mueller PR, Warshaw AL (1992) Early surgical debride-
    ment of symptomatic pancreatic necrosis is beneficial irrespective of infection. Am J Surg
    163:105–109
14. Warshaw AL (1996) What to do about sterile pancreatic necrosis? Pancreas 13:223–225
15. Tsiotos GG, Luque-de Leon E, Sarr MG (1998) Long-term outcome of necrotizing pancreatitis
    treated by necrosectomy. Br J Surg 85:1650–1653
16. Echenique AM, Sleeman D, Yrizarry J, et al (1998) Percutaneous catheter-directed debride-
    ment of infected pancreatic necrosis: results in 20 patients. J Vasc Interv Radiol 9:565–571
17. Freeny PC, Hauptmann E, Althaus SJ, Traverso LW, Sinanan M (1998) Percutaneous CT-guided
    catheter drainage of infected acute necrotizing pancreatitis: techniques and results [see com-
    ments]. AJR Am J Roentgenol 170:969–975
18. Baril NB, Ralls PW, Wren SM, et al (2000) Does an infected peripancreatic fluid collection or
    abscess mandate operation? Ann Surg 231:361–367
19. Oria A, Ocampo C, Zandalazini H, Chiappetta L, Moran C (2000) Internal drainage of giant
    acute pseudocysts: the role of video-assisted pancreatic necrosectomy. Arch Surg 135:136–141
20. Carter CR, McKay CJ, Imrie CW (2000) Percutaneous necrosectomy and sinus tract endos-
    copy in the management of infected pancreatic necrosis: an initial experience. Ann Surg
    232:175–180
21. Gagner M (1996) Laparoscopic treatment of acute necrotizing pancreatitis. Semin Laparosc
    Surg 3:21–28
22. Gambiez LP, Denimal FA, Porte HL, Saudemont A, Chambon JP, Quandalle PA (1998) Retro-
    peritoneal approach and endoscopic management of peripancreatic necrosis collections.
    Arch Surg 133:66–72

Invited Commentary

Beat Gloor, Markus W. Büchler

The key principles, as mentioned by Dr. Dellinger – prompt debridement when
infection is diagnosed and, if at all, late debridement in patients with sterile
necrosis – certainly represent today's "gold standard" in the surgical management of patients with severe acute pancreatitis. Although we agree with the key
message of this chapter we take a somewhat different position regarding the
following issues:

The Use of Antibiotics in Patients with Severe Acute Pancreatitis

A meta-analysis of all prospective randomized trials investigating the use of prophylactic antibiotics in patients with necrotizing pancreatitis revealed that prophylactic antibiotics reduce the infection rate of necrotic tissue and reduce mortality, provided antibiotics with appropriate activity and pharmacokinetic
characteristics are given [1]. In accordance with the results of this meta-analysis,
we support a routine antibiotic prophylaxis in all patients with necrotizing pancreatitis. Of course, it must be remembered that antibacterial therapy carries the
risk of promoting fungal infection and selecting multiresistant organisms. We
addressed this issue in an analysis of 103 patients receiving an antibiotic prophy-

laxis with Imipenem/Cilastatin for 14 days [2]. The important findings of this study were that:

a) the occurrence of multiresistant organisms is a rare finding (3 of 103 patients) and,

b) fungal infection, if treated adequately, does not carry an increased risk for a negative outcome [2].

Nevertheless, we agree with the author that further data from randomized controlled trials are necessary to define the optimal duration and choice of antibiotic agents in patients with severe acute pancreatitis.

Treatment of Patients with Sterile Necrosis

It is abundantly clear that many – probably most – patients found to have areas of sterile pancreatic necrosis will heal successfully without debridement [3, 4]. It is indeed a matter of controversy which subgroup of patients with sterile necrosis should undergo surgical debridement. We proposed a treatment strategy according to the status of infection. The death rate in a group of 86 patients with necrotizing pancreatitis was 1.8 % (1/56) in those with sterile necrosis managed without surgery, and 24 % (7/29) in patients with infected necrosis. However, in that series two patients whose infected necrosis could not be diagnosed in a timely fashion died while receiving nonsurgical treatment. Thus, an intention-to-treat analysis (nonsurgical treatment) revealed a death rate of 5 % (3/58) with conservative management versus 21 % (6/28) with surgery [4]. From such data we learn that patients with sterile necrosis have to be reexamined continuously, if fine needle aspiration does not prove infection and the patient is not improving, despite correct intensive care treatment. Such patients, especially if organ failure is present, need to be treated surgically (i.e., as if they were infected) and the intervention, as outlined by Dellinger, should be postponed to the third or fourth week after onset of the disease.

Algorithm

Because of the foregoing arguments, we would like to present a similar but simpler algorithm for the management of patients with severe acute pancreatitis (Diagram 2). First, disease stratification should be done according to disease severity. As outlined above, we recommend routine antibiotic treatment for up to 14 days. According to our experience, such a policy delays the occurrence of pancreatic infection, thereby allowing intervention later in the course of the disease when surgery can be performed with less morbidity. In addition, if the first intervention can be performed late, when the distinction between viable and necrotic tissue is easier, only one surgical intervention is sufficient for the vast majority of patients undergoing surgery, and further interventions usually can be reduced to percutaneous procedures.

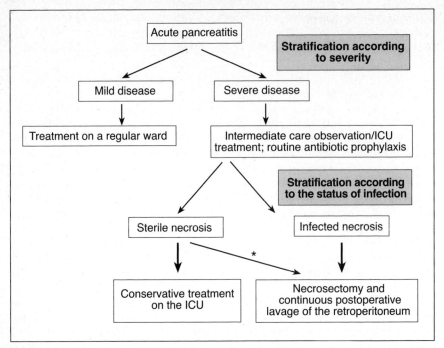

Diagram 2. Stratification, according to disease severity and then according to the status of infection, represents the key element in the management of patients with acute pancreatitis. *A minority of patients with sterile necrosis, not responding to optimal ICU treatment, benefit from surgical intervention

References

1. Golub R, Siddiqi F, Pohl D (1998) Role of antibiotics in acute pancreatitis: a meta-analysis. J Gastrointest Surg 2:496–503
2. Gloor B, Müller AC, Worni M, Stahel FP, Redaelli C, Uhl W, Büchler MW (2001) Pancreatic infection in severe pancreatitis: the role of fungus and multi-resistant organisms. Arch Surg 136:592–696
3. Warshaw AL (2000) Pancreatic necrosis: to debride or not to debride – that is the question. Ann Surg 232:627–629
4. Büchler MW, Gloor B, Müller CA, Friess H, Seiler CA, Uhl W (2000) Acute necrotizing pancreatitis: treatment strategy according to the status of infection. Ann Surg 232:619–626

Editorial Comment

Moshe Schein

Dr. Dellinger's methodical review emphasized the many remaining controversies while Dr. Gloor and Professor Büchler reiterated their simple but logical (and based on extensive personal experience) approach.

I do not agree entirely with Dr. Dellinger suggestion that "the choice of specific incision is better left to the experience and preference of the operating surgeon." I think the choice of incision does matter and may influence eventual results. The site of infected necrosis can be approached either from the front, transperitoneally, or extraperitoneally – via a flank incision. The latter allegedly prevents contamination of the peritoneal cavity and could decrease the incidence of wound complications. This "blind" technique, however, is associated with a higher risk of injury to the transverse colon and of retroperitoneal hemorrhage; it makes proper exploration and necrosectomy difficult. I prefer therefore a transperitoneal approach through a long transverse incision (Chevron), which offers generous exposure of the entire abdomen. A midline incision offers adequate exposure but interferes with the small bowel in cases where planned reoperations or laparostomy are subsequently necessary. In our experience, a transverse laparostomy protects the small bowel and prevents exposure fistulas; a transverse laparostomy usually contracts spontaneously, leaving smaller abdominal wall defects, which do not need the major reconstruction required in patients treated with a midline vertical laparostomy. The extraperitoneal routes are valuable in rare instances when the process is localized to the pancreatic tail, on the left side, or to its head, on the right. These routes are more often used to evacuate localized "sequestra" of necrotic fat during subsequent reoperations.

I want to mention that patients with severe acute pancreatitis occasionally develop intra-abdominal hypertension due to the swelling of the pancreas and adjacent retroperitoneal tissues, and to peripancreatic fluid collections and associated intestinal ileus. Surgeons should be aware that this hypertension may result in an abdominal compartment syndrome, which would necessitate an emergency abdominal decompression early in course of the disease [1].

Thankfully, the contributors ignore the outdated term of "pancreatic abscess" which is still used in the community to erroneously describe infected pancreatic necrosis. Pancreatic abscess is a well-demarcated collection of pus – representing an infection of a residual sequestrum of necrotic fat, or an infected pseudocyst – rarely occurring late in the course of the disease or after its surgical management. Pancreatic abscess is thus a relatively benign complication of acute pancreatitis and easily manageable with percutaneous drainage.

The optimal management of severe acute pancreatitis requires understanding of its natural history and a lot of patience. During the early phases of the disease, we have to patiently avoid operation and look for infection. Later on, when called to operate on necrotic and infected complications we have to patiently debride what is debridable, re-debride if and when necessary, and spare the adjacent vital structures.

John Marshall

I believe that the operative approach depends on the timing of intervention (early vs. late) and the anatomic location of infection as defined by CT scan. A midline incision provides better exposure to the pelvis if this is needed, and facilitates the creation of stomas. A retroperitoneal approach is better for a well-demarcated, mature, and localized process. Laparoscopy has the additional advantage of permitting visualization of areas (e.g., the lesser sac) that may not be readily visible at laparotomy. I agree with both commentators that delaying surgery to permit demarcation of viable and nonviable tissue is a key principle; when this is done, debridement can often be accomplished with a single operation. Personally I don't use CT-guided aspiration, for in a relatively stable patient with suspected retroperitoneal infection I am quite comfortable with antibiotic maintenance (the flora is usually evident from other sites), and delay surgery until there is good evidence of tissue demarcation, typically 4 weeks or longer. This approach may, however, be a bit too radical for some, even though it works well!

Reference

1. Gecelter G, Fahoum B, Gardezi S, Schein M (2002) Abdominal compartment syndrome in severe acute pancreatitis: an indication for a decompressing laparotomy? Dig Surg (in press)

18 Liver Abscesses

Iskender Sayek, Demirali Onat

Key Principles

- Liver abscesses are either pyogenic or parasitic.
- Early diagnosis and prompt treatment of the underlying cause reduce morbidity and mortality.
- Source control consists of drainage using surgical or US/CT-guided aspiration and antibiotic therapy.
- Hydatid cysts of the liver can be managed surgically as well as percutaneously. Source control can be achieved by radical or conservative procedures.

General Approach

Pyogenic Abscess

The incidence of pyogenic liver abscess ranges from 0.03% to 1.4% in autopsy studies [1]. There has been a recent shift in etiology (Table 1) with the biliary tract replacing infectious processes spreading through the portal route as the most common cause of pyogenic liver abscesses [2]. Whereas appendicitis was previously considered as the most common cause of portal venous spread of bacteria, diverticulitis, perforated ulcers, and cancers have become the leading causes of this complication.

Kupffer cells in the liver usually engulf bacteria entering the portal system. A liver abscess may form if the quantity of the organisms exceeds the phagocytic capacity of the Kupffer cells, or when the host is immunocompromised. The hepatic artery is the source of contamination in cases of systemic bacteremia such as subacute bacterial endocarditis. Pyogenic liver abscesses are most commonly located in the right lobe of the liver. Biliary obstruction from stones, strictures or

Table 1. Causes of pyogenic liver abscesses

---

1. Diseases of the biliary tract

2. Infectious process of the gastrointestinal tract

3. Hematogenous spread via the hepatic artery

4. Direct extension from an intra-abdominal pathology

5. Trauma

---

tumors leads to contamination of the bile, leading to cholangitis and multiple abscesses. In patients with Oriental cholangiohepatitis with biliary stricture, abscesses are most commonly are located in the lateral segment of the left lobe [3].

Gram-negative aerobic microorganisms (*E. coli, Klebsiella, Proteus*) are the most commonly isolated bacteria; anaerobic bacteria are rarely cultured. Abscesses are polymicrobial in 30%-50% of the cases [2-5].

Fever and chills are the most common symptoms of patients with liver abscesses; right upper quadrant abdominal pain, jaundice, weight loss, nausea, and vomiting are commonly associated manifestations. Rupture of the abscess with peritonitis may be seen occasionally. Leukocytosis, hyperbilirubinemia, hypoalbuminemia, and elevated serum alkaline phosphatase are the predominant laboratory findings [1-3].

Diagnosis

Imaging techniques are extremely helpful in the diagnosis of hepatic abscesses. Plain abdominal X-rays may demonstrate gas within the abscess cavity or elevation of the diaphragm in 10%-20% of cases. Ultrasonography – demonstrating an irregular margin and a hypoechoic lesion – is the preferred initial diagnostic method, having an 80%-90% accuracy rate in diagnosing abscesses larger than 2 cm in diameter; its utility is limited when abscesses are located in the dome of the liver [2, 3].

Computerized tomography (CT) has the advantage of detecting intrahepatic abscesses as small as 0.5 cm, an important advantage in patients with multiple small pyogenic abscesses [2]. Pyogenic abscesses on CT may appear as well-defined round or oval cavities, but may also be lobulated with poorly marginated edges. Contrast enhancement increases the ease of diagnosis. US- or CT-guided needle aspiration of the abscesses may further contribute to the diagnosis.

Magnetic resonance (MR) is a sensitive imaging method for detection of liver lesions but does not provide additional information on liver abscesses beyond that provided by CT or US. Runge et al. claimed, however, that the diagnosis of an early liver abscess is improved on delayed MR imaging with gadolinium-BOPTA [6].

Treatment

Source control in pyogenic liver abscess includes *adequate drainage, proper antibiotic therapy, and elimination of the cause of the abscess* (if identifiable) (see Diagram 1).

Drainage of pyogenic liver abscesses is the mainstay of treatment. Drainage can be accomplished either surgically or percutaneously. The operative risk to the patient, the presence or absence of coexisting primary intra-abdominal pathology, and local expertise are all factors that should be considered in selecting the optimal therapy.

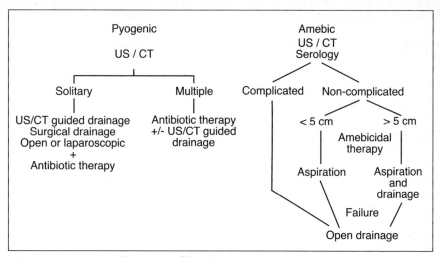

Diagram 1. Diagnosis and treatment of liver abscess

Surgical Management. Location of the abscess is important in determining the surgical approach. Abscesses located in the dome of the liver can be approached transpleurally through the bed of the 10-11th rib. This approach has the advantage of avoiding peritoneal contamination, but the disadvantage of providing only limited exposure. Recent series [5, 7] reported an overall success rate of transperitoneal surgical drainage of up to 90%. Herman et al. [5] advocated surgical drainage as the first step in septic patients when a delay in adequate drainage might be detrimental. Intraoperative ultrasonography may also be helpful in localizing abscesses deep in the liver parenchyma.

Laparoscopic drainage has also been advocated. Tay et al [8] reported 20 patients with liver abscess – of which 18 were pyogenic – treated with laparoscopic drainage. The success rate was 85%.

Percutaneous drainage of pyogenic liver abscesses was initially accomplished by needle aspiration. Dietrick [9] reported a mortality rate of 2.8% and a complication rate of 17.4% with needle aspiration alone. *US or CT directed percutaneous drainage is now considered the treatment of choice for patients who do not have a surgically correctible primary source.* The reported success rate ranges between 70%-90% [10, 11] and some consider percutaneous drainage – using multiple catheters – effective even in patients with multiple pyogenic liver abscesses [12].

As with any acute surgical disease the mortality rate is related to the severity of illness in the individual patient and his or her premorbid health. In a multivariate analysis Chou et al. [13] reported that age > 60 years, blood urea nitrogen > 20 mg/dl, serum creatinine > 2 mg/dl, total bilirubin > 2 mg/dl, and albumin < 2.5 gm/dl, were independently significant factors predicting mortality in 352 patients with pyogenic liver abscesses.

Amebic Liver Abscess

Amebiasis occurs in subtropical and tropical climates, is associated with poor sanitation, and is more common in immunocompromised hosts. Liver abscesses complicate 3%-10% of cases of amebiasis. *E. histolytica* gains access to the host by oral ingestion of contaminated food or water. After digestion of the cyst, the trophozoites are released into the gastrointestinal tract and reach the liver via the portal system. Amebic liver abscesses are usually solitary, occur more commonly in the right lobe, and are surrounded by a thin wall of compressed granulation tissue. The content of the abscess is described as resembling "anchovy paste."

The symptoms of amebic liver abscess are similar to those of pyogenic liver abscess, however, patients with amebic abscess tend to be younger and are more likely to have traveled to an endemic area [2, 14]. A history of diarrhea is present in 20%-30% of the cases. Abdominal pain, fever, hepatomegaly, and tenderness are the most frequent manifestations [15].

The diagnosis is confirmed by serologic testing. Indirect hemagglutination and gel diffusion precipitation are the most commonly used tests, and have 85%-95% sensitivity and specificity for detecting antibodies to *E. histolytica* [2]. The cysts of the protozoon are found in the stool in about one-fourth of the patients. US reveals a round or oval lesion with well-defined margins and lacking prominent peripheral echoes. CT features a low-density lesion with a smooth margin and a contrast-enhancing peripheral rim.

Secondary infection is the most common complication of amebic liver abscess, occurring in 10%-20% of patients. Abscesses located in the dome of the liver may rupture through the diaphragm, causing empyema, pleural effusion, or bronchopleural fistula, and involve the pericardium in 4%-7% of cases. Abscesses located in the inferior surface tend to rupture into the peritoneal cavity (7%-11%).

Treatment

The selection of treatment depends on the size of the abscess and the presence of complications (Diagram 1). Amebicidal drugs are the first line of treatment in uncomplicated amebic abscess. Metronidazole, the drug of choice, is effective against both the intestinal and hepatic phase: 750 mg three times a day for 7-10 days is recommended. Abscesses smaller than 5 cm in diameter respond well to metronidazole treatment. Larger abscesses require percutaneous needle aspiration. If needle aspiration combined with medical therapy fails, US or CT guided catheter drainage can be used [15]. Surgical open drainage may be indicated in complicated abscesses. But even in the case of free perforation into the peritoneal cavity, the pleura, or the pericardium, conservative treatment with an amebicidal drug has been recommended. Surgical drainage is indicated in patients with clinical evidence of peritonitis, however, the mortality increases significantly with laparotomy.

Hydatid Disease

Hydatid disease is caused by *Echinococcus granulosus* and *Echinococcus multi-locularis* (*alveolaris*). The most common cause is *E. granulosus*, which is endemic in the Mediterranean, Middle East, and South America; but international migration has led to the emergence of the disease in other countries as well. The liver is the most commonly involved organ, with hepatic disease occurring in 52%-77% of cases [16]. Liver cysts are generally asymptomatic; symptoms may occur secondary to a toxic reaction to the parasite, the local mechanical effects of the cyst (in turn dependent on the location and nature of the cyst), and complications such as rupture into the biliary tract, bronchi, or the peritoneal cavity, with resultant superinfection [17].

Diagnosis

Pain in the right upper quadrant or the epigastrium is the most common symptom, while hepatomegaly and a palpable mass are the most common findings [18]. There is no single biochemical test that definitively establishes the diagnosis of hydatid disease. In active disease specific immunoglobulin E (IgE) antibodies can be demonstrated by ELISA or radioallergosorbent test (RAST). The arc 5-antibody test is a specific immunoelectrophoretic precipitation test, and is positive in 91.1% of patients with hydatid disease [19].

Ultrasonography, with a specificity of 90%, is useful in defining the number, location, and internal structure of the cysts, and in detecting complications [20, 21]. CT provides better information about the location and the depth of cysts in the liver parenchyma, and the presence of daughter and or exogenous cysts. MRI provides good structural details of the hydatid cysts, but does not provide additional information beyond that gained by CT, and is thus not cost-effective [16, 22].

Treatment

Treatment is instituted to prevent complications such as infection, rupture of the cyst to the adjacent structures, or anaphylaxis. Despite reports of good results with percutaneous drainage and progress in medical treatment, surgery is still the treatment of choice for hydatid cysts of the liver [18, 22-24]. The aim of surgery is source control, and that can be achieved by different methods. The objectives of surgical treatment are:
- Inactivation of scolices
- Prevention of spillage of cyst contents
- Elimination of the viable elements of the cyst
- Obliteration of the residual cystic cavity

The spectrum of surgical procedures ranges from a radical resective approach (pericystectomy or hepatic resection) to a conservative approach (drainage or obliteration of the cavity, or both). Source control can be achieved by a radical approach, but only with a risk of increased morbidity. Surgical management may be performed by either a laparoscopic or open approach. The nature of the cyst, presence of complications, and the general state of the patient govern the indication for operative intervention. Small cysts (< 4 cm) located deep in the parenchyma of the liver, if uncomplicated, can be managed conservatively, because of the difficulty in approaching them.

Scolicidal Agents

Various scolicidal agents have been used for inactivation of the cyst contents [25]. Hypertonic saline solutions (3%-20%) seem to be effective in our experience. It is essential to aspirate as much of the hydatid fluid as possible before injecting the scolicidal agent into the cyst, and then to wait an adequate time before opening the cavity. Measures to prevent spillage of cyst contents should be taken. Based on experimental studies, we have advocated the prophylactic use of mebendazole or albendazole before any surgical procedure [26, 27]. Treatment modalities are given in Diagram 2.

Radical Versus Conservative Surgery

Both radical and conservative surgical approaches have been advocated. When a radical resective procedure such as total cystectomy, pericystectomy, or liver resection is undertaken, all the objectives of the surgical treatment are met. Advocates of these methods claim that postoperative complications and recurrence rates are decreased and that exogenous cysts are included within the resected material [22, 28]. De-

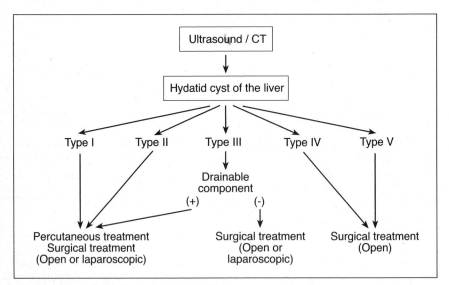

Diagram 2. Management of hydatid cysts of the liver

spite these advantages, a number of surgeons believe that major extirpative procedures, especially liver resection, represent overtreatment of a benign disease [18, 29-32]. Total cystectomy or pericystectomy should be reserved for peripherally located cysts and pedunculated cysts. Evacuation and obliteration of the cavity can be achieved by methods such as external or internal drainage, omentoplasty, capitonnage, introflexion, or capsulorrhaphy. The cavity should be explored carefully for any gross communication with the biliary tract and for the presence of exogenous cysts embedded in the pericyst. In the presence of a major biliary tract communication, common bile duct exploration and drainage may be indicated. Biliary fistulas may develop, and are treated by sphincterotomy and/or nasobiliary drainage.

Laparoscopic Approach

The laparoscopic approach can be used for surgical treatment of hydatid cysts. Total excision of the cyst, unroofing, evacuation, and obliteration of the cyst cavity have been performed laparoscopically by various authors [33-35]. The laparoscopic approach has the advantage of being noninvasive, leading to a shorter hospital stay and reduced wound complications. Moreover, the cavity of the cyst can be examined in greater detail. The disadvantages of laparoscopic approach include a limited area for manipulation, difficulty in controlling spillage during puncture, and difficulty in aspirating the thick, degenerated cyst contents, as with some Gharbi type III and IV cysts (Table 2). The location of the cyst and the presence of complications may render this method difficult in practice.

Table 2. Gharbi's classification

Type I: Pure fluid collection
Type II: Fluid collection with a split wall (Floating membrane)
Type III: Fluid collection with septa (Honeycomb image)
Type IV: Heterogeneous echo patterns
Type V: Reflecting thick walls

Percutaneous Treatment

Percutaneous treatment of hydatid cysts of the liver has become more popular over the past decade. Mueller et al. were the first to report successful percutaneous drainage of hydatid cysts [36], and several reports of good results were later published [24, 37, 38]. Based on the results of experimental and clinical studies [23, 39], we recommend percutaneous treatment for uncomplicated type I, type II, and some type III lesions.

We can conclude that the current treatment of hydatid cyst of the liver depends on the experience of the surgeon and the interventional radiologist. Based on our experience, we recommend percutaneous treatment for type I, II and some type III cysts, and surgical treatment of type IV and V cysts, unless they are completely calcified.

References

1. Mischinger HJ, Hauser H, Rabl H, et al (1994) Pyogenic liver abscess: studies of therapy and analysis of risk factors. World J Surg 18:852–858
2. Pitt HA (1990) Surgical management of hepatic abscesses. World J Surg 14:498–504
3. Donovon AJ, Yellin AE, Ralls PW (1991) Hepatic abscess. World J Surg 15:162–169
4. Gyorffy EJ, Frey CF, Silva J, McGaban J (1987) Pyogenic liver abscess. Ann Surg 206:699–705
5. Herman P, Pugliese V, Montagnini AL, et al (1997) Pyogenic liver abscess: The role of surgical treatment. Int Surg 82:98–101
6. Runge VL, Wells JW, Williams NM (1996) Hepatic abscesses: magnetic resonance imaging findings using Gadolinium-BOPTA. Investigative Radiology 31:781–788
7. Bertel CK, van Heerden JA, Sheedy PF (1986) Treatment of pyogenic hepatic abscesses: surgical vs percutaneous drainage. Arch Surg 121:554–558
8. Tay KH, Ravintharan T, Hoe MNY, et al (1998) Laparoscopic drainage of liver abscess. Brit J Surg 85:330–332
9. Dietrick RB (1984) Experience with liver abscess. Am J Surg 147:288–291
10. Barakate MS, Stephen MS, Waugh RC, et al (1999) Pyogenic liver abscess: a review of 10 years' experience in management. Aust NZ J Surg 69:205–209
11. Ch Yu S, Hg Lo R, Kan PS, Metreweli C (1997) Pyogenic liver abscess: treatment with needle aspiration. Clin Radiol 52:912–916
12. Tazawa J, Sakai Y, Maekawa S, et al (1997) Solitary and multiple pyogenic liver abscesses: characteristics of the patients and efficacy of percutaneous drainage. Am J Gastroenterol 92: 271–274
13. Chou FF, Sheen-Chen SM, Chen YS, et al (1994) Prognostic factors for pyogenic abscess of the liver. Am Coll Surg 179:727–732
14. Seeto RK, Rockey DC (1999) Amebic liver abscess: epidemiology, clinical features and outcome. West J Med 170:104–109
15. Akgün Y, Taçyýldýz ÝH, Çelik Y (1999) Amebic liver abscess. Changing trends over 20 years. World J Surg 23:102–106
16. Morris DL, Richards KS (1992) Hydatid disease. Butterworth-Heinemann, Oxford, p 23
17. Romero-Torres R, Campbell JR (1965) An interpretive review of the surgical treatment of hydatid disease. Surg Gynecol Obstet 121:851–864
18. Sayek I, Yalin R, Sanac Y (1980) Surgical treatment of hydatid disease of the liver. Arch Surg 115:847–850
19. Saidi F, Sayek I (1997) Hydatid disease of the liver. In: Sayek I (ed) Temel cerrahi, 2nd edn. Günes Kitapevi, Ankara, pp 1239–1245
20. Gharbi HA, Hassine W, Brauner MW, Dupuch K (1981) Ultrasound examination of hydatic liver. Radiology 139:459–463
21. Lewall DB, McCorkell SJ (1985) Hepatic echinococcal cysts: sonographic appearance and classification. Radiology 155:773–775
22. Mentes A. (1994) Hydatid liver disease: a perspective in treatment. Dig Dis 12:150–160
23. Akhan O, Özmen MN, Dinçer A, Sayek I, Göçmen A (1996) Liver hydatid disease: long term results of percutaneous treatment. Radiology 198:259–264
24. Khuroo MS, Wani NA, Javid G, Khan BA, Yattoo GN, Shah AH, Jeelani SG (1997) Percutaneous drainage compared with surgery for hepatic hydatid cysts. N Engl J Med 337:881–887
25. Besim H, Karayalçin K, Hamamci O, Güngör Ç Korkmaz, AI (1998) Scolicidal agents in hydatid cyst surgery. HPB Surg 10:347–351
26. Çakmakçi M, Sayek I (1992) Prophylactic effect of albendazole in experimental peritoneal hydatidosis. Hepatogastroenterology 39:424–426
27. Sayek I, Çakmakçi M (1986) The effect of prophylactic mebendazole in experimental peritoneal hydatidosis. Surg Gynecol Obstet 163:351–353
28. Magistrelli P, Masetti R, Coppola R, Messia A, Nuzzo G, Picciochi A (1991) Surgical treatment of hydatid disease of the liver: a 20 year experience. Arch Surg 126:518–522
29. Langer JC, Rose DB, Keystone JS, Taylor BR, Langer B (1984) Diagnosis and management of hydatid disease of the liver. Ann Surg 199:412–417

30. Mentes A, Yüzer Y, Özbal O, Çoker A, Ilter T, Musoglu AI (1993) Omentoplasty versus intro-flexion for hydatid liver cysts. JR Coll Surg Edinb 38:82–85

31. Ariogul A, Emre A, Alper A, Uras A (1989) Introflexion as a method of surgical treatment of hydatid disease. Surg Gynecol Obstet 169:356–358

32. Cangiotti L, Giulini SM, Muiesan P, Nodari F, Begni A, Tiberio G (1991) Hydatid disease of the liver: long term results of surgical treatment G Chir 12:501–504

33. Katkhouda N, Fabiani P, Benizri E, Moniel J (1992) Laser resection of a liver hydatid cyst un-der videolaparoscopy. Br J Surg 79:560–561

34. Alper A, Emre A, Hazar H, Özden I, Bilge O, Acarli K, Ariogul O (1995) Laparoscopic surgery of hepatic hydatid disease: initial results and early follow-up of 16 patients. World J Surg 19:725–728

35. Yücel O, Talu M, Ünalmier S, Özdede S, Gürkan A (1996) Videolaparoscopic treatment of liver hydatid disease with partial cystectomy and omentoplasty. Surg Endosc 10:434–436

36. Mueller PR, Dawson SL, Ferrucci JT, Nardi GL (1985) Hepatic echinococcal cyst: successful percutaneous drainage. Radiology 155:627–628

37. Acunas B, Rozanes I, Çelik L, Minareci Ö, Acunas G, Alper A, Arýogul O, Gökmen E (1992) Purely cystic hydatid disease of the liver: treatment with percutaneous aspiration and injec-tion of hypertonic saline. Radiology 182:541–543

38. Filice C, Pirola F, Brunetti E, Dughetti S, Strosselli M, Foglieni CS (1990) A new therapeutic approach for hydatid liver cysts. Gastroenterology 98:1366–1368

39. Akhan O, Dincer A, Gököz A, Sayek I, Havlioglu S, Abbasoglu O, Eryilmaz M, Besim A, Baris I (1993) Percutaneous treatment of abdominal hydatid cysts with hypertonic saline and alcohol: an experimental study in sheep. Invest. Radiol 28:121–127

Invited Commentary

ABE FINGERHUT

The authors have provided us with an overview of the problems related to liver abscess, whether pyogenic or parasitic in origin. They have emphasized the need for early and adequate diagnosis and work-up in order to make the least aggres-sive yet most effective means of treatment for the benefit of the patient.

Pyogenic Abscess

Source control, combined with proper antibiotic therapy, is the mainstay of treatment of uncomplicated (nonruptured) liver abscesses. The authors have reminded us of the changing etiologic patterns of liver abscesses over the last decades, with biliary tract disease having replaced disease in the distal portal system as the leading cause. Hepatobiliary and pancreatic cancer pose the problem of their proper treatment in the face of infection. Occasionally, these abscesses are secondary to chemotherapy (especially chemoembolization) and/or "mini-inva-sive" techniques (radiofrequency) which provoke tumor necrosis. Also high on the list are infections secondary to indwelling stents, which explains the changing bacteriologic spectrum encountered [1]. Another cause we see not exceptionally is posttraumatic abscesses secondary to devascularized segments of the liver, especially after nonoperative treatment [2]. Abscesses secondary to these, as well as other chronic causes treated by occasionally long-term, broad-spectrum antibiotics, may also explain the presence of fungi in some abscess cultures [1].

While percutaneous techniques offer an excellent alternative to open surgery, the two techniques have specific indications. Percutaneous drainage, combined with antibiotherapy should be the initial, and hopefully, the only management necessary in the majority of cases. Multiple, chronic, and/or abscesses having destroyed part of the parenchyma seem to be the exception to this rule, perhaps explaining why operative mortality is still high in this setting. Laparoscopic surgery may have a role to play here. Surgery should be avoided in the critically ill patient (septic shock, organ failure), in the elderly, immunocompromized patient, or in the patient with coexistent cancer. Multiple abscesses secondary to biliary tract obstruction can usually be managed successfully by drainage of the biliary tract proximal to the obstacle since most, if not all, abscesses communicate with the biliary tract. This can be accomplished either endoscopically or laparoscopically.

Causes of failure of percutaneous drainage include early (inadvertent) drain removal, obstruction due to necrotic material, displacement of the intra-abdominal extremity of the drain when large, voluminous cysts collapse, and communication with the biliary tract (requiring prolonged drainage).

Parasitic Abscess

Amebic abscesses can be treated initially, and often solely, by antibiotics; further surgical drainage is rarely indicated. We agree with the authors that in hydatid disease, Gharbi types I, II, and some III and IV cysts can be treated either percutaneously or laparoscopically [3]. A residual cavity or biliocystic fistula after unroofing surgery for hydatid disease, or difficulties in controlling bleeding and bile leaks from the hepatic parenchyma after pericystectomy, can lead to associated blood and/or bile collections, which serve as potential sources of deep suppuration and persisting bile leaks [4].

Among the adjunctive measures after surgery, special reference should be made to the only multicenter, large-scale randomized trial on the use of omentoplasty. In a randomized controlled trial conducted by the French Associations for Surgical Research [5], 53 of 115 consecutive patients (51 males and 64 females, mean age 42±16 years, range 10-80 years) with previously unoperated uni- or multilocular hydatid disease of the liver had purulent or puriform contents in their cyst(s). Deep abdominal complications developed in 2/28 patients treated by omentoplasty compared with 7/25 who did not undergo omentoplasty.

In conclusion, rather than basing the rationale for the percutaneous or surgical route on patient operative risk, we prefer to begin by percutaneous drainage of the abscess combined with antibiotics, even when the underlying cause can be cured by surgery. Laparoscopy is the second line of treatment, with surgery being reserved for failures. However, here patient status is of prime importance, for morbidity and mortality certainly increase when traditional surgery has been chosen.

References

1. Huang CJ, Pitt HA, Lipsett PA et al (1996) Pyogenic hepatic abscess: changing trends over 42 years. Ann Surg 223:600–609
2. Fingerhut A, Trunkey D (2000) Surgical management of liver injuries in adults – current indications, and pitfalls of operative and non-operative policies: a review. Eur J Surg 166: 676–686
3. Dziri C (1999) Liver hydatid disease: Tunisian experience. EAES Nice
4. Karavias DD, Vagianos CE, Bouboulis N, Rathosis S, Androulakis J (1992) Improved techniques in the surgical treatment of hepatic hydatidosis. Surg Gynecol Obstet 174:176–180
5. Dziri C, Paquet JC, Hay JM, Fingerhut A, Msika S, Zeitoun G, Sastre B, Khalfallah T, French Association for Surgical Research (1999) Omentoplasty in the prevention of deep abdominal complications after surgery for hydatid disease of the liver: a multicenter, prospective, randomized trial. J Am Coll Surg 188:281–289

Editorial Comment

The role of surgeons in the management of pyogenic, amoebic, and hydatid liver lesions is decreasing, as combined medical and percutaneous therapies become more effective. Surgeons are usually called to deal with complications of such abscesses and with the underlying causes, or when the nonoperative therapies fail.

The contributors Prof. Sayek and Dr. Onat, as well as commentator Dr. Abe Fingerhut, agree that less is usually better. Start with conservative therapy as appropriate, then percutaneous management; next comes the laparoscopic option (selectively), and finally the open surgery. The latter also should be as conservative as possible, and resective-radical procedures for hydatid cysts are rarely indicated.

A possible improvement in the laparoscopic management of hydatid disease was recently reported by Bicker at al. [1] who managed 31 patients for 52 symptomatic hydatid cysts located in the liver (49), spleen (1), and pelvis (2). Seven cysts were subdiaphragmatic and six were on the posterior aspect of the liver. Eleven patients underwent surgery for 2-5 cysts; mean cyst diameter was 8.4 cm. The main surgical maneuvers (puncture, parasite neutralization, and complete evacuation) were performed through an assembled transparent cannula, in which a vacuum was created, while its tip adhered firmly to the cyst wall. The evacuation of the cyst contents was followed by partial pericystectomy, omentoplasty, and closed-suction drainage. Mean postoperative follow-up was 49 months. Forty-one cysts contained live parasites, and 11 were secondarily infected. Complications occurred in five patients, including one who died 1 month after surgery from *Candida* sepsis. Mean hospital stay was 6 days. No evidence of recurrence was recorded during follow-up.

Reference

1. Bickel A, Loberant N, Singer-Jordan J, Goldfeld M, Daud G, Eitan A (2001) The laparoscopic approach to abdominal hydatid cysts: a prospective nonselective study using the isolated hypobaric technique. Arch Surg 136:789–795

19 Acute Mesenteric Ischemia

DANIEL P. RAYMOND, ADDISON K. MAY

Key Principles

- Maintain a high degree of suspicion: the primary goal is diagnosis prior to bowel infarction – a complication that carries a mortality of up to 90% [1, 2].
- Aggressive use of angiography to make the correct diagnosis and plan surgical intervention appropriately.
- Restoration of bowel perfusion requires not only surgical intervention but also aggressive use of invasive monitoring to assure adequate resuscitation.
- Following resection of devitalized bowel, make a plan for a second-look procedure based on the appearance of the bowel.

Etiology

Although there are a multitude of possible causes of acute mesenteric ischemia, over 95% of cases can be classified into one of four groups
- Arterial embolism (50%)
- Arterial thrombosis (25%)
- Nonocclusive mesenteric ischemia (NOMI) (20%)
- Mesenteric venous thrombosis (MVT) (<5%)

Acute arterial embolism most commonly originates from the heart as a result of atrial fibrillation, recent myocardial infarction, or valvular heart disease. Evidence of an embolic origin mandates an aggressive search for the source and therapy to decrease recurrence risks. Acute arterial thrombosis is usually associated with a preexisting stenosis, and patients will often have a history consistent with chronic mesenteric ischemia, for example weight loss, postprandial pain, and food fear [3], as well as a history of disseminated peripheral vascular disease. The pathogenesis of NOMI is complex, and felt to be related to several factors including selective vasoconstriction of the splanchnic circulation secondary to shock, ischemia-reperfusion injury, increased gut metabolic demand, and bowel distension. Mesenteric venous thrombosis is a relatively uncommon cause of splanchnic ischemia and etiologically is divided into primary and secondary MVT. Primary MVT is defined as spontaneous, idiopathic thrombosis, whereas secondary MVT is a result of a known condition that predisposes the patient to venous thrombosis – for example, hypercoagulation syndrome, cirrhosis, or cancer. The clinical presentation of mesenteric ischemia in general is vague and subtle, and differentiating the various etiologies is often challenging. (Table 1). Crampy abdominal pain that is frequently described as "pain out of proportion to exam," nausea, vomiting, diarrhea, guaiac positive stools, peritoneal signs, fever, and shock are all possible presenting symptoms of a disorder whose clinical spectrum ranges from bowel ischemia to frank necrosis. Laboratory abnormalities are similarly nonspecific, and may include leukocytosis, metabolic acidosis, elevated lactate, elevated liver enzymes, and hyperamylasemia. Similarly, biochemical abnormalities may be absent or may occur late in the course. Because of the subtle presentation and the high mortality associated with delayed recognition of acute mesenteric ischemia, the diagnosis must be considered in all patients with risk factors and acute abdominal pain.

Table 1. Differentiating causes of acute mesenteric ischemia by presentation

Etiology	Presentation	History	Examination
Arterial embolism	Abrupt onset epigastric pain	Evidence of embolic source	Pain out of proportion to physical exam
	Evidence of concurrent embolic events	Atrial fibrillation	
		Recent myocardial infarction Valvular heart disease Prior embolic events	
Arterial thrombosis	Insidious onset epigastric pain	History of chronic ischemia	Pain out of proportion to physical exam
		Weight loss	Evidence of diffuse vascular disease
		Postprandial pain Food fear History of diffuse vascular disease	
Nonocclusive mesenteric ischemia	Profound shock	Elderly ICU patient	New onset abdominal distension in sedated patient
	Exposure to splanchnic vasoconstrictors (e.g., digitalis, α-adrenergic agents)		
Mesenteric Venous Thrombosis	Insidious onset epigastric pain	Hypercoagulable state	Nonspecific
	Prolonged symptoms prior to presentation		

Radiologic Evaluation

Radiologic evaluation usually begins with a plain abdominal radiograph for a patient with abdominal pain. Although radiographs are of limited utility in the diagnosis of mesenteric ischemia, findings suggestive of mesenteric ischemia include bowel wall thickening, "thumb-printing", pneumatosis intestinalis, and portal vein gas. Completely normal radiographs, however, have been reported in up to 25% of patients with mesenteric ischemia/infarction [4, 5].

Currently the gold standard for diagnosis of acute mesenteric ischemia is angiography. When there is a high index of suspicion for mesenteric ischemia, angiography should not be delayed by other radiologic examinations. Angiographic findings are summarized in Table 2.

Table 2. Angiographic findings with acute mesenteric ischemia

Etiology	Findings
Arterial embolism	Round, smooth filling defect 3-10 cm distal to the origin of the SMA
Arterial thrombosis	Irregular obstruction at the SMA orifice often associated with collateralization and extramesenteric disease
Nonocclusive mesenteric ischemia	Diffuse narrowing of the SMA and branches, alternating arterial dilatation and narrowing ("string-of-sausages sign"), a pruned arterial tree, impaired filling of intramural vessels
Mesenteric venous thrombosis	Venous phase thrombus (poor sensitivity)

Computed tomography (CT) may demonstrate mesenteric ischemia and is an excellent means of evaluating other pathology. CT findings associated with mesenteric ischemia include mural thickening, pneumatosis intestinalis, arterial or venous thrombosis, focal lack of bowel-wall enhancement, and portal venous gas. In a retrospective study of patients with mesenteric ischemia, Smerud et al. [4] reported that 39% of patients had CT findings specific for mesenteric ischemia. Furthermore, 65% had evidence of ischemia when both radiographs and CT were combined. Conversely, 35% of patients with documented intestinal infarction had nonspecific study results (radiograph and CT). Yet, with the rapid advances in CT technology, this modality may play an increasing role in the evaluation of suspected arterial ischemia. In contrast to arterial disease, CT is the diagnostic test of choice in the evaluation of mesenteric vein thrombosis and is diagnostic in 70%-100% of cases [6, 7]. CT findings consistent with the diagnosis include portal, mesenteric, and splenic vein thrombosis, dilated collaterals, mural thickening, and pneumatosis intestinalis. MRI and duplex ultrasonography may also play increasing roles in the future, however, current use for diagnosis of acute mesenteric ischemia is of limited value.

Early Management

The primary goal of treatment of mesenteric ischemia is restoration of perfusion to prevent or limit bowel infarction. Management begins with fluid resuscitation, nasogastric decompression, optimization of hemodynamic parameters, and identification and elimination of any precipitating factors (e.g., withdrawal of splanchnic vasoconstrictors). If the patient has peritoneal signs and there is a high suspicion of mesenteric ischemia, most surgeons advocate immediate surgical exploration. There is controversy, however, over the use of preoperative angiography before peritoneal signs develop. Many authors advocate the use of angiography preoperatively if the patient is stable and services are readily available [2, 8-11] in order to make an anatomic diagnosis and direct appropriate therapy. As part of initial management, broad-spectrum antibiotics with adequate coverage of coliform species and anaerobes should be instituted. Although there are no clinical trials which support this view, it is widely accepted that mesenteric ischemia causes a breakdown in the intestinal mucosal barrier and results in endotoxemia and bacterial translocation [12-16].

In those patients with arterial embolus or thrombosis, surgical intervention is required for the restoration of perfusion. If the diagnosis of embolic acute mesenteric occlusion is made by angiography, immediate laparotomy and embolectomy is indicated. Most authors advocate embolectomy using a Fogarty catheter via a transverse arteriotomy in the proximal superior mesenteric artery after systemic heparinization [2, 5, 17]. The treatment of acute thrombotic mesenteric arterial occlusion requires immediate revascularization. Opinions differ regarding the most appropriate procedure to perform in this setting and no single technique has been shown to be clearly superior. At present other means of addressing emboli or thrombosis, including thrombolysis and angioplasty, are considered experimental.

Nonocclusive mesenteric ischemia (NOMI) and mesenteric venous thrombosis (MVT) are managed medically in the absence of peritoneal signs. Initial treatment of NOMI consists of selective infusion of splanchnic vasodilators via an angiographically placed catheter. Kaleya et al. [9] recommend continuous infusion of papaverine at 30-60 mg/h. The patient should be monitored in an intensive care unit for hypotension, which may be a sign of catheter dislodgment (papaverine infused in the SMA is mostly cleared by hepatic first pass) or clinical deterioration. Initial treatment of MVT includes immediate heparinization and intensive care unit monitoring. Subsequent therapy, however, is controversial. Successful venous thrombectomy has been described but, because recurrence rates are high, most authors recommend thrombectomy only when fresh clot is localized to the proximal superior mesenteric vein [7, 18]. Thrombolytic therapy has been reported to be successful for the treatment of MVT, either alone or in combination with venous thrombectomy. A diagnostic work-up to detect a hypercoagulable state should be undertaken and lifelong anticoagulation should be considered. Regardless of the diagnosis, if the patient develops peritoneal signs or deteriorates clinically immediate celiotomy is indicated.

Assessment of Bowel Viability

After blood flow has been restored the next step is to assess bowel viability and resect nonviable portions. A final decision regarding viability should not be made until perfusion to the bowel has been optimized by aggressive resuscitation and patient warming has been accomplished in order to prevent vasospasm resulting from hypothermia or hypoperfusion. Some authors advocate waiting 20-30 min after revascularization prior to assessing viability, and the use of intraoperative, selectively infused papaverine to diminish vasospasm [17,19]. Once perfusion has been optimized, the evaluation of viability begins with examination of the bowel. Clinical criteria, including color, arterial pulsation, and peristalsis are important factors for determining viability. There is, however, no consensus regarding the accuracy of clinical criteria alone for assessing viability. Some studies report accuracies as high as 85%-90% [20], while others report rates closer to 50% [21]. This discrepancy may be explained by a study by Bulkley et al. [22] who found that clinical judgment is 89% accurate but leads to the resection of more bowel than necessary in 46% of patients.

Clinical criteria for assessing bowel viability are notoriously inaccurate, however, several diagnostic tests can aid the surgeon in evaluating viability and limiting the extent of resection. Of these tests only fluorescein injection with Wood's lamp examination and Doppler ultrasound studies have found clinical acceptance [23]. The former test is performed by the slow intravenous injection of 1 gram of sodium fluorescein, following which the exposed bowel is illuminated with a Wood's lamp. Areas of nonfluorescence greater than 5 mm in diameter suggest nonviable bowel [2]. It is important to note that this study can only be performed once in a 48-h period. Several small studies have shown fluorescein testing to be superior to clinical judgment or Doppler ultrasound in cases of arterial pathology [22, 24, 25]. Although early experience with Doppler ultrasound appeared promising, clinical studies have failed to reveal any value of ultrasound over clinical judgment [21, 22] in the assessment of intestinal viability. Laser Doppler flowmetry (LDF), a newer technique for assessing viability, has met with early success.

"Second-Look" Procedures and Restoration of Continuity

Once bowel viability has been evaluated and infarcted bowel resected, the next critical decision is whether to restore bowel continuity. This decision should be based on the perfusion status of the bowel margins, the stability of the patient and the presence of peritonitis/suppuration [2]. Inadequate perfusion of the suture line and the presence of inflammation and suppuration greatly increase the risk of anastomotic leak. In the case of uncertainty, postponing reanastomosis is most prudent with planned reoperation after stabilizing the patient. Because intraoperative assessment of bowel viability is imperfect, it has become common practice to perform a second-look operation. There are varying opinions in the literature regarding the indications for a second-look procedure. A reasonable approach advocated by many authors [8, 17, 18, 26, 27] is to make a decision for a

second-look operation based on the appearance of the bowel at the initial laparotomy. Waiting for clinical deterioration may put a patient at unnecessary risk
as prognosis is directly related to length of ischemia. A more liberal use of second-look procedures is advocated for cases of mesenteric venous thrombosis in
which bowel viability is exceptionally difficult to evaluate [28].

Postoperative Management

Postoperative management includes invasive hemodynamic monitoring, nasogastric decompression, optimization of volume status, correction of acid/base
and electrolyte abnormalities, and antibiotic therapy. As mentioned previously,
the use of broad-spectrum antibiotics has not been rigorously tested in this patient population. Surgical Infection Society guidelines suggest that the length of
postoperative antibiotics be dictated by the degree of contamination encountered during surgery [29]. If no contamination is found then 48 h of postoperative
antibiotics is adequate (see Chap. 3). If peritoneal contamination is encountered
then the duration of antibiotic therapy is lengthened to 3-5 days. Others have recommended further shortening treatment in cases of uncomplicated ischemic
bowel to 24 h postoperatively [30]. Broad-spectrum regimens which cover coliform species and anaerobes are indicated [29,30] and nosocomial pathogens/an-
tibiotic resistance should be considered in those patients with significant prior
antibiotic exposure or prolonged hospital stays (>4 days). There are no data to
support the empiric use of antifungal agents. Certain patients, for example those
with known significant fungal colonization, long-term alkalinization of the
stomach, or broad spectrum antibiotic exposure for more than 1 week, however,
may benefit from empiric therapy until culture results return. In cases that are
managed nonoperatively, short-term, empiric, broad-spectrum antibiotic coverage (24-48 h) may be beneficial.

Currently, selective papaverine infusion remains the treatment of choice for
reducing postoperative vasoconstriction. Data supporting its efficacy have been
derived from animal models [31-33] and anecdote, although no randomized clinical trials have been performed. Since there is evidence of continued vasospasm
despite restoration of mesenteric flow, it may be reasonable to use papaverine infusion postoperatively (as described in management of NOMI) until angiographic evidence of restored splanchnic blood flow has been obtained. If a second-
look procedure is planned it is reasonable to administer papaverine until a
second evaluation of the bowel is made and bowel viability is assured.

Conclusion

The mortality rate of acute mesenteric ischemia remains high. The 70%-90%
mortality encountered commonly in the seventies has declined in some series to
40%-50% using aggressive treatment regimens, including early and aggressive
use of angiography and vasodilator therapy, however, these results are not widespread. The key to improving survival is early diagnosis; more than 90% of

patients with mesenteric ischemia diagnosed prior to the presence of peritonitis will survive. A high degree of suspicion, aggressive use of angiography and vasodilator therapy, timely surgical intervention, and participation in well-designed studies provides our best chance at improving outcomes for such critically ill patients.

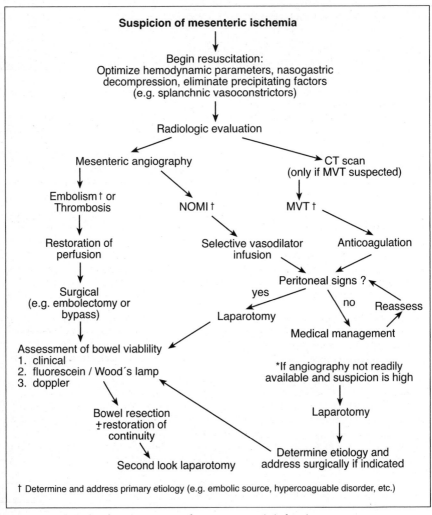

Diagram 1. Algorithm for management of acute mesenteric ischemia

References

1. Klempnauer J, Grothues F, Bektas H, Pichlmayr R (1997) Long-term results after surgery for acute mesenteric ischemia. Surgery 121:239–243
2. Montgomery RA, Venbrux AC, Bulkley GB (1997) Mesenteric vascular insufficiency. Curr Probl Surg 34:941–1025
3. Boley SJ, Brandt LJ, Sammartano RJ (1997) History of mesenteric ischemia: the evolution of a diagnosis and management. Surg Clin North Am 77:275–288
4. Smerud MJ, Johnson CD, Stephens DH (1990) Diagnosis of bowel infarction: a comparison of plain films and CT scans in 23 cases. AJR Am J Roentgenol 154:99–103
5. Eldrup-Jorgensen J, Hawkins RE, Bredenberg CE (1997) Abdominal vascular catastrophes. Surg Clin North Am 77:1305–1320
6. Boley SJ, Kaleya RN, Brandt LJ (1992) Mesenteric venous thrombosis. Surg Clin North Am 72:183–201
7. Rhee RY, Gloviczki P, Mendonca CT, et al (1994) Mesenteric venous thrombosis: still a lethal disease in the 1990s. J Vasc Surg 20:688–697
8. Bassiouny HS (1997) Nonocclusive mesenteric ischemia. Surg Clin North Am 77:319–326
9. Kaleya RN, Sammartano RJ, Boley SJ (1992) Aggressive approach to acute mesenteric ischemia. Surg Clin North Am 72:157–182
10. Boley SJ, Sprayregan S, Siegelman SS, Veith FJ (1977) Initial results from an aggressive roentgenological and surgical approach to acute mesenteric ischemia. Surgery 82:848–855
11. Bakal CW, Sprayregen S, Wolf EL (1992) Radiology in intestinal ischemia. Angiographic diagnosis and management. Surg Clin North Am 72:125–141
12. Haglund U (1994) Gut ischaemia. Gut 35[Suppl]:S73–S76
13. Herndon DN, Zeigler ST (1993) Bacterial translocation after thermal injury. Crit Care Med 21[Suppl]:S50–S54
14. Tokyay R, Zeigler ST, Traber DL, et al (1993) Postburn gastrointestinal vasoconstriction increases bacterial and endotoxin translocation. J Appl Physiol 74:1521–1527
15. Andersen LW, Landow L, Baek L, Jansen E, Baker S (1993) Association between gastric intramucosal pH and splanchnic endotoxin, antibody to endotoxin, and tumor necrosis factor-alpha concentrations in patients undergoing cardiopulmonary bypass. Crit Care Med 21:210–217
16. Schoeffel U, Baumgartner U, Imdahl A, Haering R, v Specht BU, Farthmann EH (1997) The influence of ischemic bowel wall damage on translocation, inflammatory response, and clinical course. Am J Surg 174:39–44
17. Kazmers A (1998) Operative management of acute mesenteric ischemia. Part 1. Ann Vasc Surg 12:187–197
18. Cappell MS (1998) Intestinal (mesenteric) vasculopathy. I. Acute superior mesenteric arteriopathy and venopathy. Gastroenterol Clin North Am 27:783–825
19. McKinsey JF, Gewertz BL (1997) Acute mesenteric ischemia. Surg Clin North Am 77:307–318
20. Redaelli CA, Schilling MK, Buchler MW (1998) Intraoperative laser Doppler flowmetry: a predictor of ischemic injury in acute mesenteric infarction. Dig Surg 15:55–59
21. Ballard JL, Stone WM, Hallett JW, Pairolero PC, Cherry KJ (1993) A critical analysis of adjuvant techniques used to assess bowel viability in acute mesenteric ischemia. Am Surg 59:309–311
22. Bulkley GB, Zuidema GD, Hamilton SR, O'Mara CS, Klacsmann PG, Horn SD (1981) Intraoperative determination of small intestinal viability following ischemic injury: a prospective, controlled trial of two adjuvant methods (Doppler and fluorescein) compared with standard clinical judgment. Ann Surg 193:628–637
23. Horgan PG, Gorey TF (1992) Operative assessment of intestinal viability. Surg Clin North Am 72:143–155
24. Paes E, Vollmar JF, Hutschenreiter S, Schoenberg MH, Kubel R, Scholzel E (1988) [Mesenterial infarct. New aspects of diagnosis and therapy]. Chirurg 59:828–835
25. Mann A, Fazio VW, Lucas FV (1982) A comparative study of the use of fluorescein and the Doppler device in the determination of intestinal viability. Surg Gynecol Obstet 154:53–55

26. Schneider TA, Longo WE, Ure T, Vernava AM3rd (1994) Mesenteric ischemia: acute arterial syndromes [see comments]. Dis Colon Rectum 37:1163–1174
27. Bradbury AW, Brittenden J, McBride K, Ruckley CV (1995) Mesenteric ischaemia: a multidisciplinary approach [see comments]. Br J Surg 82:1446–1459
28. Rhee RY, Gloviczki P (1997) Mesenteric venous thrombosis. Surg Clin North Am 77:327–338
29. Bohnen JM, Solomkin JS, Dellinger EP, Bjornson HS, Page CP. Guidelines for clinical care: anti-infective agents for intra-abdominal infection. A Surgical Infection Society policy statement. Arch Surg 127:83–89
30. Schein M, Wittmann DH, Lorenz W. Duration of antibiotic treatment in surgical infections of the abdomen. Forum statement: a plea for selective and controlled postoperative antibiotic administration. Eur J Surg Suppl 57:66–69
31. Dunn MM, McFall TA, Rigano WD, Peoples JB (1993) Adjunctive vasodilator therapy in the treatment of murine ischemia. Am J Surg 165:697–699
32. MacCannell KL (1986) Comparison of an intravenous selective mesenteric vasodilator with intraarterial papaverine in experimental nonocclusive mesenteric ischemia. Gastroenterology 91:79–83
33. Williams RA, Wilson SE (1980) Effect of intra-arterial vasodilators on blood flow in ischemic dog colon. Arch Surg 115:602–605

Invited Commentary

Asher Hirshberg

Acute mesenteric ischemia (AMI) presents a special challenge to the surgeon because the gut is especially vulnerable to acute ischemia, with a very narrow window of opportunity for salvage before irreversible tissue loss ensues. Both ischemia and reperfusion injury probably play a role in AMI. The key events are loss of the gut mucosal barrier function, leading to endotoxemia with bacterial translocation into the portal and systemic circulation, and a systemic inflammatory response that leads to remote organ dysfunction. The goals of source control for AMI are therefore urgent restitution of the intestinal blood supply and removal of nonviable bowel.

Clinical Contexts

Since the clinical presentation of all forms of acute mesenteric insufficiency is acute but *nonspecific* abdominal pain, a high index of suspicion as advocated by Drs. Raymond and May is not enough. This suspicion must be targeted towards identification of *clinical contexts* in which mesenteric ischemia is likely to develop. For example, in patients with superior mesenteric artery (SMA) embolism a source of emboli (such as atrial fibrillation or angiographic procedures in the proximal aorta) can usually be demonstrated. SMA thrombosis typically occurs in patients with evidence of atherosclerotic disease in other arterial systems, and a history of chronic postprandial abdominal pain and significant weight loss can be elicited in about 50% of these patients. Nonocclusive mesenteric ischemia typically occurs in the critically ill patient in an intensive care unit setting. Abdominal pain is frequently absent, vague or difficult to elicit. Unexplained clinical deterioration, abdominal distention, and especially progressive metabolic acidosis are often the only clues. While a history of portal hypertension or a hypercoagulable state may point to the possibility of mesenteric venous thrombosis, this uncommon condition is either diagnosed by CT scan (performed for another presumptive diagnosis), or more commonly during laparotomy.

Ischemic Colitis

The most common form of AMI that was not addressed by Drs. Raymond and May is ischemic colitis, which involves the smaller arteries of the large bowel. The precise pathophysiology of this condition remains unclear. The clinical context is typically an elderly patient with a recent onset of "colitis"-like symptoms and signs. Mild ischemic colitis is a nontransmural disease that presents with bloody diarrhea and abdominal pain. It usually resolves with nonoperative management. The most severe degree of ischemic colitis is transmural necrosis of the colon with peritonitis. An intermediate form of the disease, while not resulting in perforation, can lead to fibrosis and stricture formation, or to a persistent colitis that requires resection. Ischemic colitis is diagnosed by colonoscopy.

Management Algorithm

The management algorithm proposed by Drs. Raymond and May calls for radiological evaluation of all patients with AMI. In our view, when a patient presents with unequivocal signs of peritonitis, time should not be wasted on radiological studies that will not change the decision to operate. Instead, the next step in the algorithm for these patients (following appropriate fluid resuscitation and empirical antibiotics) should be a laparotomy. In all forms of AMI, peritonitis is a late sign that usually indicates the presence of transmural bowel infarction.

A "Major Trap"

The angiographic distinction between acute and chronic SMA thrombosis in a patient with acute abdominal pain is a major trap. Chronic ischemia is usually marked by well-developed collaterals with retrograde filling of the SMA beyond the occlusion, whereas in acute occlusion there is extensive nonfilling of the distal intestinal arteries beyond the occlusion. This distinction is of critical importance because, while AMI is an indication for an urgent laparotomy, chronic occlusion is not. Instead, a diligent search for another cause of acute abdominal pain is indicated.

The Operation

The etiology of AMI becomes obvious at laparotomy. An SMA embolus typically lodges distal to the takeoff of the middle colic artery, sparing the proximal jejunal branches. A minor peripheral embolus may result in only a short segment of ischemic gut. SMA thrombosis causes global midgut ischemia, which extends from the ligament of Treitz to the midtransverse colon. In nonocclusive mesenteric ischemia, bowel segments that have suffered varying degrees of insult alternate with nonischemic segments. In mesenteric vein thrombosis the bowel and mesentery are swollen, cyanotic and edematous, and the mesenteric arteries are pulsatile.

When Fogarty thrombectomy of the SMA does not restore inflow, a bypass graft must be constructed. For emergency mesenteric revascularization our preference is a quick and simple option such as a retrograde bypass from the right common iliac artery or the infrarenal aorta.

The central goal in bowel resection for AMI is to remove irreversibly ischemic intestine without removing segments that may be salvaged. The principle of planned reoperation (or "second-look" laparotomy), as discussed by Drs. Raymond and May, is the key to conserving bowel length. We use the planned reoperation principle for virtually every patient with AMI regardless of the underlying etiology.

The management of patients with nonocclusive mesenteric ischemia is frequently very frustrating. The principal modality is angiographic intra-arterial vasodilator (papaverine) infusion as advocated by Boley et al., and the algorithm is based on the patient's clinical response to this therapy in conjunction with repeat angiograms to document resolution of the arterial spasm. In clinical practice, these patients are critically ill and heavily sedated, and it is therefore not possible to base decisions on the presence or resolution of abdominal pain. Since transfer of a critically ill patient to the angiography suite is a complex and dangerous undertaking, follow-up angiograms to document resolution of the arterial spasm are also seldom a practical option. Instead, the surgeon will often find that improvised measures such as a bedside laparotomy in the ICU to assess bowel viability are less risky alternatives to the "classical" algorithm.

The very high mortality rate (approximately 50%) of patients with nonocclusive mesenteric ischemia reflects both the grave condition of these patients and the sequelae of significant delays in diagnosis.

References

1. Hirshberg A, Adar R (1999) Mesenteric insufficiency. In: Wolfe MM (ed) Therapy of digestive disorders. Saunders Philadelphia, pp 629–635
2. Boley SJ, Sprayregen S, Siegelman SS, et al (1977) Initial results from an aggressive roentgenological and surgical approach to acute mesenteric ischemia. Surgery 83:848–855

Editorial Comment

MOSHE SCHEIN

AMI is still a highly lethal condition. In a recent study from Scotland, 46 out of 57 (80%) patients suffering from acute mesenteric arterial ischemia died; only 18(32%) were accurately diagnosed before operation or death [1]. A recent review of the results from a teaching hospital in New York showed a mortality rate of 90% (unpublished results). Whether "early and aggressive" angiographic therapy with vasodilators, as advocated more than 20 years ago by Boley et al. [2], improves outcome is unknown. We do not know about anybody else who published significant clinical experience to validate Boley's results.

In order to improve results, Drs. Raymond and May, and the commentator Dr. Hirshberg, stress the following:

- To suspect/consider ischemia before intestinal gangrene develops
- To proceed with diagnostic/therapeutic angiography
- To revascularize the bowel during laparotomy
- To execute "second-look" operations

That these recommendations are considered the "standard of care" reflects the fact that AMI is a relatively common reason for malpractice claims, based on an alleged failure to make a timely diagnosis, failure to provide anticoagulant protection, and failure to prevent nonocclusive ischemic infarction being the basis [3].

The authors and the commentator did not mention that the creation of "ostomies" in lieu of an anastomosis might be advantageous in selected patients – particularly after a massive bowel resection. Observing the pink stomas may obviate the need for a relaparotomy and spare the survivor an intractable diarrhea. They also did not mention the option of angiographic thrombolysis in acute embolic mesenteric arterial ischemia. This, as published in isolated case reports [4], may be possible and successful in early cases and in the absence of peritoneal signs.

That raised intra-abdominal pressure, often caused in these patients by the swollen ischemic bowel and the associated colonic ileus, significantly decreases mesenteric blood flow has been well documented. Thus, it may be beneficial to leave the abdomen open (i.e., laparostomy) during the period leading to the second-look laparotomy.

JOHN MARSHALL

Ultrasonography can assist in the diagnosis of mesenteric venous thrombosis: marked thickening of the bowel wall from venous congestion, and the absence of peristalsis are characteristic findings.

Second-look laparotomy is an invaluable adjunct in the resolution of diagnostic uncertainty; it is most useful in patients whose cause of intestinal ischemia is NOMI, mesenteric venous thrombosis, or arterial thrombosis. Ischemia from acute inflow occlusion by an embolus or an adhesive band generally results in a sharp demarcation between viable and nonviable bowel.

Dr. Hirshberg draws attention to a commonly missed cause of acute mesenteric ischemia – embolization of plaque or thrombus during an angiographic investigation. Left colon ischemia following aortic aneurysmectomy (particularly for a ruptured aneurysm) is relatively common, and a consequence of ligation of the inferior mesenteric artery. This diagnosis should be kept in mind in the patient who has recently undergone aortic surgery.

References

1. Mamode N, Pickford I, Leiberman P (1999) Failure to improve outcome in acute mesenteric ischaemia: seven-year review. Eur J Surg 165:203–208
2. Boley SJ, Feinstein FR, Sammartano R, Brandt LJ, Sprayregen S (1981) New concepts in the management of emboli of the superior mesenteric artery. Surg Gynecol Obstet 153:561–569
3. Fink S, Chaudhuri TK, Davis HH (2000) Acute mesenteric ischemia and malpractice claims. South Med J 93:210–214
4. Kwauk ST, Bartlett JH, Hayes P, Chow KC (1996) Intra-arterial fibrinolytic treatment for mesenteric arterial embolus: a case report. Can J Surg 39:163–166

20 The Esophagus

JAIME ESCALLON, MARIA FERNANDA JIMENEZ

Key Principles

- Early diagnosis and appropriate use of diagnostic imaging
- Use of broad-spectrum antibiotics
- *Early* diagnosis – within 24 h (no associated esophageal diseases) = primary repair
- *Delayed* diagnosis – debridement and drainage, reinforced primary repair or exclusion and diversion
- Cancer, megaesophagus, caustic stenosis: one stage esophagectomy with immediate or delayed reconstruction
- Adequate postoperative drainage
- Early nutritional support

General Approach

The most common indication for source control in infections of the esophagus is mediastinitis secondary to esophageal perforation. Primary infections are rare in healthy persons, however, *Candida*, herpes simplex virus, and cytomegalovirus infections may occur in patients with compromised host defenses. Unlike secondary infections, these infections rarely need surgical intervention.

Esophageal perforation is a life-threatening condition that requires urgent diagnosis and management. Principles guiding source control methods in the management of patients with esophageal infections are often anecdotal, confusing, and poorly articulated. Thus, the physician must tailor therapy to an often-unique clinical situation based on limited experience and a paucity of solid scientific evidence.

Iatrogenic injury secondary to instrumentation is the most common cause of esophageal perforation, followed by ingestion of foreign bodies, postemetic tear (Boerhaave's syndrome), penetrating injuries, blunt trauma, caustic ingestion, and postoperative anastomotic leakage. The reported incidence of perforation during rigid esophagoscopy is 0.11%; whereas for fiberoptic endoscopy reported rates vary from 0.018%–0.03%, related to a difficult intubation, inexperienced operators, and patients with distorted anatomy. The presence of underlying esophageal disease such as carcinoma or benign stricture increases the risk of perforation. Therapeutic endoscopy is associated with higher incidence of perforation (0.9%–11%).

Infections secondary to esophageal perforation are typically polymicrobial, and yield Gram-negative, Gram-positive, aerobic, and anaerobic pathogens, as well as yeast. *Streptococcus*, *Pseudomonas*, and *Candida* are the most commonly cultured organisms.

Critical Factors and Decision Making

Several factors that influence outcome have been identified:
- Time to diagnosis
- Anatomic location
- Extent of local inflammation
- Status of residual esophagus
- Underlying esophageal disease
- The age and condition of the patient (as in any surgical emergency)

Early in the course of the disease clinical manifestations are often absent, leading to diagnostic delays in almost 50% of the patients, and resulting in increased mortality and morbidity. As a result, some propose that surgical exploration is justified in patients with a high clinical suspicion of perforation, despite normal radiological and endoscopic studies. The overall mortality associated with esophageal perforation ranges from 26% to 45%, and increases dramatically when appropriate treatment is delayed [1-3]. According to Blichert-Toft, patients operated on within 12 h of perforation had a mortality of 22%, and within the next 12 h, 36%, whereas the mortality rose to 64% if the treatment was delayed beyond 24 h. Nonoperative management resulted in an 80% rate of mortality while primary repair reduced mortality to 34% [4].

The mortality for patients under the age of 60 is significantly lower (2%) compared to that for patients aged 60 and over (33%). Cervical perforations have a more favorable outcome, probably because they are diagnosed earlier, are less likely to be associated with mediastinitis and are easier to treat. Perforations of the middle third of the esophagus (47%) and distal esophagus (59%) are associated with a higher mortality [5].

The presence of tight reflux stricture, megaesophagus, caustic stenosis, and esophageal carcinoma are unfavorable conditions for a successful repair. A mortality rate of 23% was reported in patients with perforations associated with intrinsic esophageal disease, whereas only 4% of patients died if the esophagus was normal [6]. However, others [5] have reported that overall survival was not significantly influenced by the presence of underlying esophageal disease. The history of primary esophageal disease, however, clearly influences management.

Management Options

The goal of source control in esophageal perforation is to control the ongoing contamination of the periesophageal tissue planes, to perform adequate mediastinal debridement, and to achieve wide drainage of the esophagus and the infected tissues. Treatment options range from nonoperative therapy in selected patients to immediate esophagectomy in others. The optimal approach remains controversial.

Nonsurgical therapy without drainage includes parenteral nutrition, broad-spectrum intravenous antibiotics, and gastric decompression. Oral intake can be resumed after from 15 to 52 days [7], as guided by a contrast esophagogram to document healing (see "Controversies").

Primary closure consists of exploration of the region of perforation (cervical, thoracic, or abdominal), identification and debridement of the necrotic muscle and mucosa, and approximation of the esophageal wall layers with nonabsorbable or absorbable sutures – in one or two layers [8-10]. Appropriate drainage is mandatory. Reinforcement of the primary repair can be accomplished with a pedicle flap of the pleura, muscle pedicle (diaphragm, latissimus dorsi, sternocleidomastoid), intercostal muscle, pericardial fat, or gastric fundus [9, 11, 12].

Reinforced primary repair has been advocated in early and late esophageal perforations to decrease the occurrence of fistula. The incidence of fistula after reinforced repair for patients with thoracic esophageal perforation repaired within 24 h decreases to 13% [13]. When the surgical procedure is delayed the local inflammatory reaction makes a technically satisfactory suture difficult. Pedicle flaps of pleura, intercostal muscle, pericardial fat, or gastric fundus – sutured firmly over the area of perforation and around its margins – have all been advocated [9, 12, 14]. Bringing a vascularized pedicle into a potential ischemic area can help to prevent tracheoesophageal fistula formation, especially in injuries due to high-velocity missiles [15].

Debridement and drainage of the region of perforation may be used when local inflammatory reaction precludes closure; this approach may be combined with an indwelling nasoenteric tube, feeding gastrostomy, or jejunostomy [3].

Diversion of the esophagus is accomplished by a side or end cervical esophagostomy, drainage of the thoracic esophagus, and complete occlusion or division of the esophagogastric junction; a feeding gastrostomy is created for nutritional support. The perforated esophagus is left in situ and gastrointestinal continuity reestablished after the perforation has healed [16].

Irrigation and drainage: Santos and Frater [17] advocated this technique for late esophageal perforations. After operative debridement, or under CT guidance, a chest tube is positioned at the site of perforation. Saline solution is continuously introduced through nasogastric tube proximal to perforation. The adequacy of drainage is documented by esophagoscopy or esophagography.

Esophagectomy of the perforated thoracic portion of the esophagus as initial treatment can be accomplished by a left thoracotomy or transhiatal approach. After resection, a cervical esophagostomy and closure of the cardia with feeding gastrostomy can be performed. Primary anastomosis or esophagogastrostomy are alternatives described to achieve immediate reconstruction of the gastrointestinal tract [3, 18, 14].

The site of perforation determines the surgical approach. An anterior left cervicotomy is performed for cervical esophageal perforations, whereas the upper two thirds of the esophagus is reached through a right thoracotomy. Perforations of the lower two thirds are exposed through a left thoracotomy. Abdominal perforations are repaired through an upper midline laparotomy.

As a general rule, surgical intervention is indicated for all types of esophageal perforation. It is agreed that management of a recently ruptured esophagus is direct suture with drainage of the compromised region [3, 20, 21]. This is the ideal treatment when the patient is in good condition, the perforation is discovered within 24 h, and there is no underlying esophageal disease. A water soluble contrast study is performed 7 days after repair; oral intake is resumed, and drains removed if there is no evidence of leakage.

Minor cervical mucosal disruptions or thoracic perforation in the poor risk patient can be managed by drainage alone [6]. However, even in this critical situation some authors recommend early thoracotomy and direct repair of the perforation [22].

The presence of an *underlying esophageal disease* (achalasia, cancer, benign stricture) is a critical factor in therapeutic decision making, as relief of the obstruction is a prerequisite for successful treatment of the perforation. Furthermore, reoperations on the esophagus are technically difficult and associated with inferior outcomes. Therefore, when possible, the primary disease should be treated at the time of operation. The association of esophageal perforation with a primary esophageal disease ranges from 5% (achalasia) to 25% (benign strictures) of cases. Heller myotomy for achalasia [15], and esophageal resection and anastomosis for benign strictures are recommended in patients operated for esophageal perforations. The coexistence of carcinoma, caustic stenosis or megaesophagus of achalasia precludes primary repair of the perforation. Low-risk patients are amenable to a major initial operation – one-staged esophagectomy with immediate or delayed reconstruction [19].

Controversies

The management of *late esophageal intrathoracic* perforations is controversial. Some advocate esophageal exclusion and diversion [16], others esophageal reinforcement [14], external drainage to establish an esophagocutaneous fistula, or direct repair [23, 24]. In the past, esophageal exclusion was considered the method of choice to control mediastinal and pleural infections [25], although this approach has the disadvantage that subsequent esophageal reconstruction is difficult and discomfort is prolonged. Some authors have reported successful primary resection in patients with established mediastinitis [26]. Finley et al. [24] reported no mortality in eight consecutive patients with delayed recognition (48 h to 14 days) of nonmalignant intrathoracic esophageal perforations treated with primary closure.

Another controversy is the role of *nonoperative treatment.* SIRS, shock, respiratory failure, pneumothorax, pneumoperitoneum, and extensive mediastinal emphysema are absolute indications for an emergency surgical procedure [6]. Whereas the accepted treatment for intrathoracic esophageal disruption is thoracotomy with drainage of the mediastinum and pleural space, some authors have suggested that certain patients might benefit from nonoperative management. Cameron [7] defined certain specific instances for considering nonoperative management. Patients with minimal symptoms and minimal evidence of SIRS, a well-contained esophageal disruption, and a cavity that drains well back into the esophagus, are candidates for this conservative approach (see algorithm, Diagram 1). Immediate thoracotomy and mediastinal drainage is advocated if a patient's clinical status deteriorates within 24 h.

To be successful, the treatment for esophageal perforations must be individualized according to the cause of injury, anatomic location, time of the diagnosis, underlying esophageal disease, and physiologic condition of the patient.

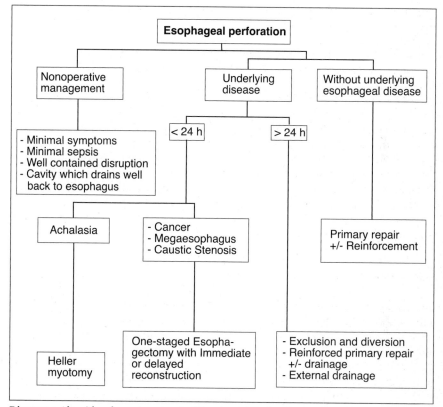

Diagram 1. Algorithm for management of Esophageal Perforation

References

1. Bergdahl L, Henze A (1978) The treatment of esophageal perforations. Scand Thorac Cardiovasc Surg 12:137–141
2. Sandrasagra FA, English TAH, Milstein BB (1978) The management and prognosis of esophageal perforation. Br J Surg 65:629
3. Skinner DB, Little AG, DeMeester TR (1980) Management of esophageal perforation. Am J Surg 139:760–764
4. Blichert-Toft M (1971) Spontaneous esophageal rupture: an evaluation of the results of treatment of 1944–69. Scand J Thorac Cardiovasc Surg 5:111–115
5. Bladergroen MR, Lowe JE, Postlewait RW (1986) Diagnosis and recommended management of esophageal perforation and rupture. Ann Thorac Surg 42:235–239
6. Michel L, Grillo HC, Malt RA (1981) Operative and nonoperative management of esophageal perforations. Ann Surg 194:57–63
7. Cameron JL, Kieffer RF, Hendrix TR, et al (1979) Selective nonoperative management of contained intrathoracic esophageal disruptions. Ann Thorac Surg 27:404–408
8. Abbott OA, Mansour KA, Logan WD Jr, et al (1970) Atraumatic so-called "spontaneous" rupture of the esophagus: a review of 47 personal cases with comments on a new method of surgical therapy. J Thorac Cardiovs Surg 59:67–83
9. Pate JW, Walker WA, Cole FH, et al (1989) Spontaneous rupture of the esophagus: a 30-year experience. Ann Thorac Surg 47:689–692
10. White RK, Morris DM (1992) Diagnosis and management of esophageal perforations. Am Surg 58:112–119
11. Dunton RF (1991) Muscle flap closure of a complicated upper esophageal disruption. J Thorac Cardiovasc Surg 101:367–368
12. Richardson JD, Martin LF, Borzotta AP, et al (1985) Unifying concepts in treatment of esophageal leaks. Am J Surg 149:157–162
13. Attar S, Hankins JR, Suter CM, et al (1990) Esophageal perforations: a therapeutic challenge. Ann Thorac Surg 50:45–49
14. Grillo HC, Wilkins EW Jr (1975) Esophageal repair following late diagnosis of intrathoracic perforation. Ann Thoracic Surg 20:387–399
15. Flynn AE, Verrier ED, Way LW, et al (1989) Esophageal perforation. Arch Surg 124:1211–1214
16. Urschel HC Jr, Razzuk MA, Wood RE, et al (1974) Improved management of esophageal perforation: exclusion and diversion in continuity. Ann Surg 179:587–591
17. Santos GH, Frater RW (1986) Transesophageal irrigation for the treatment of mediastinitis produced by esophageal rupture. J Thorac Cardiovasc Surg 91:57–62
18. Matthews HR, Mitchell IM, McGuigan JA (1989) Emergency subtotal oesophagectomy. Br J Surg 76:918–920
19. Orringer MB, Stirling MC (1990) Esophagectomy for esophageal disruption. Ann Thorac Surg 49:35–42
20. Barret NR (1947) Report of a case of spontaneous perforation of the esophagus successfully treated by operation. B J Surg 35:216–217
21. Weisel W (1952) Surgical treatment of traumatic esophageal perforations. Surg Gynecol Obstet 94:337–342
22. Loop FD, Groves LK (1970) Esophageal perforations (collective review). Ann Thorac Surg 10:571–587
23. Bradham RR, Brigdman AH, Scott SM, et al (1967) Spontaneous esophageal perforation: management of the "intermediate" phase. Ann Thorac Surg 3:6–14
24. Finley RJ, Pearson G, Weisel RD, et al (1980) The management of intrathoracic esophageal perforations. Ann Thorac Surg 30:575–582
25. Johnson J, Schwegman CW, Kirby CK (1956) Esophageal exclusion for persistent fistula following spontaneous rupture of the esophagus. J Thorac Surg 32:827–832
26. McBurney RP, Kirlin JW, Hood RR, et al (1953) One-staged esophagogastrectomy for perforated carcinoma in the presence of mediastinitis. Proc Staff Meet Mayo Clin 28:281–286

Invited Commentary

J. David Richardson

The "Time Factor"

Infections due to esophageal perforation are obviously life-threatening. My approach to these problems is certainly influenced much less by time than the authors present in their algorithm. *In fact, I really do not think that the time of perforation should enter into treatment decisions to any significant extent.* In our tertiary referral center, we often have patients transferred to our institution many days after perforation. Generally, we try to treat the patients in a similar fashion regardless of the time that they are seen after esophageal perforation.

Diagnosis

Before embarking on a discussion of treatment, I believe that several other points should be emphasized in the authors' discussion. We believe it is important to establish a definitive diagnosis of perforation. In our experience, this can almost always be done by a thin contrast study. If there is still doubt as to whether perforation has occurred, a CT scan generally can confirm the diagnosis by demonstrating microperforations with contrast extravasation; mediastinal air or periesophageal and mediastinal edema may also be identified. I would be reluctant to explore a patient based on clinical findings alone without definitive evidence of perforation. In the modern era, I think we can usually establish this diagnosis fairly readily.

Mortality Rates

The second comment regarding the authors' presentation concerns reported mortality rates. The authors quote extremely high mortality associated with perforation, particularly with delayed therapy. However, the primary reference cited was from 1971 [1]. It is my belief that these mortality rates would no longer be acceptable in the present era. Even with delayed treatment, the majority of our patients survive and that should be the norm, although occasional patients clearly will succumb to this dreaded problem.

The Condition of the Esophagus

I agree with the authors that the underlying state of the esophagus is very important. If the esophagus is presumably normal prior to the insult (such as with Boerhaave's syndrome), preservation of the esophagus should be the primary goal with attempted closure of the esophagus. If the underlying disease is cancer and an iatrogenic perforation has occurred during its diagnosis or treatment, then the patient is best treated by esophagectomy and immediate reconstruction. Anastomotic perforation of achalasia patients during pneumatic dilation can be closed and a myotomy done at 180° to the perforation as the authors suggested.

Nonoperative Management

I believe nonoperative treatment must be reserved for relatively few patients and should only be done in a very narrow set of circumstances. If contrast goes beyond the wall of the esophagus, it is my opinion that the patient should have operation and treatment of that problem – even if the contrast drains back into the esophagus from a cavity. Granted, some patients may be able to heal such a perforation nonoperatively, but I am aware of several disasters with patient deaths where this strategy was tried and subsequently failed. I have also observed significant scarring at the area of the healed perforation. Therefore, I reserve nonoperative treatment only for "microperforations" in which there may be some small tear observed in the muscle itself, but the contrast does not actually escape the confines of the esophagus.

The Operation

In patients who are treated operatively, my algorithm would focus less on time and more on the underlying state of the esophagus. If the esophagus is diseased, and return of reasonable function is not likely, then I think that the esophagus should be resected. Indications for this approach include cancer, mega-esophagus, or severe stricture in which future dilation is unlikely to result in a functional esophagus.

I believe that an attempt should be made to close *every perforation*. In addition to closure, other important management principles include debridement of infected material within the mediastinum and good tube drainage of this area. Any patient with a repair that is at high risk for breakdown is turned in a supine position, and a small abdominal incision is made to place a tube gastrostomy (unless the stomach has been brought into the chest for reconstruction) and feeding jejunostomy [2].

In my experience, primary closure of a diseased esophagus in the face of mediastinitis is extremely difficult. The key to closure of the esophagus is careful identification of the perforation. When the chest is explored, one often encounters necrotic material and a hole deep within the thorax that has bubbling, purulent secretions coming up from it. If one is inexperienced with source control of infection due to esophageal perforation, it is easy to shriek and simply place a chest tube into the area of perforation and rapidly close. In fact, if one goes as proximal into the chest as possible, it is usually possible to palpate the esophagus (if not see it directly) by locating the "esophageal stethoscope," previously placed nasogastric tube, or a dilator placed in the esophagus. Using these as guides outside the area of the primary perforation, one can usually encircle the esophagus.

With careful dissection toward the area of perforation (which is usually distal in the esophagus), the esophagus can then be mobilized out of its inflammatory bed and the perforation identified. Often it is possible to then attempt some type of direct closure. However, in my experience, primary closure often fails immediately because the sutures cut through. In that instance, I have reported extremely good results using a direct repair with a muscle flap [3]. Distal perforations are amenable to closure with a flap of diaphragm. A diaphragm flap can be mobilized posteriorly, leaving the posterior pedicle intact. I use double-arm PDS sutures to secure this pedicle in place in the esophagus and, thus, directly close the perforation. The diaphragm is then repaired primarily and the area is widely drained. If the defect can be primarily closed, I do so, and then use a muscle flap as a buttress to the repair. I find the muscle to be much sturdier than pleura, although pleura could certainly be used. I have used this technique extensively with penetrating trauma [4], occasional blunt blow-out injuries to the esophagus, many cases of Boerhaave's syndrome, and as an onlay patch for anastomotic perforations as well. In the neck, the sternocleidomastoid muscle can be used in a similar fashion. Rhomboid flaps for high thoracic perforations have been used on a couple of occasions. The use of these muscle flaps can prevent the esophageal narrowing that might come from attempted repair of defects where a major hole is present.

Esophageal Diversion?

In my opinion, esophageal diversion should be reserved only for those patients who are almost certainly going to die unless diversion is done. Esophageal diversion creates a potential disease in itself. Even if the patient survives, the closure of a cervical esophagostomy can be difficult. In my opinion, exclusion and diversion in continuity, as has been advocated by others, should never be done. The authors of this chapter state that correction of the distal obstruction is a key part of closure of the perforation. I agree with this assertion. However, the use of diversion and exclusion creates a distal esophageal obstruction by definition, and the perforation will likely never heal. Therefore, I think this is not in keeping with the principles of proper source control of esophageal perforation.

References

1. Blichert-Toft M (1971) Spontaneous esophageal rupture: an evaluation of the results of treatment of 1944–69. Scand J Thorac Cardiovasc Surg 5:111
2. Richardson JD, Martin LF, Borzotta AP, et al (1985) Unifying concepts in treatment of esophageal leaks. Am J Surg 149:157–162
3. Richardson JD, Tobin GR (1994) Closure of esophageal defects with muscle flaps. Arch Surg 129:541–547
4. Cheadle W, Richardson JD (1982) Options in management of trauma to the esophagus. Surg Gynecol Obstet 155:380–384

Editorial Comment

We agree with all authors that nonoperative treatment can be selectively employed in a well-chosen patient. When successful, it is considered a victory, but we have seen patients so treated rapidly succumbing to virulent mediastinitis. Patients with minor, instrumental injuries of the cervical esophagus are the ideal candidates for nonoperative treatment; such an approach can be only used in perforations documented as contained on contrast studies.

Dr. Richardson claims out that "even with delayed treatment, the majority of our patients survive and that should be the norm...." We have to point out, however, that in a tertiary care setting, transferred patients may represent a self selected group – those suffering from fulminant mediastinitis dying prior to transfer.

The overall message is clear: resuscitate, provide wide spectrum antibiotics, diagnose with contrast study and/or CT, operate on most patients to repair the hole, use muscle, drain widely, and reserve exclusion to the few who are in very bad shape.

21 Pleural Empyema

T. Hau, E. Förster

Key Principles

- Pleural empyema can be divided into three phases:
  a) Exudative
  b) Fibrinopurulent
  c) Organizing
- Pleural empyema may be:
  a) Para- or postpneumonic
  b) Postoperative
  c) Posttraumatic
  d) Secondary to other intrathoracic or upper abdominal infections
- Primary management of para- or postpneumonic empyemas is with antibiotics. Source control is a secondary measure whose aims are the evacuation of pus and full expansion of the lung; approaches to source control must be adapted to the stage of the disease.
- The objective of source control in postresectional empyema is to close any bronchopleural fistula and reexpand the lung, or, after pneumectomy, to stabilize or obliterate the thoracic space.

Empyema is the accumulation of pus in a preformed body cavity. Thus, pleural empyema (or empyema thoracis) is the accumulation of pus or other infectious material in the pleural space. Based on natural history, pleural empyema has been arbitrarily divided into three phases [1].

Exudative or Acute Phase

In the exudative phase, the pleural fluid is characterized by low viscosity and low cell count. There are no adhesions or loculations and the visceral and parietal pleura are freely movable against each other. Pleural fluid has a low white cell count, a pH of more than 7.2 and a glucose content of more than 60 mg/dl. The LDH level is normal.

Fibropurulent or Transitional Phase

In the fibrinopurulent phase, the pleural fluid becomes more turbid due to an increased number of polymorphonuclear cells. Fibrin is deposited, limiting the extension of the empyema, but trapping the lung. At this stage the pleural fluid has a high cell count, the pH is less than 7, the glucose content less than 40, and the LDH more than 1,000 u/dl.

Organizing or Chronic Phase

The organizing phase of empyema is characterized by the development of a pleural peel with ingrowth of capillaries and fibroblasts. The remaining pleural fluid is viscous consisting up to 75 % of cells, and expansion of the lung is severely impaired. This stage usually evolves over 4-6 weeks, but may develop in as little as 7-10 days.

Roughly 50 % of all empyemas are para- or postpneumonic, 25 % occur after operations on the lung, esophagus and mediastinum, 10 % occur after blunt or penetrating thoracic trauma, and the remainder arise secondary to generalized sepsis, tuberculosis, mycotic infections, subdiaphragmatic abscesses, and spontaneous pneumothorax [2-4]. The distinction between para- or postpneumonic and postoperative empyema is important in defining the need for source control. Para- and postpneumonic empyemas are treated primarily by systemic antibiotics, reserving surgical intervention for the secondary manifestations of the infection. For patients with postoperative empyema, the primary source, i.e., a bronchopleural fistula, is dealt with primarily by surgery.

Because patients with pleural empyema are often treated with a prolonged course of antibiotics prior to diagnosis, pleural fluid often is sterile by routine clinical culture methods. The most common organisms in parapneumonic empyema are *S. aureus, S. pneumonia,* and *S. pyogenes*; in postoperative empyema, *S. aureus* and Gram-negative rods. Anaerobic bacteria can be recovered from most empyemas as well [2–4].

Para- and Postpneumonic Empyema

Clinical signs and symptoms in the early phase of empyema are nonspecific and frequently hard to distinguish from the underlying pneumonia. However, surgical treatment depends on appropriate diagnosis and staging of the disease, therefore the diagnosis and staging of pleural empyema is based on radiologic methods and examination of the pleural aspirate. Pleural fluid accumulation occurs in 40 %-50 % of all patients with pneumonia [5]. If the pleural effusion is small and the patient responds promptly to antibiotic therapy no further measures are necessary; if not, further investigations are indicated. Radiologically, a stage I empyema is indistinguishable from a simple pleural effusion. The effusion is freely mobile on fluoroscopy or on decubitus chest X-ray, and CT scan shows no pleural thickening or loculation. The density of the fluid is below 15 Hounsfield units. The diagnosis of a stage I empyema is established either by the presence of bacteria on the Gram stain or culture, or the chemical characteristics of the pleural aspirate – pH < 7, glucose < 40 mg/dl, and LDH > 1,000 u/dl; the cell content is variable. A stage I empyema can be managed by the insertion of a large-bore chest tube (28-32 Charrière or French). Two days after the chest tube has been inserted, a chest X-ray should be taken to confirm that all fluid has been evacuated, and the pleural space completely obliterated [5, 6]. If this is not the case, it is likely that loculations have been overlooked and the patient should be treated as in phase II empyema.

In phase II empyema, thickening of the pleura and loculations can be seen on chest X-ray or computed tomography. Pleural fluid is now rich in protein and, therefore, has over 30 Hounsfield units on CT scan. In the past, treatment of a stage II empyema was thoracotomy and debridement of the pleural cavity. This procedure today can be done by the thoracoscopic approach and yields equivalent results [7, 8]. It has also been shown that thoracoscopic debridement is superior to the use of fibrinolytic agents in the treatment stage II empyema [9].

Chronic or phase III empyema is characterized by a thick pleural peel, entrapment of the lung, and thick pus, and is treated by open drainage. Drainage can either be accomplished by the resection of one to three ribs over the most dependent portion of the empyema and the insertion of several chest tubes, or by the construction of a skin flap that is inserted through the bed of a resected rib into the thoracic cavity [10]. A skin flap is easier to care for and stays open longer than a tube thoracostomy. If the wall of the empyema is unusually rigid and the lung cannot expand, especially if there is a significant restrictive impairment of pulmonary function, a decortication of the lung through an open thoracotomy should be performed, including, if possible, the removal of the entire empyema cavity (empyectomy) [11]. A thoracoplasty is hardly ever indicated in the treatment of postpneumonic empyema (Diagram 1).

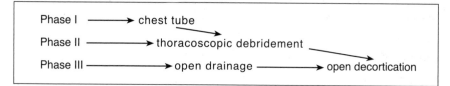

Diagram 1. Flow diagram for the treatment of para- or postpneumonic empyema. Phase I empyema usually can be treated with a chest tube, phase II empyema with thoracoscopic debridement. If chest tube drainage of a phase I empyema is not successful, thoracoscopic debridement should be done. Phase III empyema usually is treated with open drainage. If the lung does not expand open decortication is indicated as is the case if thoracoscopic debridement is unsuccessful

Postresectional Empyema

Postresectional empyema is frequently, but not always, associated with a bronchopleural fistula. Primary treatment is drainage. If the preceding operation has been a partial lung resection and no bronchopleural fistula is present, surgical treatment is similar to that of postpneumonic empyema. If, however, a fistula is present, it must be closed with a muscle flap, and if the lung does not completely reexpand after the decortication, the remaining space should be filled with transposed muscle [12] (Diagram 2). After pneumonectomy an attempt can be made to sterilize the empty thoracic cavity. To accomplish this, a rib resection is performed and the thoracic cavity is irrigated with antibiotic solution [13]. An acute bronchopleural fistula can usually be closed by resecting the bronchial stump and reclosing it primarily. The suture line should be reinforced by a pericardial, pleural, or intercostal muscle flap [12]. If a chronic bronchopleural fistula develops, it can be closed transpericardially with a stapling device [14], or the entire thoracic cavity can be obliterated by transposed muscle [15] (Diagram 3).

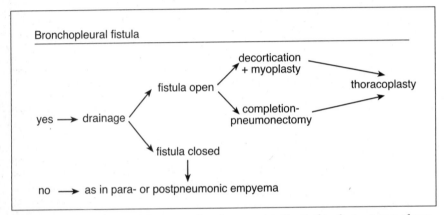

Diagram 2. Initial treatment of postresectional empyema is identical to the treatment of para- and postpneumonectomy empyema if no bronchopleural fistula is present or if the fistula closes after drainage. If the fistula remains open, either decortication and myoplasty or completion pneumonectomy can be done. A thoracoplasty is rarely indicated

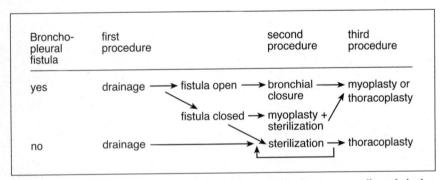

Diagram 3. Postpneumonectomy empyema is initially treated by drainage regardless of whether a fistula is present or not. If there is no fistula or the fistula closes spontaneously after drainage, sterilization of the pleural cavity can be attempted. If this is unsuccessful, a thoracoplasty may be necessary. If the fistula remains open, an attempted bronchial closure can be done. If this is unsuccessful, myoplasty or thoracoplasty is indicated

Summary

The aim of surgical treatment in pleural empyema – regardless of etiology – is evacuation of pus, full expansion of the lung, and operative source control if a surgically treatable underlying cause is present. Evacuation of pus and full expansion of the lung is accomplished by chest tube drainage, thoracoscopic debridement, open drainage or decortication, depending on the stage of the empyema. Surgical source control is necessary, albeit often difficult to achieve, in postresectional empyema with a bronchopleural fistula.

References

1. American Thoracic Society (1962) Management of non-tuberculous empyema. Am Rev Respir Dis 85:935–936
   This is a statement of the Subcommittee on Surgery of the American Drug Society about the management of non-tuberculous empyema, defining the classical phases of pleural empyema.
2. Yeh TJ, Hall DP, Ellison RG (1963) Empyema thoracis: a review of 110 cases. Am Rev Respir Dis 88:785–790
3. Snider, GL, Saleh, SS (1968) Empyema of the thorax in adults: review of 105 cases. Dis Chest 54:12–17
4. Vianna NJ (1971) Nontuberculous bacterial empyema in patients with and without underlying disease. JAMA 215: 69–75
   These two papers present large series of patients with pleural empyema. In addition to therapeutic guidelines they give a good overview of the etiology and bacteriology of the disease.
5. Light RW (1992) Management of empyema. Sem Respir Med 13167–176
   A good overview of the management, but also of the clinical manifestations and the diagnosis, of empyema.
6. Mandal AK, Thadepalli H (1987) Treatment of spontaneous bacterial empyema thoracis. J. Thorac Cardiovasc Surg 94:414–418
   An outline of the antibiotic as well as the surgical treatment of para- and postpneumonectomy empyema.
7. Sendt W, Förster E, Hau T (1995) Early thoracoscopic debridement and drainage as definite treatment for pleural empyema. Eur J Surg 161:73–76
   This is one of the first papers showing that thoracoscopic treatment of phase II empyema is feasible and yields satisfactory results.
8. Cassina PC, Hauser M, Hillejan et al (1999) Video-assisted thoracoscopy in the treatment of pleural empyema: stage based management and outcome. J Thorac Cardiovasc Surg 117:234–238
   A large series of patients with stage II and stage III empyema treated with video-assisted thoracoscopic debridement.
9. Wait MA, Sharma S, Hohn J, Dal Nogoe A (1997) A randomized trial of empyema therapy. Chest 111:1548–1551
   A randomized trial of empyema therapy showing that primary treatment with video-assisted thoracoscopic surgery is more efficient than local fibrinolytic therapy.
10. Eloesser L (1935) An operation for tuberculous empyema. Surg Gynecol Obstret 60:1096–2000
    This classic paper describes the use of a skin flap in the treatment of stage III empyema.
11. Samson PC (1971) Empyema thoracis: essentials of present day management. Ann Thorac Surg 11:210–221
    An overview of the treatment of empyema. including the indication and technique of open tube thoracostomy and decortication.

12. Pezzella A, Adebonoja SA, Hooker SG, Mabogunje OA, Conlan AA (2000) Complications of general thoracic surgery. Curr Probl Surg 37:742–858
    This short monograph gives an overview over the complications of general thoracic surgery including the space problems and pleural infections after lobectomy and pneumonectomy.
13. Clagett OT, Geraci JE (1962) A procedure for the management of postpneumonectomy empyema. J Thoracic and Cardiovasc Surg 45:141–145
    This is about the sterilization of the thoracic cavity in postpneumonectomy empyema by antibiotic irrigation.
14. Baldwin JC, Mark JBD (1985) Treatment of bronchopleural fistula after pneumonectomy. J Thorac Cardiovasc Surg 90:813–817
    Transpericardial closure of the bronchial stump with a stapling device is advocated in patients with a chronic broncho-pleural fistula after pneumonectomy.
15. Miller JI, Mansour KA, Nahai F, Jurkiewicz MJ, Hatcher CR Jr (1984) Single-stage complete muscle flap closure of the postpneumonectomy empyema space: a new method and possible solution to a disturbing complication. Ann Thorac Surg 38:227–231
    This classical paper describes the obliteration of a postpneumonectomy space in a single-stage transposition of multiple muscle flaps.

Invited Commentary

J. DAVID RICHARDSON

Hau and Förster stress that empyema can be divided into three phases: exudative, fibrinopurulent, and organizing. While this is certainly classic teaching and appears in all textbooks on thoracic surgery, I find it is often of little benefit in caring for patients with empyema. Furthermore, over-reliance on this progressive pathophysiologic concept may suggest that there is an orderly progression from one phase to another, while in fact there is not. The authors note that the organizing or chronic phase is variable in length, and I believe this point deserves double emphasis.

The problem I have with the concept of phases of empyema is that it does not apply to all etiologies causing empyemas [1]. Patients with para- or postpneumonic empyema, particularly those caused by Gram-positive organisms, may produce a thin exudative material that is amenable to drainage by thoracentesis or tube thoracostomy, if antibiotics fail. The concept of the three stages likely applies very well to this etiology of empyema. However, surgeons rarely are called to consult on this type of empyema.

Our experience with empyema caused by mixed organisms in an intensive care unit setting is much different. There is less likelihood of an exudative phase, and operative treatment may be required.

Empyema following trauma does not behave in a controlled, predictable fashion. The pathophysiology of this disease is different than that of parapneumonic empyema caused by a Gram-positive organism: blood in the pleural space from the original injury becomes infected by direct contamination from tube thoracostomy or other instrumentation, or by secondary infection from a parapneumonic or subdiaphragmatic process. If empyema is diagnosed in this setting, operative treatment should be undertaken. Tube thoracostomy is rarely effective because fibrin and pus precludes effective drainage. I support the authors' emphasis on early treatment with thoracoscopic techniques. However, I am concerned that the continued emphasis on "three phases" might lull the physician into a false sense of security that there is a prolonged period to treat the patient by nonsurgical means when, in fact, an operation is required. Prolonged delays in treating empyema make it much more likely that a thoracotomy will be required to manage the empyema, as opposed to a thoracoscopic procedure.

The authors appropriately emphasize the critical role of CT scans in diagnosing empyema and in identifying undrained collections. This is especially critical in posttraumatic and postoperative empyema.

The authors' emphasis on flap closure of bronchopleural fistulas is entirely correct in my opinion. On the other hand, I have never encountered or seen an acute bronchopleural fistula that was successfully reclosed primarily. If lung tissue remains, it is imperative that the lung be freed from any entrapping peel to allow it to expand and fill the thoracic space. Although the use of antibiotic solution to free the thoracic space of infection has been discussed for years, I have rarely seen that be successful, either – perhaps because the technique has not been properly employed. Our unit has had much better results with the staged approach the authors recommend, of open drainage and dressing changes, followed eventually by muscle transposition to close the space.

Reference

1. Richardson, JD, Carrillo, E (1997) Thoracic infection after trauma. Chest Surg Clin N Am 7:401–427

22 Soft Tissue Infections

Seong K. Lee, Jan K. Horn

Key Principles

- Soft tissue infections can be classified as either simple or necrotizing.
- Necrotizing soft tissue infections (NSTI) generally involve the subcutaneous tissue, fascia, or deeper tissues. Therefore, an NSTI may not be readily apparent on external inspection of the skin.
- Patients with a history of blunt or penetrating trauma, diabetes mellitus, illicit parenteral drug use, burns, bites, stings, recent surgery, immunologic deficiency, or soft tissue contamination are at risk for NSTI.
- Initial management of NSTI includes administration of antibiotics, hemodynamic monitoring and physiologic stabilization, treatment of electrolyte/acid-base imbalances, and correction of coagulopathy.
- Treatment consists of urgent surgical exploration with drainage and debridement of nonviable or infected tissue. Wounds require frequent inspection until one is assured that tissues remain viable and infection is no longer spreading.

General Approach

Infection can involve all layers of soft tissues. The severity of infection can range from a simple cutaneous infection to widespread necrosis of skin, muscle, and bone. While infections of the soft tissues are common, and can usually be managed with medical therapy, clinicians should be aware of the less commonly seen invasive infections that are potentially fatal.

Soft tissue infections can be classified as simple localized processes or serious necrotizing infections. Examples of simple soft tissue infections include: cellulitis, carbuncle, furuncle, erysipelas, impetigo, suppurative flexor tenosynovitis, and folliculitis [1]. Necrotizing soft tissue infections (NSTI) are associated with tissue destruction caused by pathogen-induced vascular thrombosis. Specific patterns of infection have been described, for example, Fournier's gangrene (perineal infection), Meleney's gangrene (streptococcal gangrene), and clostridial myonecrosis [2]; however, it is not clear that these represent distinct pathologic processes. To avoid confusion, this chapter will define as NSTI all infections involving multiple layers of soft tissue. Nomenclature regarding the depth of soft tissue involvement for such infections is displayed in Table 1 [3].

Typically, simple soft tissue infections begin with localized erythema and pain. Cutaneous lesions, minor trauma, or any area of skin breakdown may precede such infections. In patients with a competent immune system, normal host

Table 1. Layers of the soft tissues and common infections involved [2]

Anatomical layer	Infection
Epidermis	Erysipelas Impetigo Folliculitis Furunculosis Carbunculosis
Dermis	Abscess Cellulitis
Subcutaneous fat (e.g., Camper's fascia), nerves, and vessels	Panniculitis
Superficial fascia (e.g., Scarpa's fascia) Deep fascia (e.g., aponeurosis, fascia lata)	Necrotizing fasciitis
Muscle and tendon	Myonecrosis (Clostridial and non-Clostridial) Tenosynovitis
Bone	Osteomyelitis

defenses contain the initial infection to a limited area of cellulitis or abscess, and treatment with antibiotics and abscess drainage commonly provides resolution. Tetanus prophylaxis should be administered in any patient with a potentially contaminated wound.

If a local infection continues without treatment, spread with deep invasion may occur. Extensive destruction of tissues can occur without obvious external signs. By the time patients present with a clinically manifest NSTI, appropriate interventions must immediately be performed in order to prevent the devastating spiral of systemic sepsis and death [4]. The focus of this chapter will be the diagnosis and management of NSTI.

NSTI can exist as a complication of cellulitis, panniculitis, burns, bites, osteomyelitis, or contamination by foreign bodies from blunt or penetrating trauma. This disease can affect any area of the body but most commonly involves the extremities, perineum, or buttocks [3]. Direct injection of either contaminated needles or other foreign substances mixed with illicit drugs has been an increasing cause of NSTI in urban centers [5, 6]. Other causes include ulcers, decubiti, abscesses, contaminated postoperative wounds, and internal infections such as diverticulitis or strangulated hernia [6].

The reported mortality of NSTI ranges between 6%-48% [5], and is increased when care is delayed either as a result of patient transfer or misdiagnosis [7, 8]. Diabetes, malnutrition, peripheral vascular disease, comorbid disease, HIV infection, or an immunocompromised state are all risk factors for NSTI [6, 9]. When more than three risk factors exist, mortality may exceed 50% [10].

The diagnosis of NSTI is made more difficult by the paucity of signs and symptoms at presentation (Table 2). Short of an operative exploration, there is no standard test to diagnose NSTI, and clinicians must rely upon judgment and a high index of suspicion. External clinical clues to deeper tissue involvement in-

Table 2. Presenting signs of necrotizing soft tissue infections [5]

Sign	Percentage
Pain	100
Erythema	77
Induration	43
Swelling	20
Fluctuance	20
Necrosis	10
Bullae	3
Crepitance	3

clude persistent edema out of proportion to erythema, fluctuance, and gas [1] in the subcutaneous tissues – often identified on plain films or by palpating crepitance over the wound. As the disease progresses, skin blistering occurs followed by ecchymosis (purpura fulminans) and skin necrosis [1, 11].

NSTI spread along tissue planes within layers of fascia and muscle [1, 12]. When fluctuant and erythematous tissues are encountered, adequate examination of the underlying fascia or muscle is critical [5, 11]. Infiltration with local anesthesia facilitates placement of a small incision to expose the superficial fascia and muscle compartments. Discolored fascia or malodorous watery drainage suggests the diagnosis of NSTI [11, 12]. Needle aspiration of tissues may be misleading when no organisms are found and is not recommended as a diagnostic maneuver. Computerized tomography, magnetic resonance imaging and ultrasound have all been reported to yield further evidence of gas in the tissue planes, fluid collections, tissue edema, and inflammation [5, 13]. These adjuncts can occasionally be useful, but should not delay surgical exploration.

Systemic infection and bacteremia occur late in the course of NSTI. Patients are usually febrile and appear toxic. Laboratory abnormalities are nonspecific and can include an elevated leukocyte count and derangements of serum electrolytes [7]. Systemic hypotension and sepsis can progress rapidly. Patients with NSTI may occasionally present in septic shock, making the diagnosis of a local process even more difficult [14].

Microbiology

A wide range of bacteria and fungi have been associated with NSTI, including *Clostridia* and *Streptococci* (Group A *Streptococci* are extremely virulent) alone or in combination with other bacteria [2, 12]. Mixed infections may also occur with *Staphylococcus*, *Bacteroides*, and *Peptostreptococcus* in combination with one or more facultative anaerobic species or other Gram-negative bacilli such as *E. coli*, *Enterobacter*, *Proteus*, and *Klebsiella* [2]. The rate of mixed infections has been reported to be as high as 80 % [6, 15]. Synergy between organisms in mixed infections may encourage bacterial growth or elaboration of factors promoting the spread of infection. Virulence appears to correlate with the production of specific procoagulants and tissue proteases by invading organisms. Fungal infections involving *Mucormycosis* or *Aspergillus* can also present with necrotic lesions. Infections with *Vibrio* may occur in patients exposed to a marine environment [4].

Antibiotics

Broad-spectrum antibiotic therapy should be employed in treating NSTI. Combination therapy should be started immediately, then modified by the results of subsequent wound or blood cultures. Special attention should be given to anaerobic coverage. Common regimens include a maximal dose of penicillin with either an aminoglycoside or third generation cephalosporin to cover Gram-negative bacteria, along with either clindamycin or metronidazole for anaerobes [4, 13]. Other options include broad-spectrum antibiotics such as imipenem, or variations of penicillinase-resistant antibiotics.

Operative Treatment

Once a diagnosis of NSTI is suspected, surgical exploration and debridement should be performed urgently. Surgery is both diagnostic and therapeutic because the early clinical differentiation of the entities encompassing NSTI can be difficult. During operative debridement, necrosis is easily identified by the lack of bleeding from involved tissues, and by the finding of fascial planes that separate easily with little resistance [3, 6]. Classically, necrotizing fasciitis is an infection involving the superficial fascia without direct involvement of the skin or deep muscle [1, 12]. The fascia typically appears yellow-gray and may be liquefied [16]. Compartment syndrome, requiring extensive fasciotomy, may develop as a result of circumferential swelling. If the muscle is infected, the typical findings include purulent material or gas between the fibers. Fat necrosis (panniculitis) is usually focal and should also be widely debrided. Complete removal of nonviable tissue is mandatory. Superficial tissue and skin may not be initially involved, but may subsequently become gangrenous and require removal as nutrient vessels thrombose [6, 10, 16]. Since retained broken needles are common with illicit drug users, blunt digital dissection of tissues should be avoided. Open management of the resulting wounds is preferred to avoid resuppuration. When the infection involves an extremity, appropriate splints should be applied and the affected extremities elevated. Gram stain by touch prep or frozen section biopsy of the debrided tissue can be used to confirm that margins are free of infection [9, 17, 18]. Tissue and fluid should be cultured for aerobic, anaerobic, and fungal organisms to assist in the refinement of antibiotic regimens [12].

Reconstruction is a secondary consideration during the initial debridement phase. Patients should be scheduled for a repeat exploration with possible further debridement within 12-24 h. In general, this should be conducted in the operating room under general anesthesia, as bedside examination is generally too painful for the patient and may not allow for adequate wound inspection. Tissues and fascia should be carefully inspected with particular attention to wound boundaries and overlying skin, since areas of NSTI can persist after an inadequate initial debridement or with disease progression [16]. Amputation may be necessary if tissue destruction portends a useless extremity or if infection threatens spread to the torso [15].

Supportive Care

Resuscitation following operative intervention should be continued in a monitored intensive care unit. Treatment of acidosis, dehydration, and hemodynamic instability may all become necessary. Ventilatory support and close hemodynamic monitoring are mandatory. Septic shock and multiorgan failure with a systemic inflammatory response is a common complication of the disease process. Nutritional support should also be initiated as soon as possible, preferably through the enteral route.

Controversies

Fecal Diversion?

In general, fecal diversion for perineal wounds is not required unless complex wounds fail to heal because of persistent soiling [15]. Indications for the performance of a diverting ostomy include an infected sphincter, colonic or rectal perforation, incontinence, large nonhealing wounds, and certain conditions of immunocompromise [14].

Hyperbaric Oxygen?

When available, hyperbaric oxygen (HBO) therapy can be used as an adjuvant to surgical therapy. Proponents of HBO point to the advantages of hyperoxia, including improved phagocytosis of leukocytes, eradication of anaerobes, reduction of tissue edema, stimulation of fibroblast growth, and increased collagen formation [3]. HBO may be of some benefit in patients with *Clostridial* myonecrosis [15]. While anecdotal reports suggest that HBO therapy can decrease mortality in certain patients, evidence from prospective randomized trials is lacking [19]. Regardless of the decision to incorporate HBO therapy, its use should not preclude or delay early surgical debridement.

Critical Factors and Decision Making

Patients with suspected NSTI require operative exploration and evaluation of infected tissues. Obvious necrotic infections need urgent operative debridement and postoperative intensive care unit monitoring with planned reexploration within 24 h. Broad-spectrum antibiotics should be initiated early, and then tailored based upon culture results and clinical response [17]. At the time of reexploration, further serial debridement should be undertaken of all necrotic areas involved. Reconstruction and closure of large wounds should not be considered until all infection has cleared and wounds have become mature.

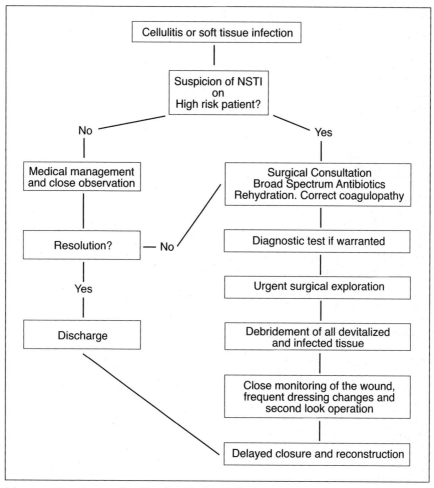

Diagram 1. Management algorithm for soft tissue infections

References

1. Lewis RT (1998) Soft tissue infections. World J Surg 22:146–151
   Classification of soft tissue infections including review of necrotizing soft tissue infections.
2. Hill MK, Sanders CV (1998) Skin and soft tissue infections in critical care. Inf in Crit Care II 14:251–262
   Review of bacteriology of infections occurring in the ICU.
3. Green RJ, Dafoe DC, Raffin TA (1996) Necrotizing fasciitis. Chest 110:219–229
   Review of necrotizing fasciitis including figure reference and extensive bibliography.
4. Singh G, Ray P, Sinha K, Adhikary S, Khanna SK (1996) Bacteriology of necrotizing infections of soft tissues. Aust NZ J Surg 66:747–750
   Detailed bacterial profile of 55 patients with NSTI.
5. Callahan TE, Schecter WP, Horn JK (1998) Necrotizing soft tissue infection masquerading as cutaneous abscess following illicit drug injection. Arch Surg 133:812–818
   Retrospective analysis of 30 cases of NSTI from parenteral drug use.
6. Bosshardt TL, Henderson VJ, Organ CH (1996) Necrotizing soft-tissue infections. Arch Surg 131:846–854
   Review of 45 patients with NSTI demonstrating parenteral drug use as an increasing cause.
7. Wall DB, De Virgilio C, Black S, Klein SR (2000) Objective criteria may assist in distinguishing necrotizing fasciitis from nonnecrotizing soft tissue infection. Am J Surg 179:17–21
   Retrospective review of necrotizing vs. non-necrotizing soft tissue infections in which WBC > 14, serum Na < 135 and, BUN > 15 predicted NSTI.
8. Bilton DB, Zibari GB, McMillan RW, Aultman DF, Dunn G, McDonald JC (1998) Aggressive surgical management of necrotizing fasciitis serves to decrease mortality: a retrospective study. Am Surg 64:397–401
   Retrospective comparison of aggressive surgical debridement vs. delayed therapy demonstrating a significantly decreased mortality with aggressive therapy.
9. McHenry CR, Piotrowski JJ, Petrinic D, Malangoni MA (1995) Determinants of mortality for necrotizing soft-tissue infections. Ann Surg 221:558–565
   Large review of NSTI with identification of delay to operation significantly increasing mortality.
10. Francis KR, Lamaute HR, Davis JM, Pizzi W (1993) Implications of risk factors in necrotizing fasciitis. Am Surg 59:304–308
    Retrospective review of risk factors in patients with NSTI in which more than three factors increased mortality over 50%.
11. Ward RG, Walsh MS (1991) Necrotizing fasciitis: 10 year's experience in a district general hospital. Brit J Surg 78:488–489
    Review of 14 patients with necrotizing fasciitis with analysis of factors involved with mortality.
12. Giuliano A, Lewis F, Hadley K, Blaisdell FW (1977) Bacteriology of necrotizing fasciitis. Am J Surg 134:52–57
    Classic review of 16 patients with necrotizing fasciitis with focus on bacteriology and culture results.
13. Beauchamp NJ, Scott WW, Gottlieb LM, Fishman EK (1995) CT evaluation of soft tissue and muscle infection and inflammation: a systemic compartmental approach. Skeletal Radiol 24:317–324
    Description and review of multiple soft-tissue infections as diagnosed using computerized tomography.
14. Laucks S (1994) Fournier's gangrene. Anorec Surg 74:1339–1352
    Review of Fournier's gangrene including anatomical descriptions of perineal fascial planes and description of treatment.
15. Elliott D, Kufera JA, Myers R (1996) Necrotizing soft tissue infections. Ann Surg 224:672–683
    Large review of 198 cases of NSTI with extensive analysis and strategies for management.

16. Schecter W, Meyer A, Schecter G, Giuliano A, Newmeyer W, Kilgore E (1982) Necrotizing fasciitis of the upper extremity. J Hand Surg 7:15–20
    Retrospective review of 33 cases of necrotizing fasciitis of the upper extremity with operative and diagnostic descriptions.
17. Elliott D, Kufera JA, Myers R (2000) The microbiology of necrotizing soft tissue infections. Am J Surg 179:361–366
    Large retrospective review of 198 cases of NSTI focusing on bacteriology and antibiotic used in treatment.
18. Nolan T, King L, Smith R, Gallup D (1993) Necrotizing surgical infection and necrotizing fasciitis in obstetric and gynecologic patients. South Med J 86:1363–1367
    Review and case presentation of necrotizing fasciitis in obstetrical and gynecologic patients with recommendations of early colostomy.
19. Brown DR, Davis NL, Lepawsky M, Cunningham J, Kortbeek J (1994) A multicenter review of the treatment of major truncal necrotizing infections with and without hyperbaric oxygen therapy. Am J Surg 167:485–489
    Retrospective review of patients with NSTI who received hyperbaric oxygen therapy with those who did not, demonstrating a 12 % increase in survival with its use.

Invited Commentary

H. HARLAN STONE

- Although the classification of soft tissue infections as presented is acceptable, my personal preference has been to use a different organization of categories. *Cellulitis* is a diffuse inflammatory response without areas of necrosis during its earliest phases, is confined to tissue superficial to the deep enveloping fascia, generally is caused by Gram-positive cocci, and is almost uniformly responsive to beta lactam antibiotics.
- *Abscess,* on the other hand, represents a central area of liquefied necrotic material that, in turn, is surrounded by a halo of cellulitis. In general, the infection has been confined by the freshly established granulating wall. Host defenses have limited the process, so all that is needed is drainage. Antibiotics are indicated only if there has been an attendant bacteremia, and only until the abscess has been drained. Responsible pathogens include Gram-positive cocci, Gram-negative rods, or a mixed flora which may also include anaerobes.
- *Phlegmon* is a process that is made up of innumerable small abscesses that have been compartmentalized by soft tissue structures resistant to bacterial enzymatic digestion. Treatment is the same as for an abscess, except that the intervening septi must be divided to create a single confluent cavity. At times it is more practical to excise the entire inflammatory process, such as with sigmoid colectomy for diverticulitis.

A more serious infection is that which causes frank tissue necrosis. If the process involves those planes superficial to the deep enveloping fascia, then spread is along the equivalent of Scarpa's fascia (*Necrotizing fasciitis*). It can be recognized at a relatively early stage because of thrombosis of the perforating vessels, which nourish the more superficial tissues – the skin and subcutaneous fat. If caused by a single pathogen, either the aerobic *Streptococcus* or *Pseudomonas* is the usual culprit. Most, however, are caused by a mixed flora and may be promoted by microbial synergy, for example in infections caused by anaerobic *Streptococci* (*Peptostreptococcus*) in combination with *Staphylococcus aureus,* as described first by Meleney. Other soft tissue infections result from fusospirochetes or marine Vibrios. Most, however, yield a polymicrobial mixture of aerobic Gram-negative rods in symbiosis with a large array of anaerobes. Treatment consists of antibiotic therapy appropriate for the offending bacteria until the process can be excised. Management is the same as described in the chapter from that point on.

Gangrenous infection below the deep enveloping fascia *Necrotizing myosiitis,* appears late and often has no obvious wound, or the penetrating site is some innocuous form of trauma. Management here is similar to that used in necrotizing fasciitis, except that generously wide excision of skin and subcutaneous tissue seldom is necessary. Gas gangrene is the classic example and is certainly the most fulminant.

In infections caused by toxic material introduced by a poisonous snake, spider, or scorpion, the primary site is excised as soon as possible. If an antitoxin is available, certainly it warrants administration.

Finally, hyperbaric oxygen therapy has no proven benefit and is indeed a form of late twentieth century alchemy.

23 Diabetic Foot

Daniel Vega, Kristine West, Jose M. Tellado

Key Principles

- *Diabetic foot* is a syndrome involving pain, deformation, inflammation, infection, ulceration, and tissue loss of the foot in diabetic patients.
- Neuropathy, ischemia, and infection are the principal pathogenic factors.
- Clinical features are neuropathic and ischemic ulcers and infection.
- Diagnosis should identify and grade neuropathology, osteopathy, and vascular pathology.
- Treatment involves relieving weight from the ulcerated area, treating infection, and restoring arterial perfusion.

General Approach

Diabetic foot is a clinical syndrome involving pain, deformation, inflammation, infection, ulceration, and tissue loss of the foot in diabetic patients.

Pathophysiology

The predominant cause is sustained hyperglycemia [1], although diabetic foot lesions frequently result from two or more risk factors occurring together (Diagram 1). In the majority of patients, diabetic peripheral neuropathy plays a central role [2]; up to 50 % of patients with type 2 diabetes have neuropathy and are at risk of developing the syndrome. Neuropathy leads to an insensitive and subsequently deformed foot with an abnormal walking pattern and, in conjunction with limited joint mobility, can result in abnormal biomechanical loading of the foot. Initially a callus is formed, but ultimately the skin breaks down. In addition, minor trauma may precipitate a chronic ulcer. Regardless of the primary cause, the patient continues walking on the insensitive foot, impairing subsequent healing. Minor trauma in the setting of peripheral vascular disease may result in a painful, ischemic foot ulcer [3]. However, in patients with both neuropathy and ischemia (neuroischemic ulcer), symptoms may be absent despite severe peripheral ischemia. Microangiopathy is rarely a primary cause of an ulcer.

Once neuropathy develops, other aggravating factors, including infection and ischemia, play a major role, the former provoking extensive tissue damage, and the latter delaying the healing process.

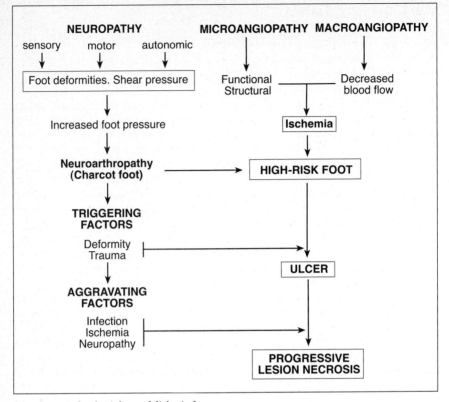

Diagram 1. Pathophysiology of diabetic foot

Clinical Features

Patients at risk for developing diabetic foot suffer from neuropathy (dysesthesia, paresthesia, hyperesthesia or anesthesia) or dermopathy (cutaneous dryness, ungal alteration, and atrophy of the subcutaneous cellular tissue) [5].

Neuropathic ulcers usually occur on the plantar surface of the foot, or in areas overlying a bony deformity. Ulcerations come in three different forms: typical rounded ulcers, a periulcerative callus, and painless ulcerations. Arterial perfusion in such cases may be adequate with normal peripheral pulses [4].

Occasionally patients present with asymptomatic spontaneous tarsometatarsal fractures. The radiological findings include periosteal and osteolytic bone reaction. More advanced stages, the so-called global arthropathy (Charcot's joints), are defined by the presence of plantar tarsal subluxation and loss of medial conductivity of the foot caused by displacement of the calcaneoastragaloid joint, which can be associated with luxation of the tarsometatarsals [5].

Neuroischemic ulcers are more common on the tips of the toes or the lateral border of the foot. Initial necrosis is dry but may become wet, particularly if it becomes infected [6].

The Infected Diabetic Foot

Not all neuropathic foot ulcers are infected. Infection is suggested by local inflammation, purulent drainage, sinus-tract formation, or crepitation. The severity of cellulitis may range from a mild, localized infection to a limb-threatening, necrotizing process with fasciitis [7]. Foot ulcers can be divided into superficial lesions that do not threaten the limb and deeper, limb-threatening ulcers. Fever, chills, and leukocytosis are absent in two thirds of patients with limb-threatening infection, which may include deep abscesses, extensive soft tissue infection, or metastatic infection involving remote sites. Hyperglycemia is a common sign of limb- or life-threatening infection. Erythema, swelling, and warmth in a non-ulcerated foot may indicate acute Charcot's disease rather than infection.

Most mild infections are caused by aerobic Gram-positive cocci such as *Staphylococcus aureus* or streptococci. Deeper, limb-threatening infections are usually polymicrobial and caused by aerobic Gram-positive cocci, Gram-negative bacilli (e.g., *Escherichia coli, Klebsiella* species, and *Proteus* species), and anaerobes (e.g., *Bacteroides* species and *Peptostreptococcus*). The pathogenic role of coagulase-negative *Staphylococci, Enterococci,* and *Corynebacterium* species is often difficult to discern, particularly when they are cultured along with more virulent organisms [8].

Clinically uninfected ulcers should not be cultured. The results of superficial swab cultures of an open wound are unreliable. If cultures are warranted, percutaneous needle biopsy, deep aspiration, or open debridement and tissue biopsy should be performed in order to identify the infecting bacteria [9-13]. The Wagner Scale is a useful clinical classification system for diabetic ulcers. It classifies the severity depending on the depth of the ulcer, infection grade and degree of gangrene (Table 1).

Diagnosis

Diagnosis of the diabetic foot must identify and grade all elements of pathophysiology: neuropathology, osteopathy, and vascular pathology.

Table 1. Classification of diabetic foot (from [13])

Grades	Clinical features
0	Normal foot. Variable degree of neuropathy. Joint deformities. Foot at risk.
1	Superficial ulcer, nonaffecting soft tissue. Cellulitis.
2	Noncomplicated deep ulcer, producing osteitis.
3	Complicated deep ulcer, including deep infection, osteomyelitis and abscess.
4	Limited necrotizing gangrene (digital, plantar, heel).
5	Extended gangrene.

A simple technique can identify patients who have lost protective sensation. A nylon monofilament is pressed against the skin to the point of buckling. Patients who cannot feel the monofilament are at risk for ulceration and require special care [14].

The diagnosis of osteomyelitis is difficult, since plain radiographs are neither sensitive nor specific. Differentiating between diabetic osteoarthropathy and osteomyelitis is difficult. The ability to reach bone by gently advancing a sterile surgical probe has a high specificity and positive predictive value in diagnosing osteomyelitis, but the sensitivity of this technique is low [15]. Combining plain radiography with a probe for bone is a reasonable initial approach to the diagnosis of osteomyelitis [3].

Vascular assessment should include palpation of pulses (pedal, tibial posterior, popliteal, and femoral), and evaluation of asymmetries in temperature, coloration, and capillary-venous refilling. In the absence of pulses, the Hemodynamic Functional Exam providing information regarding the Doppler velometric curve and ankle pressure, should be performed. Values lower than 1.2–1.0 on the leg/arm blood pressure gradient indicate the presence of vascular pathology [16]. However, in some diabetic patients, this index may be normal due to calcification of the medial arterial layer. Finally, an angiographic study is indicated when surgical revascularization treatment is contemplated.

Treatment

General Principles

The most effective approach to prevent the appearance of symptomatic neuropathy is to maintain normal blood glucose levels, as reflected by HbA1C levels, under 7.5%.

Optimal treatment requires that weight bearing be eliminated. Foot ulcers commonly fail to heal simply because patients continue to put weight on their feet. Because prolonged absence of weight-bearing on the affected foot is usually unrealistic, devices are required that reduce pressure at the site of the ulcer while allowing ambulation. Small shallow ulcers have been treated successfully with felted foam inserts. However, the total-contact cast is the optimal device for protecting neuropathic ulcers during ambulatory management [3]. This device is designed to distribute pressure over the entire surface of the foot and lower leg and thereby protect the site of the ulcer. The cast should be removed 24–48 h after application to assess the adequacy of the fit. Another cast is then applied and changed every week thereafter. Healing generally occurs in 8–10 weeks.

Local treatment should be carried out according to the degree of ulceration (Wagner Scale). For a *Grade 0* ulcer, education and adoption of prophylactic measures have been demonstrated to prevent ulceration and infection [19]. For *Grade 1* ulcers, the priority is to decrease pressure over the ulcerated area; usually infection is not yet present. Infection is frequently present in *Grade 2* ulcers, therefore, it is necessary to obtain samples for culture and sensitivity. Early debridement of fistulous tracts is effective, and must be done independent of the blood perfusion to the foot. Infections of *Grade 3,* are usually extensive and debridement should be performed in the operating room. Treatment of diabetic foot osteomyelitis is summarized in Diagram 2. For *Grades 4 and 5* ulcers, amputation is generally needed.

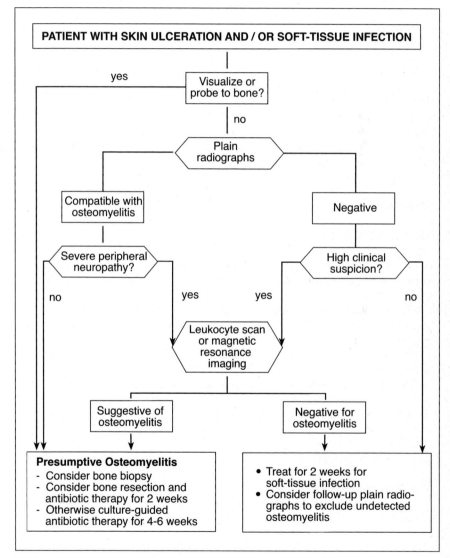

Diagram 2. Diabetic foot osteomyelitis

Table 2. Antibiotic treatment of diabetic foot

Non-limb-threatening
  No hospital admission
  Previously untreated; limited in extent
  Oral regimen (Cephalexin, Clindamycin, Amoxicillin-clavulanate)

Limb-threatening infection
  Chronic, recurrent
  Hospital admission
  Parenteral regimen [Ampicillin-sulbactam, Piperacillin-tazobactam, ticarcillin-clavulanate or clindamycin+ (ceftriaxone/cefotaxime or fluoroquinolone or aztreonam)]

Life-threatening infection/Osteomyelitis
  Septic, severe
  Parenteral regimen [(Imipenem-cilastatin, meropenem or trovafloxacin) + Vancomycin]

Antibiotic Therapy

Antibiotics should be administered once appropriate specimens have been obtained for culture (Table 2). The choice of regimen should be based on the suspected pathogens. Infections can be classified as non-limb-threatening, limb-threatening, or life-threatening for the purpose of empiric selection of an antibiotic regimen [17]. Aminoglycosides should generally be avoided in favor of less nephrotoxic antibiotics. Fluoroquinolones, which lack adequate activity against Gram-positive and anaerobic pathogens, should not be used empirically as single agents. If the infection does not respond adequately to treatment, the antimicrobial agent should be changed according to the culture results.

For non-limb threatening ulcerations, outpatient care using oral antibiotics such as cephalexin, clindamycin, or amoxicillin-clavulanate is appropriate if the patient is previously untreated and the ulceration is limited in extent [11]. Limb-threatening infections are classified as chronic or recurrent, requiring hospital admission and parenteral antibiotics. Severe infections are life-threatening and require parenteral antibiotics [18].

The optimal duration of antimicrobial therapy after surgical debridement of infected bone has not been established. Traditionally, a regimen of 4-6 weeks of parenteral antibiotic therapy has been recommended. If all infected bone has been removed by digital or ray amputation, a 2- to 3-week course of antibiotics directed at residual soft tissue infection is reasonable [3].

Surgical Treatment

Local Wound Care

Dry Clean Ulcers

Wound care includes debridement of callus, application of sterile dressings, and frequent inspection. Dry dressings are used in casts; otherwise, saline-moistened sterile gauze is applied and changed two to three times a day. Occlusive dressings also appear to be satisfactory. The efficacy of topical growth factors has not been conclusively established. Topical iodine preparations, astringents, and hydrogen peroxide interfere with the healing of the wound. Foot soaks and whirlpool therapy are rarely effective and may lead to further skin maceration or wound breakdown [19]. When healing has occurred, weight bearing is gradually introduced and increased with the use of accommodative footwear to protect the wound.

Infected Ulcers

Sharp debridement, usually in the operating room, allows for thorough removal of all necrotic material and diminishes the bacterial load, and so promotes healing [12]. All necrotic bone, plus a small portion of the uninvolved bone, soft tissue, and devascularized structures, should be excised, and the degree of penetration of the infection should be established. Curettage of any exposed or remaining cartilage is important to prevent this avascular structure from becoming a nidus of infection.

The use of moist dressings on clean, granulating wounds improves the wound environment [20]. The dressings not only provide protection against further bacterial contamination but also maintain moisture balance, optimize the wound pH, absorb fibrinous fluids, and reduce local pain. A variety of dressings are currently available that can be targeted to specific characteristics of the wound. However, moist normal-saline dressings are probably sufficient for the majority of wounds [21]. These inexpensive dressings are highly absorptive of exudative drainage and maintain the moist environment.

With extensive wound infections and rampant cellulitis, use of a topical antimicrobial agent such as sulfadiazine or mupirocin may be help to reduce the bacterial load and serve as a chemical barrier to exogenous pathogens. Caution in the use of such medications is warranted to avoid selecting resistant organisms and preventing wound drainage [18].

Amputation

Between 30 % and 50 % of diabetics with critical ischemia will reach this terminal phase. It is crucial to obtain hemodynamic, angiographic data, and systemic tests, in order to properly plan the necessary level for amputation. In well-perfused feet the amputation level can be "functional", at either the digital or transmetatarsal level. Major amputations are necessary in extremities with critical ischemia, with or without gangrene, after hemodynamic and angiographic parameters indicate no possibility of revascularization [22].

Minor Amputations

Toe Amputation

Tissue resection is minimal leaving a functioning foot.

Indications

Lesions located in the distal phalanges – well-demarcated dry gangrene, neuropathic ulcers, or osteomyelitis – with healthy skin in the base of the toe, to cover the wound.

Contraindications

- Gangrene or infection that includes the soft tissue of the proximal phalanges
- Septic arthritis of the metatarsophalangeal joint
- Cellulitis that penetrates the foot
- Involvement of the interdigital space
- Intense pain in the remaining toes

Technique

A "racquet" shaped incision is recommended. The tissues should be severed from the incision line directly down to the shaft of the phalanx and dissection of tissues should then continue proximally as close to the bone as possible, to avoid the possibility of damaging the digital vessels laterally and thus compromising the blood supply to the flaps and other digits.

Transmetatarsal Toe Amputation

Indications

Lesions involving the proximal phalanges and the metatarsophalangeal joint.

Contraindications

- Septic arthritis of the metatarsophalangeal joint
- Cellulitis that penetrates the foot
- Involvement of the interdigital space

Technique

A "racquet" shaped incision is recommended. The head of the metatarsal should then be removed with nibbling forceps preventing damage to the surrounding tissues. The bone should be nibbled back until the soft tissues fall in to cover approximately half of the cut end of the bone. Tendons should be pulled down with forceps, severed, and allowed to retract. The incision should not be sutured but rather packed lightly with ribbon gauze, to limit bleeding, and allowed to heal by secondary intention.

Atypical Foot Amputations

Atypical amputations involve the removal of all necrotic soft tissue and affected bony structures. The limit of bony resection must be located in the distal part of the metatarsal, since a more proximal line of amputation does not result in a functional foot. If a more limited amputation cannot be performed, it is better to proceed with a below-knee amputation. The skin is usually left open so that healing is by secondary intention.

Transmetatarsal Amputation

Transmetatarsal amputation includes all phalanges and the head of metatarsal bones, preserving acceptable function without the need for a complex process of rehabilitation.

Indications

Lesions that include several toes and the interdigital spaces.

Contraindications

• Extensive deep fascial infection

Technique

A dorsal midmetatarsal transverse incision is made. Metatarsal bones are divided 1-2 cm proximal to the skin incision. The plantar flap is brought forward over the metatarsals and cut to the appropriate length to allow closure without tension.

Major Amputations

Below-Knee Amputation

Indications

• Failure of transmetatarsal amputation
• Gangrene of the foot that invades the metatarsal region and precludes amputation at this level

Contraindications

• Extensive gangrene of the leg
• Patient who is unlikely to benefit from a below-knee prosthesis

Amputation: Long Posterior Flap Technique

The stump should be as short as possible to maximize the chances of healing but long enough to allow optimal use of a below-knee prosthesis. The level of the bony section is marked at approximately 13-15 cm distal to the knee joint line. The midmedial and midlateral line of the lower leg is marked at the same point, and the two points are connected over the anterior aspect of the leg. The apex of the posterior flap is approximately 15 cm distal to this line. The flap is based on half the circumference of the leg to maximize the blood supply from above. The muscle of the anterior and lateral compartments is divided to expose the fibula, ligating the anterior tibial vessels. The fibula is divided with a lateral bevel 1.5 cm proximal to the tibial line. The tibia is divided with an anterior bevel and the lower leg removed by dissecting the posterior flap away from the bones. The bulk of the flap should be reduced by complete removal of the soleus muscle, which does not contribute to the blood supply of the flap.

Above-Knee Amputation

Indications

- Failure of healing below the knee
- Patient who is certain not to benefit from a below-knee prosthesis

The site of division of the femur should not be more than 12 cm from the knee joint line to allow room for the knee mechanism in the prosthesis. The minimum length of stump that can be used to fit an above-knee prosthesis is 7.5 cm below the adductor muscle insertion. If the amputation must be shorter than this and it is hoped eventually to fit a prosthesis, a hip disarticulation should be performed, as this allows better fitting of a prosthesis and reduces weight.

The bone end should be rounded off and covered by suturing the deep fascia of the posterior flap, with its attached muscles, to the same structures anteriorly.

Guillotine Amputation

Indicated when the infection has destroyed the architecture and function of the foot. Consists of a cross-section, over the malleolus and perpendicular to the axis of the leg, of the skin, soft tissues and bones. Once the infection is controlled a conventional amputation is performed.

Controversies

- The efficacy of topically growth factors has not been conclusively proven [23, 24]. The addition of G-CSF to the treatment does not reduce the duration of antibiotic administration, duration of hospital stay, or need for amputation in diabetic foot infection [25].
- Topical iodine preparations, astringents, and hydrogen peroxide interfere with the healing of the wound [26, 27]. In a double-blind randomized trial, topical hyperbaric oxygen was not beneficial [28].
- Treatment of osteomyelitis has traditionally included aggressive surgical debridement or limited amputation of infected bone (Diagram 2). A 10- to 12-week course of antibiotics has been reported to cure pedal osteomyelitis with-

out the need for surgical debridement [17, 29]. However, these studies included patients in whom the diagnosis of osteomyelitis was based solely on plain X-rays and technetium bone scans, and the conclusions may not be relevant to patients with more advanced disease. At present, it is difficult to recommend a single approach to the diagnosis and treatment of pedal osteomyelitis in diabetic patients, and clinical judgment is required. Patients with limb- or life-threatening infections must undergo early aggressive drainage and debridement of all necrotic tissue, including bone. In some patients with less serious infections, a cycle of prolonged antimicrobial therapy may be a reasonable approach [3].

Critical Factors and Decision Making

- Blood sugar control retards the progression of neuropathy, the most important risk factor for ulceration.
- Early detection of the loss of protective sensation and implementation of strategies to prevent ulceration will reduce the rates of limb-threatening complications. Education in foot care, proper footwear, and close follow-up are required to prevent or promptly detect neuropathic injury.

General principles	Antibiotic therapy	Surgical treatment
• Metabolic control • Grade 0 Preventing and education of patients Vascular and radiological assessment • Grade 1 Antibiotic therapy Relief of pressure Bone removal if necessary Revascularization if necessary • Grade 2 Debridement • Grade 3 Hospital admission Surgical debridement • Grade 4 Minor amputation • Grade 5 Major amputation	1. **Non-limb-threatening** - Outpatient care - Previously untreated. Limited in extent. - Oral regimen (Cephalexin, Clindamycin, Amoxicillin-clavulanate) 2. **Limb-threatening infection** - Chronic recurrent. - Hospital admission. - Parenteral regimen [Ampicillin-sulbactam, Piperacillin-tazobactam, ticarcillin-clavulanate or clindamycin + (ceftriaxone / cefotaxime or fluorquinolone or aztreonam)]. 3. **Life-threatening infection** - Septic, severe - Parenteral regimen [(Imipenem-cilastatin, meropenem or trovafloxacin) + Vancomycin]. 4. **Osteomyelitis**	• Local wound care - Dry clean ulcers - Infected ulcers • Amputations Minor - Toe - Transmetatarsal digital amputation - Transmetatarsal - Atypical amputation Major - Below-knee amputation - Above-knee amputation - Guillotine amputation

Diagram 3. Principles of treatment of diabetic foot treatment

- If ulceration occurs, removal of pressure from the site of the ulcer and careful management of the wound will allow healing in most cases. The failure to heal despite these measures should prompt a search for associated arterial insufficiency.
- If infection is present, appropriate antimicrobial therapy combined with immediate surgical intervention, including revascularization when necessary, will increase the chances of saving the limb.

References

1. Hatary Y (1987) diabetic peripheral neuropathy. Ann Int Med 107:546–559
2. Asbury AK (1988) Understanding diabetic neuropathy. N Engl J Med 319:577–578
3. Caputo GM, Cavanagh PR, Ulbrecht JS, Gibbons GW, Karchmer AW (1994) Assessment and management of foot disease in patients with diabetes. N Engl J Med 331:854–860
4. Edmonds Management of the diabetic foot (1990) Critical Ischaemia 1:5–13
5. Tawn DJ, O'Hare JP, O'Brien IAD, et al (1988) Bone scintigraphy and radiography in the early recognition of diabetic osteopathy. Br J Radiol 61:273–279
6. European Working Group on Critical Leg Ischaemia (1992) Second European consensus document on chronic critical leg ischaemia. Eur J Vasc Surg 6 Suppl A:1–32
7. Lipsky BA, Pecoraro RE, Wheat LJ (1990) The diabetic foot: soft tissue and bone infection. Infect Dis Clin N Am 4:409–432
8. Wheat JL, Allen SD, Henry M, et al (1986) Diabetic foot infections: bacteriologic analysis. Arch Inter Med 146:1935–1940
9. Sapico FL, Witte JL, Canawati HN, Montgomerie JZ, Bessman AN (1984) The infected foot of the diabetic patient: quantitative microbiology and analysis of clinical features. Rev Infect Dis 6:Suppl 1:S171–S176
10. Knox R, Dutch W, Blume P, Sumpio B (2000) Diabetic foot disease. Int J Angiol 1:1–6
11. Joshi N, Caputo GM, Weitekamp MR, Karchmer AW (1999) Infections in patients with diabetes mellitus. N Engl J Med 341:1906–1912
12. Steed DL, Donohoe D, Webster MW, Lindsley L (1996) Effect of extensive debridement and treatment on the healing of diabetic foot ulcers. J Am Coll Surg 183:61–64
13. Wagner FWJr (1981) The dysvascular foot: a system for diagnosis and treatment. Foot Ankle 2:64–122
14. Bloom S, Till S, Sönken P, et al (1984) Use of biothesiometer to measure individual vibration thresholds and their vibration in 519 non-diabetic subjects. BMJ 288:1793–1795
15. Grayson ML, Gibbons GW, Balogh K, Levin E, Karchmer AW (1995) Probing to bone in infected pedal ulcers: a clinical sign of underlying osteomyelitis in diabetic patients. JAMA 273:721–723
16. Fitzgerald DE, Carr J (1977) Peripheral arterial disease: assessment by arteriography and alternative non-invasive measurements. Am J Roentgenol 128:385–388
17. Lipsky BA (1997) Osteomyelitis of the foot in diabetic patients. Clin Infect Dis 25:1318–1326
18. Sumpio BE (2000) Foot ulcers. New Engl J Med 343:787–793
19. Apelqvist J, Bakker K, Van Houtum WH, et al (2000) International consensus and practical guidelines on the management and the prevention of the diabetic foot. Diabetes Metab Res Rev 16Suppl 1:S84–S92
20. Bergstrom N, Bennett MA, Carlson CE, et al (1994)) Treatment of pressure ulcers. Clinical practice guidelines, no. 15. Rockville, Md., Agency for Health Care Policy and Research (AHCPR publication no. 95–0652):1–102
21. Resources in wound care, directory (1999) Adv Wound Care 12:155–223
22. American Diabetes Association: Clinical Practice Recommendations (1997) Foot care in patients with diabetes mellitus. Diabetes 20:Suppl 1

23. Steed D, Goslen JB, Holloway GA, et al (1992) Randomized prospective double-blind trial in healing chronic diabetic foot ulcer: CT-102 activated platelet supernatant, topical versus placebo. Diabetes Care 15:1598–1604
24. McGrath MH (1990) Peptide growth factors and wound healing. Clin Plast Surg 17:421–432
25. Yonem A, Cakir B, Guler S, Azal O, Corakci A (2001) Effects of granulocyte-colony stimulating factor in the treatment of diabetic foot infection. Diabetes Obes Metab 3:332–337
26. Lineaweaver W, Howard R, Soucy D, et al (1985) Topical antimicrobial toxicity. Arch Surg 120:267–270
27. Kucan JO, Robson MC, Heggers JP, Ko F (1981) Comparison of silver sulfadiazine, povidone-iodine and physiologic saline in the treatment of chronic pressure ulcers. J Am Geriatr Soc 29:232–235
28. Leshe CA, Sapico FL, Ginunas VJ, Adkins RH (1988) Randomized controlled trial of topical hyperbaric oxygen for treatment of diabetic foot ulcers. Diabetes Care 11:111–115
29. Bamberger DM, Daus GP, Gerding DN (1987) Osteomyelitis in the feet of diabetic patients: long-term results, prognostic factors, and the role of antimicrobial and surgical therapy. Am J Med 83:653–660

Invited Commentary

YENUMULA P. REDDY, SATISH C. KHANEJA

Foot infections in a diabetic population are cared for by a variety of specialists including physicians, podiatrists, general surgeons, and vascular surgeons. It is estimated that 35% to 40% of the diabetic foot ulcers will result in a major amputation within 3 years [1].

Diagnosis

The authors have appropriately emphasized preventive measures, the mainstay in extremity preservation in a diabetic population. However, once infection sets in, prompt and complete treatment is mandatory to avoid its devastating consequences.

At the outset a decision needs to be made: is the blood supply to the foot normal, indeterminate, or inadequate? A clearly palpable, bounding dorsalis pedis or posterior tibial pulse will exclude ischemia. It is worth emphasis that the presence of a femoral or popliteal pulse does not exclude leg or foot ischemia in a diabetic patient. Obvious signs of ischemia are generally recognized, but the difficulty is in the group with marginal blood supply where the extremity is at risk in the presence of infection.

We classify acute infections in patients with normal blood supply into three broad groups:
1. Superficial cellulitis
2. Deep-seated infection
3. Potentially life-threatening infection

The clinical problem lies in differentiating superficial cellulitis from deep-seated, limb-threatening infection. When one encounters an inflamed, swollen toe in a diabetic patient, this distinction is not so obvious and the onus is on the clinician to ensure that a deep-seated infection with possible involvement of bone or tendons does not exist. Because this distinction is often unclear at the time of initial presentation, we recommend initial therapy with broad-spectrum antibiotics and extensive use of imaging, including CT scan or MRI and bone scan. The extent of the necrotic tissue, involvement of joints, and the presence of gas in the soft tissues is well delineated with the CT scan, while MRI is both sensitive and specific in detecting osteomyelitis. In cases where MRI is inconclusive, triple phase isotope bone scan using [111]indium-tagged WBC is helpful in detecting osteomyelitis [2].

Antibiotics

The choice of an appropriate antibiotic agent depends on the causative microbes. The optimal method of obtaining specimens for isolating pathogens is controversial. The portal of entry of an ulcer is often contaminated. Thus, the ideal method of isolating representative pathogens is by deep tissue biopsy where the chance for contamination is minimal. Belief that antibiotic selection can be based on superficial wound swab culture may lead to under-treatment. Our policy is to treat all infections with broad-spectrum antibiotics; in cases where the skin is intact, therapy is continued empirically until the clinical response and imaging studies exclude deep-seated infection. Superficial cellulitis that does not resolve in 2-3 days suggests deep tissue infection. In patients with open wounds, we perform a deep tissue biopsy prior to starting antibiotics, and coverage is changed as necessary. There is a compelling need for prospective studies correlating cultures from superficial wound, deep tissue and bone [3]. The choice of antibiotic is based on microbial etiology, severity of infection, presence or absence of osteomyelitis, vascular status of the limb, etc. Of these, vascular status of the limb is particularly important, since the antibiotic must reach the site of infection before it can act on bacteria. Agents that penetrate into tissues effectively such as fluoroquinolones and ampicillin/sulbactam are good choices in this context. In the presence of osteomyelitis, imipenem/cilastatin and ampicillin/sulbactam are both effective with cure rates of 81% and 85% respectively [4].

Source Control

Surgical treatment is the mainstay of treatment for limb and life-threatening infections. Meticulous debridement of all infected and necrotic tissues including the interfascial planes, where the infection can track quite extensively, is crucial. If the bone or joint space is involved, it must be removed, accounting for the classical amputations – *ray amputation of toe,* if the infection is confined to individual toe, and *transmetatarsal amputation,* if the whole of the forefoot is involved. Any uninvolved medial or lateral digit – even if only a single digit – should be preserved, no transmetatarsal amputation performed. In the presence of palpable pedal pulses, these procedures can be safely accomplished without the fear of nonhealing. However, if there is gangrene involving a major portion of the foot, or if extensive debridement is required, a major amputation – preferably below knee, or even above knee, depending on the condition of the leg – is recommended.

A complete debridement and a good blood supply are necessary at the site of amputation. When clinically appropriate, it is preferable to undertake a lesser amputation and accept the need for revision, rather than perform a higher amputation at the outset. Following debridement, we leave all the wounds open, as the failure rate with primary closure is high. Wounds are also left open following major amputations, and guillotine amputation is the procedure of choice in the presence of spreading cellulitis. Deep seated infections are treated with drainage, debridement of all nonviable tissues and, with the wound left open, covered with skin grafts or tissue flaps as necessary.

Revascularization

Revascularization has an important role in the source control of infection in the diabetic foot. It helps to control infection by improvement of circulation, and it increases delivery of antibiotics to the infected tissues. Arterial insufficiency is present in 20 % of diabetic patients with lower extremity ulceration [5]. When pedal pulses are not palpable, demonstration of biphasic flow in the pedal arteries using arterial Doppler is helpful in excluding ischemia. The traditional ankle/brachial index can be spuriously high in diabetic patients. If there is evidence of ischemia, angiography is mandatory in planning further treatment. Customary signs of infection in an ischemic foot may be absent, and a seemingly innocuous infection in the presence of ischemia has devastating consequences. Aggressive revascularization, usually a femoral or popliteal artery bypass to the peroneal or tibial, or even plantar, arteries (using vein grafts) is the approach of choice. Correction of inflow in the iliac, femoral, or popliteal artery alone, in the presence of distal obstruction, is unlikely to achieve control of infection. Aggressive use of in situ or reversed vein bypass appears to be a reasonable option. Patients with severe infection are debrided immediately and revascularization is undertaken expeditiously, generally within 2-3 days. Waiting for the infection to resolve completely in an ischemic foot before revascularization can be devastating. Under these circumstances, the revascularization procedure itself helps to control the infection by providing good blood supply and delivering antibiotics.

While extremity salvage is the main objective of treatment, a common-sense approach should prevail when treating patients who are nonambulatory, with nonfunctional limbs, and nonreconstructable distal vessels. A high amputation is safe in these cases.

Osteomyelitis

Another controversial issue is the treatment of osteomyelitis in the absence of clear indications for surgery such as necrosis, gangrene, or abscess. Medical therapy alone, using long-term antibiotics is successful in 53%-87% of cases [6]. In patients with osteomyelitis of the phalanx and metatarsal head, limited amputation may be more cost-effective. In retrospective studies comparing early limited amputation and long term antibiotics, future above knee amputation rates were significantly lower in patients managed surgically when compared to those managed medically (13% vs. 28%) [7].

Foot infections in diabetic patients will continue to challenge the clinicians for some time. It is important that we develop more precise staging and classification systems to simplify treatment algorithms.

References

1. Lipsky BA (1997) Osteomyelitis of the foot in diabetic patients. Clin Infect Dis 25:1318–1326
2. Struk DW, Munk PL, Lee MJ, et al (2001) Imaging of soft tissue infections. Rad Clin North Am 39:277–303
3. Pellizer G, Strazzabosco M, Presi S, et al (2001) Deep tissue biopsy vs superficial swab culture monitoring in the microbiological assessment of limb-threatening diabetic foot infections. Diabet Med 18:822–827
4. Grayson ML, Gibbons GW, Habershaw GM et al (1994) Use of ampicillin/sulbactam versus imipenem/cilastatin in the treatment of limb-threatening foot infections in diabetic patients. Clin Infect Dis 18:683–693
5. Krasner D (1998) Diabetic ulcers of the lower extremity: a review of comprehensive management. Ostomy/Wound Manage 44:56–75
6. Calret HM (2001) Infections in diabetes. Infect Dis Clin N Am 15:407–421
7. Tan JS, Friedman NM, Hazelton-Miller C, et al (1996) Can aggressive treatment of diabetic foot infections reduce the need for above-ankle amputations? Clin Infect Dis 23:286–291

24 Hand Infections

ROGER SAADIA

Key Principles

- Determine nature and extent of infection.
- Institute appropriate antimicrobial treatment.
- Perform surgical debridement and drainage, if necessary.
- Institute early measures to preserve hand function.

General Approach

Nature and Extent of Infection

It is important to differentiate between the early stages of infection and the formation of an abscess. In the former, nonoperative measures are usually sufficient to abort the progression towards purulence, while in the latter surgical drainage is required.

Classically, hand infections can be classified according to their anatomic location. A simplified classification is provided (Table 1).

Fingertip Infections

A *paronychia* [1] is an infection of the lateral soft tissue fold surrounding the fingernail. Acute paronychia is most commonly caused by penetrating trauma,

Table 1. Anatomical classification of hand infections

Infections of the fingertip
Acute paronychia
Chronic paronychia
Felon
Deep subfascial space infections
Subaponeurotic space
Thenar space
Midpalmar space
Hypothenar space
Interdigital (web) space
Parona's space
Flexor tenosynovitis
Finger tenosynovitis
Radial or ulnar bursa tenosynovitis

nail biting or manicures. *Staphylococcus aureus* is the usual infecting organism. Chronic paronychia is an entirely different and much more difficult disease to treat. It usually occurs in hands repeatedly exposed to moist or alkaline environments and is commonly found in bartenders, housekeepers, and swimmers. *Candida albicans* is cultured in 95 % of cases. A *felon* [1] is a subcutaneous abscess of the distal pulp of the fingertip. Penetrating trauma, sometimes sufficiently inconsequential to have been forgotten, is the main cause. The clinical picture is characterized by rapid onset of throbbing pain and swelling of the entire pulp. *S. aureus* is usually the causative organism, but opportunistic mixed organism infections are being increasingly encountered in immunocompromised patients.

Deep Subfascial Spaces

Infections of the potential *deep subfascial spaces* [2] comprise about 10 % of hand infections. These infections are characterized clinically by painful swelling over the site of the infection. Pitfalls in their evaluation include underestimation of the amount of pus collected in these spaces and the differentiation between cellulitis and abscess. "Collar button" (hour-glass shaped) abscesses may be found in web space infections. *Pyogenic flexor tenosynovitis* [3] is a closed space infection of the finger or thumb flexor tendon sheath, or the radial and ulnar bursae. If unrecognized and treated too late, this condition can result in significant morbidity and loss of function. The classic clinical presentation was described by Kanavel [4] a century ago. The clinical signs include tenderness over the course of the entire sheath, a semi-flexed posture of the affected digit, pain on passive extension, and symmetrical swelling of the entire finger. The etiology is penetrating injury and the most common infecting bacteria are *Staphylococcus* and *Streptococcus* species.

Human Bite Infections

Human bite infections are particularly virulent, and a relatively common problem [5]. There are four basic mechanisms:
1. Self-inflicted wounds from nail biting or sucking a bleeding wound
2. Traumatic amputations of a finger
3. Full thickness bites
4. The clenched-fist injury sustained when the patient strikes the mouth and teeth of another person, impaling the areas over the third, fourth or fifth metacarpal heads; as a result, penetration of several spaces within the hand occurs

The complex flora of the human mouth adds to the challenge of treating these injuries. There may be 100 million organisms per milliliter of saliva and over 42 species of bacteria [6]. However, not all organisms are pathogenic. The most commonly isolated bacteria are *Staphylococcus, Streptococcus, Eikenella corrodens* and anaerobes.

Antimicrobial Treatment

All patients with a traumatic hand infection should have appropriate tetanus prophylaxis. Early, acute fingertip infections can be treated with a few days of an
antistaphylococcal antibiotic. In chronic paronychia, antifungal ointment is often
prescribed but is generally unsuccessful; surgical eponychial marsupialization is
usually effective. When surgical drainage of an abscess is required, adjunctive antibiotic treatment is given for several days postoperatively, first intravenously then
orally. In most cases, an antistaphylococcal cephalosporin like cephazolin is adequate. However, Gram stain and cultures and sensitivities should be obtained routinely and treatment adjusted accordingly. Aerobic and anaerobic cultures are adequate for uncomplicated cases. Specialized stains, including fungal or atypical
mycobacterial cultures or biopsy studies, are ordered in unusual infections such as
those occurring in diabetics, in immunocompromised patients, and in those with
chronic infection. Hand infections in diabetics tend to be more aggressive and are
complicated by delayed wound healing. Gram-negative bacilli are causal organisms
in a high proportion of these patients and it is therefore recommended that initial
therapy include an aminoglycoside. In human bite infections, current antibiotic recommendations include penicillin to cover anaerobes and *Eikenella corrodens*, and
a cephalosporin for *staphylococci*. Of note, *Eikenella corrodens* is resistant to oxa-
cillin, methicillin, nafcillin, most aminoglycosides, and clindamycin. It is sensitive to
penicillin G, ampicillin, carbenicillin, and tetracycline [5]. Another antibiotic option
for human bite infections is ampicillin-sulbactam or amoxicillin-clavulanic acid [7].

Surgical Treatment

When the diagnosis is made early, within 24-48 h of injury, during the cellulitic
phase, conservative treatment with hand elevation and antibiotics may be sufficient.
The infection must be monitored and, in the absence of rapid improvement,
surgical treatment must be considered. Once an infection has progressed to the
stage of suppuration, adequate debridement and drainage of pus are indicated.

Several principles of surgical treatment need to be followed [7]. Even seemingly minor fingertip infection requires well-equipped facilities and appropriate
instruments. Adequate anesthesia may be regional (axillary, wrist, or finger
block) or general. Infiltration of local anesthetic into an infected area is contraindicated. A tourniquet is used and the arm is elevated but not exsanguinated prior
to elevation. Operative exposure is planned to allow wide opening of the infected
space. Straight incisions heal better than curved ones. Superficial staphylococcal
abscesses heal well with simple drainage and irrigation. Deep or polymicrobial
infections may require additional debridement of devitalized tissues. Intraoperative saline irrigation may be performed with a bulb syringe or pulsatile
device. Incisions are left open to heal by secondary intention; they are lightly
packed with a moist dressing and the hand is splinted in a bulky dressing and
elevated. Constricting bandages should be avoided. The wound should be re-
inspected at 24-48 h and dressings at the bedside should be continued two or three
times a day. The patient is encouraged to soak the hand daily in sterile water or

a mild antiseptic. In the absence of improvement after 2-4 days, adjustment of the antibiotic regimen or reexploration for a purulent collection is considered. Catheter irrigation is often used in the treatment of acute pyogenic flexor teno-synovitis, and has the advantage of limiting the incision and therefore promoting more rapid healing and rehabilitation. The catheters are left in situ postopera-tively for a variable period of time.

Preservation of Hand Function

Preservation of function is an extremely important component of the treatment. Hand elevation should be started immediately in order to decrease edema. Early active motion assists in minimizing edema and avoiding the formation of tendon adhesions, joint contractures, and stiffness. When available, the expertise of a hand therapist is invaluable postoperatively to instruct the patient and supervise the graded introduction of activity as the pain decreases. The early incorporation of the hand and extremity into daily activities is encouraged to improve motion and strength and avoid neglectful disuse.

Controversies

Controversies of operative technique are beyond the scope of this text. Open treat-ment of the wound versus primary closure is still being debated. A minority of surgeons make a plea for primary closure over a drain, or the insertion of a catheter for continuous wound irrigation with sterile isotonic saline [8], at a rate of 100 ml/h for 24-48 h. The claimed advantages of this technique are improved mechanical cleansing of the infected cavity and primary wound healing.

Critical Factors and Decision Making

Adequate decision making in the treatment of hand infections includes the following steps:
- Correct diagnosis of the nature of the infection: typical versus atypical, cellulitis versus abscess
- Identification of host factors: healthy versus immunocompromised
- Identification of the anatomic site of the infection
- Appropriate use of antibiotics either alone or in combination with operative treatment
- Extent of exploration of the presumed site of infection and adequacy of debride-ment
- Management of the wound: open versus primary closure
- Interpreting failure to improve postoperatively: inappropriate adjunctive anti-biotic treatment versus inadequacy of surgical drainage

For septic arthritis of the hand, see Chap. 27.

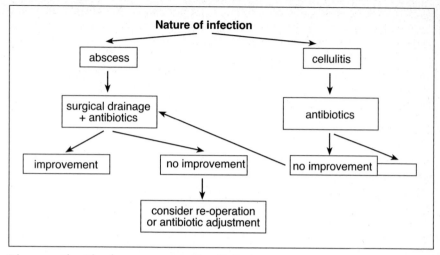

Diagram 1. Algorithm for management of hand infections

References

1. Jebson PJL (1998) Infections of the fingertip: paronychias and felons. Hand Clin 14:547–555
2. Jebson PJL (1998) Deep subfascial space infections. Hand Clin 14:557–566
3. Boles SD, Schmidt CC (1998) Pyogenic flexor tenosynovitis. Hand Clin 14:567–578
4. Kanavel AB (1905) Study of acute phlegmons of the hand. Surg Gynecol Obstet 1:221–235
5. Faciszewski T, Coleman DA (1998) Human bite infections of the hand. Hand Clin 14:683–690
6. Shields C, Patzakis MJ, Meyers MH, et al (1975) Hand infections secondary to human bites. J Trauma 15:235–236
7. Hausman MR, Lisser SP (1992) Hand infections. Orthop Clin N Am 23:171–185
8. Neviaser RJ (1988) Infections. In: Green DP (ed) Operative hand surgery, 3rd edn. Churchill Livingstone, New York, pp 148–156

Invited Commentary

WERNER WEISSENHOFER

The author has pointed out that the unique nature of hand infections arising from the distinctive anatomical structures of the hand necessitates special concepts of treatment and surgical techniques.

It is important to note that there are differences in the volar and dorsal aspect of the hand. The volar aspect is divided by a multitude of delicate but rigid fibrous bundles reaching down from the skin to the aponeurosis of the hand and the periostium of the digits and metacarpals; whereas the skin of the dorsal aspect of the hand is loosely bound to the deeper structures, creating a large potential space. Thus, dorsal infections often present as abscesses and are treated accordingly. Nevertheless, due to lymphatic drainage of the volar aspect towards the dorsum of the hand the collateral dorsal edema may be just a symptom, while the actual site of infection is on the volar aspect.

Although the author states that surgical intervention has to be timely, it must be emphasized that the earliest possible intervention has to be chosen, i.e., during the initial inflammatory phase, when swelling, reddening, and pain starts. Liberal opening of tendon sheath, debridement, and rinsing, using anatomically correct incisions are essential. The rinsing intra- and postoperatively may be augmented by antiseptics like povidone iodine.

I would also like to add a few technical points: In approximately 85 % of cases of flexor tenosynovitis, the radial and the ulnar sheath connect at the wrist, and therefore an infection of the thumb will result in a V-shaped infection spreading to the fifth finger and vice versa. Even the felon – seemingly easy to treat – presents pitfalls due to longitudinal fibrous divisions of the fingertip. These divisions may lead to infections of the flexor tendon sheath and undetected infection of the collateral side. These considerations influence the choice of methods of anesthesia. General anesthesia is preferred; if regional anesthesia is used the finger block should rarely be considered due to limitations in possible exposure.

All the entities mentioned by Dr. Saadia have symptoms in common with rare diseases like necrotizing fasciitis, mycetomas, syphilitic lesions, and Hanson's disease (a synonym of leprosy). To prevent misdirected operative approaches, careful evaluation of each case history is to be recommended.

Recommended Reading

1. Murray PM (1998) Septic arthritis of the hand and wrist. Hand Clin 14:587–597
2. Tsai E, Failla JM (1999) Hand infections in trauma patients. Hand Clin 15:373–386

Editorial Comment

The vast majority of hand infections seen in the community are "minor," but those that present to the surgeon in the emergency room are far from being so. The novice tends to underestimate the potential significance of hand infection which often leads to procrastination, which in turn may result in loss of function, and even loss of tissue and disfiguration.

The same surgeon who assessed the hand on admission and prescribed initial conservative therapy ought to examine the hand 6-8 h later. At reexamination the hand must be fully exposed. Has the pain decreased? Is the swelling reduced? Can the patient move his or her fingers? Lack of improvement, either subjective or objective, suggests that there is deep pus or necrotic tissue. In our experience, the persistence of extreme local tenderness to pressure commonly indicates that this is the point of deep, undrained pus. An initial improvement, however, does not indicate that a subsequent operation will not be necessary: the antibiotics may only localize the infection into a drainable abscess.

Deep palmar infections are in fact a variant of necrotizing fasciitis (Chap. 22): at exploration of those deep spaces one does not find much formed pus but the gray, flimsy, necrotic tissue typical of necrotizing soft tissue infections. And finally, one has to remember that the hand and the fingers are composed of multiple compartments subjected to the risks of acute compartment syndrome. Tense-swollen fingers and hands, with loss of sensation and/or motor function, should be thus urgently decompressed.

25 Head and Neck Infections

María F. Jiménez, Jaime Escallon

Key Principles

- Head and neck infections are generally controlled without surgical drainage. Progression to abscess indicates the need for intervention to achieve source control.
- The clinician must identify infection, and define the topographic diagnosis of the disease and the need for prompt and aggressive treatment.
- A purulent collection or cellulitis in a fascial space of the head and neck requires drainage for source control of the infectious process.

General Approach

Infections occurring in the head and neck range from mild to severe, may be acute or chronic, and can lead to potentially life-threatening complications. Modern techniques of diagnosis and treatment have significantly reduced the need for surgical intervention. Mediastinal and thoracic extension of head and neck infections are rare but occasionally occur.

Head and neck infections are characterized by distinctive anatomic properties: easy healing due to abundant vascular supply, and predictable routes of extension to the central nervous system (following a retrograde rich venous drainage and lymphatic channels), or into the mediastinum through the communicating fascias of the neck. Prediction of the routes of extension can help in determining the best route of surgical drainage.

The upper gastrointestinal tract has both an abundant resident flora and the defense mechanisms to protect the host from these organisms. Odontogenic infection, local surgical procedures, cancer, and immunosuppression alter the equilibrium, potentially leading to life-threatening problems.

It is important to understand the anatomy of the fascia and spaces to predict the potential routes of dissemination of infection and avoid iatrogenic injuries. The fascia of the neck is divided into superficial and deep layers. The subcutaneous tissue of the head and neck comprises the superficial fascia and encloses the platysma in the neck, the muscles of facial expression, and the epicranial muscles in the scalp. The deep cervical fascia is divided into anterior, middle, and posterior layers investing the vessels, nerves, muscles, and viscera in the neck. The prevertebral fascia divides into two layers lateral to the transverse process. The anterior layer is called the alar fascia. The deep cervical fascia communicates with the superior mediastinum (pretracheal layer) and the posterior mediastinum (prevertebral fascia). The potential space between the alar and prevertebral fascia is known as the dangerous space through which infections of the head and neck can easily access the thoracic cavity. The ability of the fascia to contain infection depends on the thickness of the membrane. The carotid sheath, the prevertebral, and pretracheal fascias are characteristically strong membranes, whereas the buccopharyngeal fascia is poorly defined.

Cervical space infections are classified according to their anatomic location. Scott proposes one classification (of many) of the spaces of the neck:
1. Superficial compartment
2. Floor of the mouth
   a) Sublingual space
   b) Submandibular space
   c) Submental space
3. Masticator space
   a) Temporal space
   b) Submasseteric space
   c) Superficial pterygoid space
4. Parapharyngeal space
   a) Deep pterygoid space
5. Parotid compartment
6. Paratonsillar space

Infection of the *submandibular compartment* usually arises from odontogenic infections. The treatment includes antibiotics, dental extraction, and extraoral surgical drainage to obtain dependent drainage. Incision is made below the inferior margin of the abscess avoiding injury to the facial artery and vein and the marginal mandibular branch of the fascial nerve. Infection of *sublingual space* originates from lower molars, surgical trauma, or inflammation of the sublingual and/or submandibular glands. Dependent drainage of the abscess is best achieved by an extraoral incision. Infection of the *masticator compartment* originates most frequently as a result of infection involving the third molar. This space communicates with the submandibular and lateral pharyngeal spaces. Infection can also extend into the orbit. The treatment includes a course of antibiotics before considering surgical drainage [1, 8]. The *parapharyngeal compartment* is an inverted cone shaped space with its base at the skull, extending inferiorly to the hyoid bone. Infections from the parotid, pharynx, and tonsilar region or from dental pathology can extend into this space. A CT scan is necessary for accurate diagnosis and to determine the extent of the involvement. Source control of the infection must be performed through an external approach because of the possibility of a pseudoaneurysm of the carotid artery. The *retropharyngeal compartment* encloses the esophagus, trachea, and thyroid gland. It can communicate with the prevertebral space and thus infection can extend into the superior mediastinum. Lymphadenitis in children, endoscopic instrumentation, or trauma to the pharynx can result in retropharyngeal space infection. Dependent drainage is achieved by an extraoral approach with a horizontal incision in the carotid triangle of the neck in adults, whereas the preferred approach in children is transpharyngeal. The causes of infection of the *visceral* and *carotid sheath compartments* include intravenous drug use and esophageal perforation. Infections in both spaces can readily extend to the mediastinum; direct surgical drainage is necessary to control the problem.

Infections such as *suppurative sialoadenitis* and *cervical necrotizing fasciitis* represent a challenge for diagnosis and source control. *Acute suppurative sialoadenitis* includes parotitis and infections in the submandibular gland. Abscess formation in the parotid is difficult to diagnose clinically because of the dense investing fascia of the gland. When antibiotics fail to control the infection, CT scanning and surgical drainage is indicated; the optimal approach is direct drainage of the abscess using an incision parallel to the branches of the facial nerve as far anteriorly as is feasible to avoid potential injury to the main trunk of the nerve. *Chronic submandibular gland sialoadenitis* is generally the result of obstruction produced by a ductal stricture or stone. Stones should be removed from the duct by an intraoral approach if located within 2 cm of the ductal orifice. If located further posteriorly, the options are to treat expectantly if the symptoms are mild, or to perform a formal submandibular gland excision if severe infection is present. *Cervical necrotizing fasciitis* is a rare soft tissue infection that occurs mainly in compromised hosts following various minor procedures and local infections. The initial appearance of the skin resembles cellulitis or erysipelas. However, the patient is toxic and presents clear systemic manifestations of sepsis. Early aggressive surgical debridement is the most important element of therapy after hemodynamic stabilization. Delayed diagnosis and limited or inadequate resection results in higher mortality, as suggested in early reports [2] and more recent retrospective cohort studies [3].

Critical Factors and Decision Making

Information from the history, physical examination, and radiological studies is integrated to identify severe infections such as cervical necrotizing fasciitis or mediastinitis, the source and predictable routes for the extension of the infection, and the need for adequate airway control. The possibility of associated airway obstruction, generally within 24 h of hospitalization, has to be kept in mind. Retropharyngeal abscess, lateral pharyngeal abscess, bilateral sublingual and submandibular cellulitis (Ludwig's angina) can produce airway obstruction, and necessitate endotracheal intubation or tracheotomy. Patients with signs of partial airway obstruction (sore throat, labored breathing, changes in voice quality, or tachypnea) should be considered for intubation. Patients with trismus or elevation of the floor of the mouth require an emergent procedure. If the cords are not visualized, oral intubation is discouraged and intubation with the use of fiberoptic laryngoscope should be considered. Blind nasoendotracheal and retrograde intubation should be discouraged. A surgical airway is recommended for patients requiring an emergent airway, or when other measures of intubation fail [4].

In a logistic regression analysis of patients with severe deep neck infections, Chen et al. [5] found that the presence of an underlying disease, neck swelling, and delayed diagnosis were all associated with a higher risk for the development of lethal complications. Others have reported a more severe clinical course and poorer diagnosis in immunocompromised hosts such as diabetics [6].

In addition to the timing, it is important to determine the exact location and the extent of the abscess in order to determine the optimal placement of the incision. Generally it is easy to identify the cause of the infection. However, in some cases the etiology is difficult to determine. Dental radiographs help to determine the etiology of odontogenic infection. Soft tissue X-ray films provide information regarding extension of the process to the sinuses or to the retropharyngeal region. CT scanning is the single most effective tool to differentiate cellulitis from abscess. Magnetic resonance imaging (MRI) is as sensitive as CT, but not as specific for collections. Labeled white blood cell scanning [7] has helped to define the magnitude of the disease, but does not play a significant role in acute infections.

The traditional approach to peritonsillar abscess has been immediate or delayed tonsillectomy because of the high rate of recurrence (up to 25%), failure to control the source of infection, and the frequent presence of bilateral infection. However, some authors have advocated drainage of the abscess alone, by incision or aspiration with an 18-gauge needle [8]. Tonsillectomy is considered for patients with previous peritonsillar abscess, repeated episodes of acute or chronic tonsillitis, systemic toxicity, or airway obstruction [9].

Changing Practices and Controversies

Traditionally, source control of head and neck fascial space infections was indicated only in the presence of a defined abscess. However, recent literature supports incision and drainage of an infectious process when areas of cellulitis are located in potentially dangerous tissue planes, or in patients with clinical signs of severe infection [10]. Surgical management of fascial space infections generally requires a generous incision and adequate drainage of the area performed in the operating room with the patient under general anesthesia. The treatment must include the removal of the cause as early as possible to prevent recurrence. Incisions in the skin or mucosa should be placed in healthy skin and positioned to achieve dependant drainage, preserving important anatomic structures and minimizing cosmetic sequelae. Drains should be left in place until the drainage becomes minimal. For multiple deep space infections multiple incisions are required.

Recent diagnostic and therapeutic advances such as fiberoptic sinus endoscopy and better understanding of the physiology of the sinuses has changed the surgical approach to paranasal infections. The aim of therapy is to relieve the cause of the obstruction of the middle nasal meatus more than to control the secondary infection. Treatment of acute sinusitis includes decongestants and empiric antibiotics. Failure to show response after 24-48 h of treatment indicates the presence of an abscess and the need for external drainage.

Conclusion

Evidence-based support defining optimal approaches to source control for patients with head and neck infections is limited. The applicability of guidelines derived from this methodology is highly influenced by a number of factors best evaluated by a consultant experienced in the process of surgical decision making in infections. The formulation of general principles does not lead necessarily to an easy implementation of treatment algorithms.

References

1. Peterson LJ (1993) Odontogenic infections. In Cummings CW (ed) Otolaryngology: head and neck surgery, vol 2, 2nd edn. Mosby-Year Book, St Louis
2. Zide MF, Limchayseng LRG (1991) Complications of head and neck infections. Oral Maxillofac Surg Clin N Am 3:355–405
3. Majeski JA, Alexander JW (1983) Early diagnosis, nutritional support, and immediate extensive debridement improve survival in necrotizing fasciitis. Am J Surg 145:784–787
4. Bilton BD, Zibari GB, McMillan RW, et al (1998) Aggressive surgical management of necrotizing fasciitis serves to decrease mortality: a retrospective study. Am Surg 64:397–400
5. Chen MK, Wen YS, Chang CC, et al (1998) Predisposing factors of life-threatening deep neck infection: logistic regression analysis of 214 cases. J Otolaryngol 27:141–144
6. Chen MK, Wen YS, Chang CC, et al (2000) Deep neck infections in diabetic patients. Am J Otolaryngol 21:169–173
7. Lalwani AK, Kaplan MJ (1991) Mediastinal and thoracic complications of necrotizing fasciitis of the head and neck. Head Neck 13:531–539
8. Schechter GL, Sly DE, Roper AL, et al (1982) The changing face of treatment of peritonsillar abscess. Laryngoscope 92:657–659
9. Holt GR, Tinsley PP (1981) Peritonsillar abscess in children. Laryngoscope 91:1226–1230
10. Flynn TR (1991) Odontogenic infections. Oral Maxillofac Surg Clin N Am 3:311–340

Invited Commentary

Lorne E. Rotstein

Drs. Jimenez and Escallon have done an excellent job in elucidating the key issues in source control in this anatomical area, as there is a paucity of evidence-based guidelines for this site. The anatomical complexity of the head and neck makes decision-making additionally difficult.

The authors have correctly described the most common sources for development of infections in the head and neck, i.e., the teeth, salivary glands, paranasal sinuses, oropharyngeal mucosa, and tonsils, but it is important to emphasize that inadequate or delayed recognition of the source and delay in initiation of antibiotic treatment is overwhelmingly the cause of abscess development. Further, with dental infection as the commonest cause of deep cervical space infection, the role of the dentist in diagnosis and early drainage of periapical abscesses and extraction of unsalvageable carious dentition is substantial, and should be appreciated by the surgeon who cares for patients with infections of the head and neck [1].

The anatomical description of the fascias of the neck in this chapter helps in understanding the route of progression of head and neck infections. It underscores that the fascial compartmentalization of the neck is a key factor in progression, but conversely that it may delay clinical diagnosis of abscess formation, impair adequate surgical drainage, and so result in life-threatening airway obstruction or mediastinitis. All suspected cervical space infections should be expeditiously imaged by CT, and operated upon if the imaging shows any suspicion of infection.

The section on airway management in this chapter is useful for the clinician and the potential difficulties in airway control cannot be overemphasized. The authors state the obvious, but it bears repeating that trismus precludes oral intubation and so fiberoptic laryngoscopic intubation is an alternative. However, the surgeon must be aware that preexistent glottic edema or minor injury to the glottis at the time of attempted fiberoptic intubation can result in immediate and complete airway obstruction and the surgeon must be present and prepared to perform an emergency cricothyrotomy or tracheostomy [2].

The bibliography for this chapter is short and reflects the fact that there is a lack of sound evidence in this area to guide treatment decisions. Treating surgeons therefore are unfortunately forced to fall back on clinical experience in the process of surgical decision making in the source control of head and neck infections.

References

1. Lawson W, Blitzer A (1993) Odontogenic infections. In: Bailey BJ (ed) Head and neck surgery – otolaryngology. Lippincott, Philadelphia
2. Stone DJ, Gal TJ (2000) Practice guidelines for management of the difficult airway. In: Miller J (ed) Anesthesia, 5th edn. Churchill Livingstone, New York

26 Vascular Graft Infections

MICHAEL S. DAHN

Key Principles

- Ideally, diagnostic evaluation of suspected graft sepsis should identify the presence or absence of infection, ascertain the offending organism, and define the extent of involvement, to determine the extent of graft removal and debridement. No single modality can accomplish these goals, although CT scanning is currently the most useful test. Diagnostic angiography serves a supplementary role, allowing the definition of target vessels, which may be useful for extra-anatomic reconstruction in the event of graft removal.
- Infections due to methicillin-resistant *Staphylococcus aureus* (MRSA) and *Pseudomonas aeruginosa* are more virulent. Total graft removal is more frequently required for infections involving these organisms. Infections due to *S. epidermidis* are more localized and can frequently be managed with partial graft removal followed by extra-anatomic or in situ reconstruction.
- Repeated radical debridement of the tissues surrounding an infected graft as well as debridement of all infected arterial tissue is pivotal for the control of a graft infection.
- Graft preservation is becoming increasingly popular to avoid extensive extirpative procedures in association with complex extra-anatomic reconstructions in frail patients.
- Arterial stents are an infrequent but potentially catastrophic source of sepsis.

Introduction

The occurrence of vascular graft infections remains a major complication in vascular reconstructive procedures. Fortunately, they are uncommon (1.0 %-2.6 %) but when they occur, they have been associated with a high mortality rate (25 %-88 %) [1, 2]. The diagnosis, control, and eradication of graft infections present difficult challenges and there is no clear consensus on their management.

Clinical Presentation and Diagnostic Methods

The clinical presentation of vascular infections depends on the anatomic location of the process. In extracavitary locations, infections may be diagnosed by physical signs such as progressive groin swelling, persistent erythema, the presence of a pulsatile mass, or a draining sinus. In contrast, intracavitary graft infections may be asymptomatic or present with much more subtle findings, including malaise, back pain, fever, and gastrointestinal bleeding. Generally, radiographic studies are performed in order to confirm a clinical suspicion.

CT scanning is the most effective diagnostic study for establishing this diagnosis. Factors that support the diagnosis include persistent perigraft fluid or gas, perigraft soft tissue attenuation (suggesting edema), pseudoaneurysm formation, and proximate bowel-wall thickening [3]. All of these changes, except pseudoaneurysm formation, may be present normally in the early postoperative period, making it difficult to differentiate graft infection from normal operative site changes. Following abdominal aortic procedures, retroperitoneal air should largely be reabsorbed by 7-10 days, but in rare instances, may last as long as 4 weeks. Perigraft fluid collections and hematomas should have resolved by approximately 3 months following the original procedure [4]. Persistent air and fluid collections beyond these time periods should be regarded as suspicious and CT- and/or ultrasound-guided needle aspiration of the fluid collections should be considered. Needle aspiration is a valuable diagnostic tool since a positive aspirate not only confirms the diagnosis but also identifies the bacteria causing the infection, allowing for specific antibiotic therapy. A negative aspirate, however, cannot exclude a graft infection since *Staphylococcus epidermidis* may be difficult to culture. Extracavitary (e.g., groin) hematomas tend to persist for longer periods compared to retroperitoneal hematomas, so these CT guidelines may not be applicable to other tissue regions. Although CT evaluation is considered highly accurate in identifying graft infections, reported sensitivities vary over a wide range (56%-94%). The lowest ranges of sensitivities tend to be associated with low-grade infections in which the clinical manifestations of the septic process are minimal. Thus, clinical judgment plays a significant role in making this diagnosis [3, 5].

Additional modalities that may contribute to the diagnostic work-up include magnetic resonance imaging (MRI) and gallium and radiolabeled white blood cell nuclear imaging. Although little data exist describing the MRI appearance of the postoperative prosthetic graft after surgery, some observations have been reported for the retroperitoneum. MRI can define periprosthetic fluid collections to an extent similar to CT, but it can also distinguish subacute and chronic hematomas from nonhemorrhagic fluid collections. Signal intensities in T1- and T2-weighted spin-echo sequences progressively decline after aortic reconstruction until they reach their lowest values 24 weeks after surgery because of fibrosis. Abscesses and necrotic material give relatively high signal intensities in T2-weighted spin-echo sequences, in contrast to chronic hematomas, which give low signal intensities [6]. Unfortunately, MRI may have difficulty in unequivocally identifying gas in the retroperitoneum.

Nuclear imaging of vascular grafts may be performed with gallium 67, indium 111-labeled white blood cells, or technetium-99m-hexamethazine-labeled white blood cells [7-9]. All of these scintigraphic methods have been reported to exhibit high (greater than 90%-95%) sensitivities and specificities. However, gallium imaging is sometimes clouded by hepatic and splenic tracer uptake, surgical incision uptake, and the presence of gallium in the gastrointestinal tract. Furthermore, gallium scans take 48-72 h to perform. Indium and technetium scans appear to be comparable; however, technetium is cheaper, more readily available and somewhat faster at reaching a diagnostic conclusion. Although these methods are accurate, it must be kept in mind that all of them have been reported to exhibit both false positives and negatives. A notable benefit of radionuclide imaging lies in the ability of these studies to reveal the extent of infection in a prosthesis. Thus, the operative planning and the management of an aortic bifurcation graft infection may be improved when the extent of prosthesis involvement can be determined before exploration. The identification of only a portion of graft involvement may increase the options for revisionary surgery.

Finally, when a draining sinus is present at an operative site, low-pressure injection of contrast material to produce a sinogram may be a useful approach in the assessment of the extent of infection since the contrast will dissect to areas of poor graft incorporation.

Microbiology and Antibiotic Therapy

Empiric antibiotic therapy for arterial graft infections should be chosen based upon knowledge of the expected pathogens. Table 1 lists the common organisms isolated from extracavitary graft infections. The distribution of organism types included 43 % pure Gram-positive and 21 % pure Gram-negative cultures, while 36 % of cultures yielded a mixed growth of Gram-positive and Gram-negative organisms [10]. In view of this diversity, the common practice of using a first-generation cephalosporin as initial empiric therapy for graft infections should be abandoned. Furthermore, the role of methicillin-resistant Staphylococcus aureus (MRSA) in vascular infections is increasing, further stressing the importance of careful antibiotic selection. A recent review of infrainguinal graft infections reported that 100 % of S. aureus infections seen at that institution over the preceding 5 years were caused by MRSA [11]. Therefore, initial therapy must provide both MRSA and Gram-negative coverage until final cultures become available. Combination therapy using vancomycin with antipseudomonal coverage such as ticarcillin-clavulanic acid or ceftazidime provides satisfactory coverage. Aminoglycosides provide adequate Gram-negative coverage, but carry the risk of toxicity associated with this group of antibiotics. Newer Gram-positive agents such as

Table 1. Common organisms cultured from extremity arterial graft infections in order of decreasing frequency [10]

Staphylococcus aureus
Staphylococcus epidermidis
Pseudomonas aeruginosa
Streptococcus faecalis
Escherichia coli
Streptococcus viridans
Proteus mirabilis

quinupristin/dalfopristin or linezolid provide effective MRSA therapy and may be substituted for vancomycin.

The surgical management of infected grafts is partially dictated by the microbiology of the infecting organisms. MRSA and *Pseudomonas aeruginosa* are particularly virulent pathogens. Although management of an infected graft may consist of a variety of approaches ranging from complete graft preservation to total graft excision, the presence of these two organisms provides increased support for total graft removal. However, clinical experience in this area is somewhat mixed, reaffirming that culture results should not be the sole criterion determining graft management. For example, Chalmers et al. [11] reported that the only mortalities observed in patients with infrainguinal graft infections involved MRSA as the infecting organism. In contrast, Calligaro et al. [12] found *Staphylococcus aureus* to exhibit no greater virulence than other Gram-positive or Gram-negative bacteria, although his report did not specify the resistance patterns of these infections. With respect to Gram-negative bacteria, Calligaro and other authors have shown that *Pseudomonas aeruginosa* is associated with significantly higher mortality and treatment failure rates during attempts at controlling graft infection, and that the presence of this organism should influence the practitioner toward total graft excision [12-14]. However, other authors have successfully treated *Pseudomonas* graft infections using complete graft preservation, indicating that a conservative approach may still remain a therapeutic option if extra-anatomic reconstruction is impossible or a graft excision is considered catastrophic [12,15].

Source Control

Clinical management of the infected vascular graft requires a comprehensive approach, including accurate diagnosis, appropriate antibiotic administration, and optimization of cardiovascular support to correct any systemic physiologic derangements associated with the septic process. Additionally, if the patient is critically ill, primary amputation and graft removal without reconstruction may be the most effective approach. This choice requires clinical judgment based upon an assessment of the patient's frailty and the extent of the systemic stress.

In the absence of critical illness and urgency, the specific operative management will largely be determined by the anatomic extent of involvement and possibly the pathologic organism responsible for the infection (*vida supra*). Although therapy is frequently categorized depending upon whether the infectious process is intra- or extracavitary, management usually consists of one of three approaches: complete graft preservation, partial graft removal, or total removal.

Complete Graft Preservation

Although the traditional approach to the infected arterial graft has been total excision followed by extra-anatomic bypass reconstruction, there is increasing interest in selective graft preservation [16]. Enthusiasm for this latter approach is driven by the risk associated with graft removal. Complete graft excision may require a difficult dissection followed by a complex revascularization procedure for attempted limb salvage, and is associated with a high mortality rate (9%-36%) and a high limb loss rate (27%-79%) [16]. In contrast, graft preservation is reported to offer a lower risk and amputation rate, particularly in patients who are chronically ill and less likely to tolerate difficult extra-anatomic bypass procedures. However, this approach is not universally applicable and requires careful patient selection. Calligaro et al. [16] reported that 43% of patients with extracavitary (including aortofemoral graft limb) arterial graft infections could be managed conservatively. This report recommends graft preservation only if it is *patent, the anastomoses are intact, and the patient does not exhibit systemic sepsis* [17]. Management consists of repeated, aggressive operative wound debridement of all infected tissue including any exudative peels or films that may be adherent to the wound or graft. Local wound care involves application of wet-to-moist dressings, which are changed at least three times per day in an intensive care unit environment until the anastomosis is covered by granulation tissue or a muscle flap. The use of a dilute antibiotic or povidone-iodine solution to moisten the dressings is recommended and the occurrence of wound hemorrhage or the development of systemic sepsis signals the need to change the management protocol [17]. This approach was associated with a hospital mortality rate of 12% and an amputation rate in survivors of 13% [16-18]. When the graft infection involves an infrapopliteal graft segment, the results are significantly inferior. Under these circumstances, mortality and limb loss rates climb to 19% and 27%, respectively. Nonetheless, it must be recognized that the limited number of outflow target vessels present in these patients also limits the use of alternative methods [19]. Additionally, as noted earlier, when *Pseudomonas* was found to be present in the wound, selective graft preservation was successful in only 40% of patients compared to 71% of those in whom *Pseudomonas* was not present.

Conservative treatment of intracavitary (retroperitoneal) aortic graft infections has also been advocated as a therapeutic option in high-risk patients [20]. However, even supporters of graft preservation approaches recommend that aortic graft excision be combined with extra-anatomic bypass, in contrast to the management of extracavitary infections where graft preservation may be preferred in selected patients. The contraindications to aortic graft preservation include systemic sepsis, anastomotic complications, and the presence of immune system disorders. Management consists of CT-guided or operative drainage of the periaortic space, followed by instillation of antibiotic-containing irrigant for an extended period (3 weeks) until the effluent becomes sterile [20, 21]. Using this approach, 65% of patients were reported to be cured and the mortality rate remained low at 18.6%.

Partial Graft Excision

Partial graft removal is most appropriate for the management of an aortofemoral graft that becomes infected in a single limb at the groin level. Removal of the involved limb with extra-anatomic bypass reconstruction carries less morbidity compared to total graft excision. The key aspect of this approach is establishing the extent of infection in order to ensure that the proximal aortic shaft remains sterile. Radionuclide or CT scanning may be helpful in this assessment, but the ultimate evaluation requires direct graft inspection via an extraperitoneal operative approach through the lower abdomen. Graft incorporation and absence of local infectious signs encourage the surgeon to proceed with division of the proximal femoral limb followed by extra-anatomic bypass. Management of the infected groin can then be performed through a separate incision, being careful to first close all other sites in order to protect the newly routed conduit. The incidence of recurrent graft infection has been reported to be as high as 44%, indicating that there is still significant hazard using this approach [22].

Aggressive local control of an infected wound (groin or otherwise) can also be combined with in situ graft replacement using prosthesis [23] or autogenous superficial femoral vein (SFV) [24, 25]. Use of an in situ prosthetic replacement may only be useful in infections caused by organisms such as *Staphylococcus epidermidis* having intrinsically low virulence [26], for example, when *S. epidermidis* is cultured or when the wound or graft culture remains persistently negative, suggesting infection by an indolent *S. epidermidis*. Partial graft removal with SFV replacement has been used either entirely in situ or as a femoral-femoral crossover graft in the case of an aortofemoral single limb graft removal.

Total Graft Excision

Traditional management of an infected graft involves total graft excision followed by revascularization with autogenous tissue and/or extra-anatomic bypass. More limited alternative approaches, as mentioned in "Partial Graft Excision", have been advocated because of the high morbidity and mortality associated with total graft excision, since the physiologic insult associated with intracavitary graft explantation is so great. However, a major argument in support of total aortic graft removal is the high mortality (50%) associated with persistent uncontrolled sepsis that may occur following unsuccessful partial graft removal [27].

Additional management issues that must be considered in relationship to aortic graft removal are:
- Whether graft removal or reconstruction should be synchronous or staged
- Whether reconstruction should be in situ or extra-anatomic
- Whether autogenous or prosthetic materials should be used for reconstruction

The mortality associated with aortic graft removal has largely been linked to the ensuing ischemic stress. Although some patients can tolerate delayed revascularization because of the presence of an extensive preexisting collateral network, this fortunate circumstance is present in a minority of patients who are not identifiable with certainty in advance. Reilly et al. [28] have reported that preliminary extra-anatomic bypass followed by immediate or staged (delayed by 2-31 days) aortic graft removal is associated with an improved mortality (~25%) compared with a traditional approach of infected graft removal followed immediately by extra-anatomic bypass (43%). In critical situations, such as acute hemorrhage from a ruptured pseudoaneurysm or aortoenteric fistula, the initial procedure, however, should be aortic exploration and graft removal. When extra-anatomic bypass is performed in advance of graft removal, initial concerns have included possible bacterial seeding of the newly placed bypass prosthesis, thrombosis of the extra-anatomic conduit due to flow competition with the aortic graft, and risk of hemorrhage from the infected graft during the waiting period prior to its removal. However, these concerns have not been borne out provided that satisfactory antibiotic coverage is given and early graft removal (~ 5 days) is accomplished [27-29].

In situ aortic reconstruction has been advocated for aortic graft infection and graft enteric fistula. Excellent results have been reported when debridement of the periaortic tissue and aortic wall is accomplished. However, this approach should not be used for patients with perigraft abscesses. Complete 360° autogenous coverage of the new graft with omentum, sartorious or rectus femoris muscle is believed to be an essential component of the operation. Patients treated by in situ graft replacement are reported to exhibit mortality rates as low as 8 %. Reinfection rates are similar to those of patients undergoing extra-anatomic bypass (~ 20 %), with a trend toward lower infection rates when rifampin-impregnated grafts are used [30].

Alternative graft materials for in situ aortic reconstruction include autogenous SFV [31] and fresh or cryopreserved aortic allografts [32, 33]. Both materials have been utilized in small series in which low mortality rates (10 %-18 %) were reported. Furthermore, harvesting of the SFV does not appear to result in signs and symptoms of severe venous insufficiency.

A similar general approach has been utilized for infected infrainguinal grafts. Incomplete excision, as noted above, has been associated with high rates of reoperation for persistent sepsis, and more than 50 % of deaths are associated with uncontrolled sepsis [34]. This statistic has spurred interest in complete removal of all involved prosthetic material for extracavitary grafts as well. Again, this should be accompanied by complete debridement of all infected tissues. If the limb is severely ischemic after graft removal, reconstruction should be attempted using autogenous material if available. However, if no autogenous material is present, extra-anatomic reconstruction with another synthetic graft should be considered.

Endoluminal Stents

The infection rate associated with transluminal angioplasty in association with stent deployment remains unknown. However, because a large number of stents are implanted annually for the treatment of occlusive vascular disease (probably more than 50,000 per year), even a low incidence of infection may translate into a large number of arterial infections. The presenting features of infected stents can be quite subtle, and include localized pain, swelling, and minor erythema of the ipsilateral leg several days following iliac or femoral stent deployment. These infections can become very aggressive, as signaled by the development of a purpuric rash in the vascular distribution served by the stented vessel. This latter sign forecasts a very complicated, rapidly progressive course of generalized systemic sepsis with multiple organ dysfunction and a very high mortality rate [35]. Almost invariably, *Staphylococcus aureus* is the responsible organism, indicating that these infections represent technical complications of the procedure. In order to avoid these catastrophic events, emphasis must be placed upon careful skin preparation and implementation of a strict sterile technique. Administration of prophylactic antibiotics during peripheral angioplasty remains an uncommon practice, but should be considered since stent deployment involves the implantation of a prosthetic device. Experimental studies [36, 37] have shown that intravascular stents remain susceptible to transient bacteremias for up to 4 weeks following deployment and that prophylactic antibiotics are effective in protecting these devices from contamination during the period surrounding implantation. The susceptibility of a stent infection may be magnified by the associated vascular damage and local hematoma, which occurs following disruption of the vascular surface integrity during the angioplasty procedure.

Evidence of an infected stent should initiate a plan for its removal. These infections are occasionally characterized by a necrotizing angitis, which occurs at the site of the stent placement with erosion through the vessel. An infected pseudoaneurysm may result, serving as a septic focus and producing cardiovascular instability if it ruptures. Operative exploration of the stent with resection of the local vessel and pseudoaneurysm remains the treatment of choice. Subsequent limb preservation efforts may require a difficult judgment decision since these patients are frequently critically ill and uncontrolled systemic infection makes extra-anatomic reconstruction hazardous.

Controversies

The major controversy in the management of vascular graft infections is whether infected arterial conduits should be completely removed, or whether local conditions can be improved sufficiently to permit in situ retention of a preexisting or newly placed graft. Contemporary series using the conventional approach of staged graft excision with extra-anatomic bypass continue to report mortality rates of 20%, amputation rates of 20-29% and reinfection rates of 20%. Significantly, recent reports utilizing graft preservation methods and aggressive local care principles report mortality rates of 8%-12%, amputation rates of 0%-13% and reinfection in 22% of cases [16, 30]. However, these more conservative management approaches have not been fully adopted by all practitioners. Additional factors that may influence the decision for conservative management techniques include:
a) The cost of prolonged hospitalization for local wound care.
b) The ability to diagnose graft infection promptly, since a delay in diagnosis may worsen local and systemic conditions and thus contribute to worsening clinical outcomes using conservative therapy. These issues are worthy of consideration as this field progresses.

Critical Factors and Decision Making

Numerous treatment options are available for the management of the infected vascular graft. However, none of these are unequivocally superior. Guidelines that appear to be applicable for most infected grafts are as follows:
- CT scanning is the most valuable diagnostic study in demonstrating the presence of a graft infection. Supplementary tests such as radiolabeled WBC scintigraphy and sinography may help to define disease extent. However, there is no definitive tool to assess infected grafts and clinical judgment plays a major role in decision-making.
- Complete debridement of infected tissue surrounding an infected graft is a vital treatment component irrespective of the specific protocol for graft management.

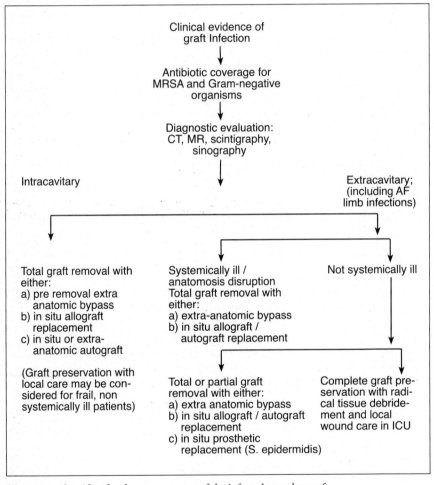

Diagram 1. Algorithm for the management of the infected vascular graft

- Selected patients may be treated with complete or partial graft preservation, provided that the infection is localized without complicating features at the anastomosis such as pseudoaneurysm.
- Patients with systemic sepsis or hemorrhagic complications generally require total graft excision.

The algorithm in Diagram 1 summarizes the management options available for the care of the patient with an infected graft.

References

1. Calligaro, KD, Veith FJ (1991) Diagnosis and management of infected prosthetic aortic grafts. Surgery 110:805–813
2. Lorentzen JE, Nielsen OM, Arendrup H, et al (1985) Vascular graft infections: an analysis of sixty-two graft infections in 2411 consecutively implanted synthetic grafts. Surgery 98:81–86
3. Low RN, Wall SD, Brooke JR, et al (1990) Aortoenteric fistula and perigraft infection: evaluation with CT. Radiology 175:157–162
4. Qarfordt PG, Reilly LM, Mark AS, et al (1985) Computerized tomographic assessment of graft incorporation after aortic reconstruction. Am J Surg 150:227–231
5. Piano G (1995) Infections in lower extremity vascular grafts. Surg Clin North Am 75:799–809
6. Spartera C, Morettini G, Petrassi C, et al (1990) Role of magnetic resonance imaging in the evaluation of aortic graft healing, perigraft fluid collection, and graft infection. Eur J Vasc Surg 4:69–73
7. Lawrence PF, Dries DJ, Alazraki N, Albo D (1985) Indium 111-labeled leukocyte scanning for detection of prosthetic vascular graft infection. J Vasc Surg 2:165–173
8. Fiorani P, Speziale F, Rizzo L, et al (1993) Detection of aortic graft infection with leukocytes labeled with technetium-99 m-hexametazime. J Vasc Surg 17:87–96
9. Harris KA, Kozak R, Carroll SE, et al (1989) Confirmation of infection of an aortic graft. J Cardiovasc Surg 30:230–232
10. Calligaro KD, Veith FJ, Schwartz ML, et al (1995) Recommendations for initial antibiotic treatment of extracavitary arterial graft infections. Am J Surg 170:123–125
11. Chalmers RTA, Wolfe JHN, Cheshire NJW, et al (1999) Improved management of infrainguinal bypass graft infection with methicillin-resistant Staphylococcus aureus. Br J Surg 86:1433–1436
12. Calligaro KD, Veith FJ, Schwartz ML, et al (1992) Are Gram-negative bacteria a contraindication to selective preservation of infected prosthetic arterial grafts? J Vasc Surg 16:337–346
13. Conn JH, Hardy JD, Chavez CM, Fain WR (1970) Infected arterial grafts: experience in 22 cases with emphasis on unusual bacteria and technics. Ann Surg 171:704–714
14. Geary KJ, Tomkiewicz ZM, Harrison HN, et al (1990) Differential effects of a Gram-negative and Gram-positive infection on autogenous and prosthetic grafts. J Vasc Surg 11:339–347
15. Kwaan JHM, Connolly JE (1981) Successful management of prosthetic graft infection with continuous povidone-iodine irrigation. Arch Surg 116:716–720
16. Calligaro KD, Veith FJ, Schwartz ML, et al (1994) Selective preservation of infected prosthetic arterial grafts. Ann Surg 220:461–471
17. Calligaro KD, DeLaurentis DA, Veith FJ (1996) An overview of the treatment of infected prosthetic grafts. Adv Surg 29:3–16
18. Budny PJ, Fix RJ (1991) Salvage of prosthetic grafts and joints in the lower extremity. Clin Plastic Surg 18:583–591
19. Calligaro KD, Veith FJ, Dougherty MJ, De Laurentis DA (1996) Management and outcome of infrapopliteal arterial graft infections with distal graft involvement. Am J Surg 172:178–180

20. Pistolese GR, Ippoliti A, Tuccimel I, Lorido A (1997) Conservative treatment of aortic graft infection. Eur J Vasc Endovasc Surg 14 (Suppl A):47–52
21. Lawrence PF (1995) Management of infected aortic grafts. Surg Clin North Am 75:783–797
22. Bunt TJ (1994) Treatment options for graft infection. In: Bunt TJ (ed) Vascular graft Infections. Armonk, Futura Publishing
23. Bandyk DF, Bergamini TM, Kinney EV, et al (1991) In situ replacement of vascular prostheses infected by bacterial biofilms. J Vasc Surg 13:575–583
24. Sladen JG, Chen JC, Reid JDS (1998) An aggressive local approach to vascular graft infection. Am J Surg 176:222–225
25. Snyder SO, Wheeler JR, Gregory RT, et al (1987) Freshly harvested cadaveric venous homografts as arterial conduits in infected fields. Surgery 101:283–291
26. Becquemin JP, Qvarfordt P, Kron J, et al (1997) Aortic graft infection: is there a place for partial graft removal? J Vasc Endovasc Surg 14 (SupplA):53–58
27. Ricotta JJ, Faggioli GL, Stella A, et al (1991) Total excision and extra-anatomic bypass for aortic graft infection. Am J Surg 162:145–149
28. Reilly LM, Stoney RJ, Goldstone J, et al (1987) Improved management of aortic graft infection: the influence of operative sequence and staging. J Vasc Surg 5:421–431
29. Meyer T, Schweiger H, Lang W (1999) Extra-anatomic bypass in the treatment of prosthetic vascular graft infection manifesting in the groin. Vasa 28:283–288
30. Young RM, Cherry KJ, Davis PM et al (1999) The results of in situ prosthetic replacement for infected aortic grafts. Am J Surg 178:136–140
31. Claggett GP (1994) The neoaortic iliac system operation for infected aortic prostheses. In: Bunt T J (ed) Vascular graft infections, Armonk, Futura Publishing, p. 277–284
32. Kieffer E, Bahnini A, Koskas F, et al (1993) In situ allograft replacement of infected infrarenal aortic prosthetic grafts: results in forty-three patients. J Vasc Surg 17:349–355
33. Vogt PR, Turina MI (1999) Management of infected aortic grafts: Development of less invasive surgery using cryopreserved homografts. Ann Thorac Surg 67:1986–1989
34. Martens RA, O'Hara PJ, Hertzer NR, et al (1995) Surgical management of infrarenal arterial prosthetic graft infections: Review of a thirty-five year experience. J Vasc Surg 21:782–791
35. Latham JA, Irvine A (1999) Infection of endovascular stents: an uncommon but important complication. Cardiovasc Surg 7:179–182
36. Thibodeaux LC, James KV, Lohn JM, et al (1996) Infection of endovascular stents in a swine model. Am J Surg 172:151–154
37. Paget DS, Bukhari RH, Zayyat EJ, et al (1999) Infectibility of endovascular stents following antibiotic prophylaxis or after arterial wall incorporation. Am J Surg 178:219–224

Invited Commentary

Frank Veith

The chapter on the management of vascular graft infections, which is clearly and concisely written by Dr. Dahn, provides an excellent contemporary overview of this topic. Because the chapter so carefully describes the graft-preserving techniques employed by Keith Calligaro and myself over the last 25 years, it is difficult to find elements within Dr. Dahn's views with which I am in disagreement. However, it is important to point out that many experts within the field of vascular graft infection are still uncomfortable with the concept of leaving an infected graft – either partially or totally – in place.

Three decades ago, standard practice mandated the removal of all infected prosthetic grafts used in the arterial circulation. Our work (Calligaro et al.) and that of Kwaan and Connolly – referenced in Dr. Dahn's chapter – clearly established that infected prosthetic arterial grafts could be salvaged. Prerequisites for successful salvage included extensive debridement and excision of all infected perigraft tissue, the maintenance of flowing arterial blood within the portion of infected graft that was to be preserved, and most importantly, evidence that the infected graft-to-artery anastomosis had not broken down with either hemorrhage or false aneurysm formation. When these requirements were fulfilled, two-thirds to three-quarters of infected prosthetic arterial grafts could be salvaged and more extensive graft excisional procedures were avoided.

We have successfully employed this approach not only with extracavitary grafts but also with infections of entire aortic grafts when systemic or local circumstances precluded standard graft excisional treatment or autologous replacement, as advocated by Dr. Clagett [1, 2]. We have now had six patients in whom extensive drainage and debridement, coupled with systemic antibiotics and antibiotic irrigation, resulted in cure of aortic graft infections in circumstances precluding more traditional forms of treatment. Several of these patients have now been followed up over 10 years so that this form of nonexcisional treatment can be applied selectively to aortic graft infections in extremely difficult circumstances as well.

Although we originally presented our graft-preserving techniques for infected arterial reconstructions years ago [3-5], these graft-sparing methods were not generally accepted. Even when our 20 years of experience with them was reported, considerable skepticism was expressed.

When an occluded infrainguinal prosthetic arterial graft becomes infected, most of that graft must be excised. This can be accomplished by leaving a residual button of the graft with flowing blood beneath it on the patient's artery. In some instances, this technique can be used when a graft originates from the common femoral artery, thereby preserving flow through that artery to the deep femoral artery and avoiding the extensive ischemia that would result if the common femoral artery proximal and distal to the origin of the infected graft were excised or oversewn [3].

Finally, on a historical note, although the classic requirement for total excision of all infected grafts was based on a 1963 article by Shaw and Baue [6], early work by Carter, Cohen and Whalen [7] had suggested that some infected grafts could be preserved with appropriate local therapy (extensive debridement and local antibiotic irrigation), as subsequently described and advocated by our group [3, 4, 5, 8].

Despite the controversy which still remains regarding how best to manage infected prosthetic arterial grafts, and even though some of these can be managed by less traumatic graft preserving techniques, all would agree that an infected arterial graft is a serious problem that may pose a threat to a patient's life and limb and that taxes the vascular surgeon's patience and ingenuity.

References

1. Clagett GP, Bauers BL, Lopez-Diego MA et al (1993) Creation of a new aortoiliac system from lower extremity deep and superficial veins. Ann Surg 218:239–249
2. Clagett GP, Valentine RJ, Hagino RT (1997) Autogenous aortoiliac/femoral reconstruction from superficial femoral-popliteal veins: feasibility and durability. J Vasc Surg 25:255–266
3. Calligaro KD, Veith F, Gupta SK et al (1990) A modified method for management of prosthetic graft infections involving an anastomosis to the common femoral artery. J Vasc Surg 11:485–492
4. Calligaro KD, Veith FJ, Schwartz ML et al (1994) Selective preservation of infected prosthetic arterial grafts: Analysis of a 20-year experience with 120 extracavitary infected grafts. Ann Surg 220:1069–1079
5. Veith FJ (1979) Surgery of the infected aortic graft. In: Bergan JJ, Yao JST (eds) Surgery of the aorta and its body branches. New York, Grune and Stratton, pp 521–533
6. Shaw RS, Baue AE (1963) Management of sepsis complicating arterial reconstructive surgery. Surgery 53:75–79
7. Carter SC, Cohen A, Whalen TJ (1963) Clinical experience with management of the infected Dacron graft. Ann Surg 158–249–251
8. Samson RH, Veith FJ, Janko GS et al (1988) A modified classification and approach to the management of infections involving peripheral arterial prosthetic grafts. J Vasc Surg 8:147–153

Editorial Comment

Moshe Schein

What is true for all types of surgical infections applies also to vascular infections – the best results are obtained by prevention. For example, distal bypasses with prosthetic material, proximal to severely ischemic-infected feet, are doomed to be infected and should be avoided. The order of words in the motto "life before limb" is occasionally confused by vascular surgeons and should be reemphasized. Attempts to save an ischemic limb, which contains an infected graft (probably nonindicated from the beginning), which was anastomosed proximal to poor outflow – in a bedridden patient – cannot be defined as heroic but rather as archaic. Thus, a box with "urgent primary amputation" has to feature prominently on Dr. Dahn's otherwise comprehensive algorithm.

General surgeons should be reminded that the so-called suspected groin abscess developing a few days after transfemoral cardiac catheterization or angiography commonly represents an acute infected femoral pseudoaneurysm. This should be resected under proximal control. Arterial reconstruction is best delayed (or may prove unnecessary) if intraoperative Doppler studies indicate adequate blood flow to the foot.

Prosthetic grafts are faster and easier to insert than autologous ones and in general replacing vessels provides the vascular surgeon with that special sense of satisfaction familiar to anyone who enjoys plumbing. But as stressed here by Dr. Veith, treating the ensuing graft infections is not such great fun. [Editors may allow themselves an occasional sarcastic note].

27 Bone and Joints

R. Jan, A. Goris

Key Principles

- Remove all dead tissue and scar tissue.
- Provide optimal soft tissue conditions around the infected area.
- Stabilize infected fractures, mobilize infected joints.
- Antibiotics are only complementary treatment and do not replace sound surgical practice.

Infections of bones and joints are major complications of trauma and surgery, and carry a potential of high morbidity and even mortality if not treated promptly and expertly.

Definitions

The word "osteomyelitis" is commonly used to encompass a variety of infections of bone tissue. Two distinct conditions can be identified: hematogenous osteomyelitis and osteitis.

Osteomyelitis is an infection of bone and/or bone marrow, occurring in juvenile patients, especially within the metaphysis of long bones, which results from hematogenous spread of organisms, typically *Staphylococcus aureus*. Bone marrow is surrounded by trabecular bone. Any infection in this area will lead to the formation of an abscess, with limited possibility of spontaneous perforation drainage.

Osteitis is an infection of bone tissue and/or bone marrow, occurring as a result of an open fracture or bone surgery. Trabecular bone is a dense structure with a poor blood supply, rendering it sensitive to infection. Once infection is established, it can only be eliminated by increased resorption of bone. When infection is present in a nonunited fracture, any residual movement within the fracture will lead to increased bone resorption as well as to activation of the infection.

Septic arthritis is an infection within a joint, most commonly the result of a perforating injury or joint puncture. While the joint capsule (synovia) is richly vascularized, the cartilage has no blood supply and is dependent for its metabolism on a convective supply of oxygen, glucose, and other nutrients from the synovia. Immobilization of the affected joint will therefore compromise the survival of the chondrocytes, as well as promote joint stiffness and even ankylosis.

Chronic infections of bone and joints result from delayed or inadequate treatment of acute infections. They are characterized by the presence of a large amount of richly vascularized scar tissue. On the other hand, tissue PO_2 in these areas is extremely low [1], providing for poor healing conditions.

Acute Hematogenous Osteomyelitis

Classic acute hematogenous osteomyelitis occurs in juvenile patients. The most frequent sites are the proximal tibia, the femur, the pelvis, and the calcaneus. *Staphylococcus aureus* is the causative microorganism in 90% of the cases. In infants, *Haemophilus influenza*, streptococcal species and *E. coli* may be isolated.

Osteomyelitis may also occur in immunocompromised adults, in whom fungi or mycobacteria may be the pathogens involved. In patients with chronic infections (i.e., endocarditis, urinary tract infections, pressure ulcers), hematogenous osteomyelitis may occur at distant osseous sites. Osteomyelitis in patients with sickle cell disease is another distinct clinical presentation.

The acute phase of osteomyelitis is characterized by high fever and severe pain localized at the level of the metaphysis of a long bone. Typically, the patient recently had furunculosis or another *Staphylococcus aureus* infection. Initially, there may be no clear signs of inflammation on the affected extremity, as the infection is contained within the medulla. Radiography will remain unrevealing for about 2 weeks, as osteolysis requires the prolonged action of osteoclasts. Bone scans may show changes earlier, with a high sensitivity, but a lower specificity. Ultrasound examination may reveal subperiosteal pus. Leukocyte count, erythrocyte sedimentation rate, and especially C-reactive protein (CRP) are elevated at an early stage. A technetium 99m methylene diphosphonate bone scan is performed to assess the location(s) and extent of the process. MRI may also provide valuable information.

Diagnosis is established by needle aspiration of pus from the focus and bacterial culture. Obtaining an antibiogram (sensitivity profile) is mandatory for directing antibiotic treatment. Blood cultures should be performed, particularly in infants.

Treatment of the juvenile form consists principally of antibiotics (flucloxacillin and fusidic acid) for 4-6 weeks [2]. When pus is present on echography or aspiration, or when there is no improvement with antibiotics alone, surgery is indicated. Burr holes are made in the metaphysis of the bone, at the level of the intramedullary abscess for decompression and drainage.

Fungal osteomyelitis is treated by Amphotericin B, mycobacterial osteomyelitis by long-term antituberculous multiple drug therapy.

Posttraumatic Osteitis

Posttraumatic osteitis results from a compound fracture or bone surgery.
Various presentations can be identified, for example:
- Acute osteitis after a compound fracture
- Acute phlegmonous infection of the marrow cavity after nailing of long bone
- Chronic osteitis (Fig. 1)

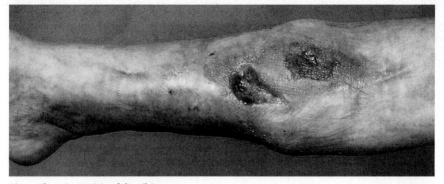

Fig. 1. Chronic osteitis of the tibia

Contamination of an open fracture may involve unusual microorganisms. The patient may have fallen into a pond or ditch and the wound can be contaminated by various aqueous bacteria. Foot infections from penetrating wounds are associated with infection by *Pseudomonas* species.

Contamination may further occur during the operative procedure with bacteria entering the wound from the skin of the patient, the operative team, or the hospital environment.

The first clinical signs are often masked by the signs and symptoms of inflammation caused by the primary injuries, by the administration of antibiotics, or by the effects of anti-inflammatory and analgesic drugs.

The leukocyte count, erythrocyte sedimentation rate, and CRP are elevated at an early stage. Radiography will remain unrevealing for the first few weeks, although bone scans may show changes earlier. A technetium-99m methylene diphosphonate bone scan is performed to assess the location and extent of the process. Gamma scintigraphy performed 4 and 24 h after IV administration of technetium-99m human immunoglobulin is highly sensitive and reasonably specific for diagnosing and localizing low grade, chronic osteitis [3]. MRI is gaining in popularity as a diagnostic tool in musculoskeletal infections.

Bacterial cultures (aerobic and anaerobic) and sensitivity should be obtained to direct antibiotic treatment. In addition to pus, tissue biopsies should be obtained and cultured. Methicillin-resistant *S. aureus* is often found in chronic osteitis, because of previous failed antibiotic treatment.

Principles of treatment depend in part on the clinical presentation.

In all forms, early and vigorous removal of all dead soft tissue and bone is mandatory. Operation may result in significant blood loss, because of the hyperemia of inflammation. Excision of all old scar tissue is required to provide for optimal healing conditions. Within the resulting wound, one or more strings of gentamicin beads or resorbable collagen sponges with antibiotics are applied [4] and the wound is loosely closed. An alternative approach is to install a continuous irrigation and closed drainage system in the infected area; however, this is cumbersome and messy.

The resulting soft tissue defect may require secondary closure with a rotation flap or a free revascularized tissue transplantation to provide for optimal soft tissue conditions around the infected area (Fig. 2). Bone defects may be treated by

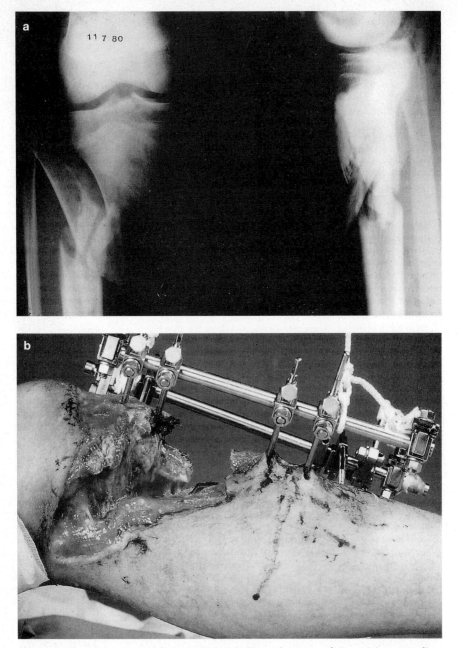

Fig. 2a-e. a X-ray of compound fracture proximal tibia, with severe soft tissue injury, complicated by gas gangrene. Condition at transferral from other hospital. Note air in soft tissues. **b** Condition after debridement and application of external fixator. **c** Open wounds were first closed by split skin grafts. **d, e** Photography and X-ray. Final result after application of free revascularized graft from the iliac crest, including skin, subcutaneous tissue, muscle and bone

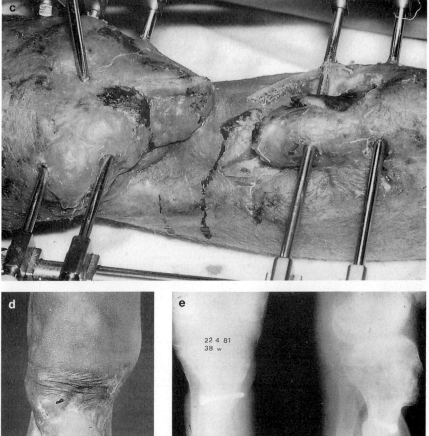

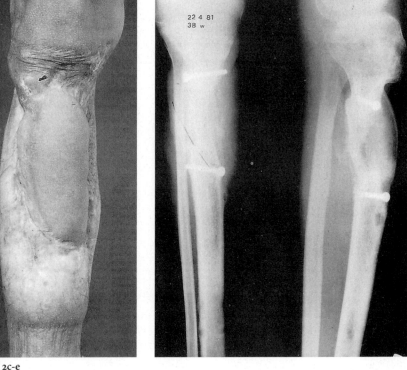

Fig. 2c-e

cancellous bone grafting, free revascularized bone transplantation, or by the Ilizarov technique.

Infected fractures should be optimally stabilized, usually with an external fixator. If a stable internal fixation device (i.e., a plate) is already present, it should be left in place. If intramedullary osteosynthesis is complicated by severe intramedullary infection, the intramedullary rod should be removed, the bone marrow cavity gently reamed to clear it of all debris, a string of gentamicin beads left within the bone marrow cavity, and an external fixator applied to provide for immobilization.

Chronic infection within the bone marrow cavity following intramedullary osteosynthesis, especially after reaming, may result in the formation of extensive intramedullary sequestra (Fig. 3). This condition requires an approach as described in the preceding paragraph.

Antibiotics are adjuvant therapy and in no way replace sound surgical practice. The choice of an antibiotic regimen should be guided by the antibiogram. A combination of quinolones and rifampin is recommended for the treatment of *Staphylococcus aureus* osteitis [5]. Antibiotic treatment is generally continued for 6 weeks.

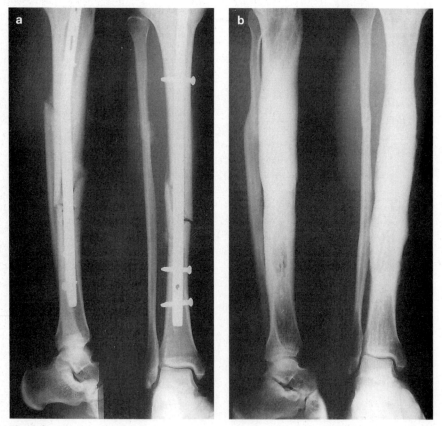

Fig. 3a, b

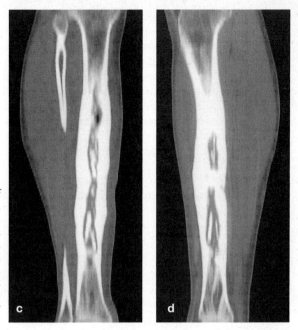

Fig. 3a-d. a Chronic osteitis of tibia after a closed fracture, treated by a reamed intramedullary nail. Only a fistula was present. **b** One year later, after nail-removal. Excessive, dense cortical bone, suspicion of sequestrum. **c, d** CT scan at time of b shows extensive sequestra within the marrow cavity

Septic Arthritis

Septic arthritis of the hand and wrist is relatively uncommon. The most common cause is penetrating trauma resulting from a clenched fist injury or a human or animal bite. Cats have sharp teeth and a bite to a finger may easily penetrate the skin and extensor tendon into a metacarpal-phalangeal or interphalangeal joint. The common causative microorganism is *Staphylococcus aureus*, but streptococcal species, *Haemophilus influenza*, *Pseudomonas aeruginosa*, *Serratia* species, and *Mycobacterium marinum* may also occur in specific clinical settings [6].

Local symptoms include swelling and redness around the affected joint, hydrops, an antalgic positioning of the joint in a slightly flexed position, extreme pain on moving the affected joint, and circumferential pain on external palpation of the joint.

In the hand, septic arthritis must be differentiated septic tenosynovitis. In the latter, there is pain on external pressure along the entire length of the affected tendon sheet and all movements of the affected finger and adjacent joints are painful.

In the metatarsal joint, the differential diagnosis includes gout; however, fever and other general signs of infection are absent. Rheumatoid arthritis may mimic septic arthritis and septic arthritis may complicate rheumatoid arthritis.

The best clinical results are obtained by prompt accurate diagnosis, surgical drainage, and joint debridement. For large joints, arthroscopic debridement with rinsing of all debris and fibrin is preferred. Appropriate antibiotics are administered and early postoperative range of motion exercises started. For human bite injuries, administration of a betalactam antibiotic with betalactamase-inhibitor is suggested [7].

Experimental studies suggest that periarticular injection of lactoferrin, which reduces articular inflammation in septic arthritis in mice, without promoting bacterial survival, may have a role in clinical management [8].

When the diagnosis is established late (2-3 weeks after the onset of the disease), the synovia has undergone substantial alterations and synovectomy is required, followed by temporary immobilization with an external fixator until acute signs of infection have resolved. Subsequently, motion exercises are started. When the articular surface is severely damaged, an arthrodesis should be considered.

Acknowledgments. The authors thank Dr. J. Biert and Dr. R. Severeijnen for valuable advice.

References

1. Francek UK, Bollinger A, Huch R (1984) Transcutaneous tension and capillary morphologic characteristics and density in patients with chronic venous incompetence. Circulation 70:806–811
2. Lane-O'Kelly A, Moloney AC (1995) Acute haematogeneous osteomyelitis. Evaluation of management in the 1990's. Ir J Med Sci 164:285–288
3. Machens HG, Pallua N, Becker M, et al (1996) Technetium 99m human immunoglobulin (HIG): a new substance for scintigraphic detection of bone and joint infections. Microsurgery 17:272–277
4. Klemm KW (1993) Antibiotic bead chains. Clin Ortop 295:63–76
5. Lew DP, Waldvogel FA (1999) Use of quinolones in osteomyelitis and infected orthopaedic prosthesis. Drugs 58:85–91
6. Murray PM (1998) Septic arthritis of the hand and wrist. Hand Clin 14:579–587
7. Bunzli WF, Wright DH, Hoang AT, Dahms RD, Hass WF, Rotschafer JC (1998) Current management of human bites. Pharmacotherapy 18:227–234
8. Guillan C, McInnes IB, Vaughan D, Speekenbrink AB, Brock JH (2000) The effects of local administration of lactoferrin on inflammation in murine autoimmune and infectious arthritis. Arthtritis Rheum 43:2073–2080
9. Recommended reading: AO principles of fracture management. Rüedi TH P, Murphy WM (eds) Thieme, Stuttgart

Invited Commentary

Bradford Henley

Dr. Goris has provided a succinct review of bone and joint infections related to trauma and surgery. This contribution begins with definitions. Though hematogenous osteomyelitis is differentiated from osteitis, these conditions are quite similar in their histopathology in that both exhibit an inflammatory process involving bone. Perhaps it is useful to differentiate them by their osseous location, as this distinction may aid in one's treatment decisions. Goris suggests that osteomyelitis be thought of as an infection of metaphyseal (trabecular and richly vascular) bone, usually occurring in juvenile patients. Morrisey and others [1, 2] have demonstrated that bacteria have a predilection to infect metaphyseal regions after trauma. On the other hand, Goris suggests that osteitis be considered an infection of cortical (haversian and less well vascularized) bone, primarily in adults. He infers that osteitis is most commonly seen in the posttraumatic and postsurgical clinical settings due to direct inoculation in contrast to hematogenous spread. The implication is that metaphyseal osteomyelitis infections, especially in juveniles, may be treated by antibiotic therapy alone, but in the presence of a medullary abscess (or dead bone) surgical drainage may be indicated. In contrast, to heal cortical posttraumatic osteitis infections, surgical debridement and/or resorption of dead bone (sequestra) with concomitant adjunctive antibiotics is usually required.

For both types of bone infections, the common etiological factors and causative organisms are described, as are the routine diagnostic modalities. C-reactive protein titers are very helpful in evaluating patients with infections as acute phase reactants rise and fall more quickly than the white blood cell count and the erythrocyte sedimentation rate. Of the imaging studies described, triphasic technetium-99 diphosphonate bone scans are sensitive for detecting bone and joint infections, though false-negative scans may occur in newborns. Correlation of flow findings (first phase) with blood pool and bone image phases [2, 3] is important. Magnetic resonance imaging (MRI) is gaining in both popularity and importance as a diagnostic imaging tool in musculoskeletal infections. Despite the cost and the adverse effect of large metallic implants on image quality, MRI is sensitive and specific and is without radiation exposure.

Cierny and colleagues [3] have stressed the importance of patient evaluation in determining the physiological status (classification) of the host. A patient with a normal physiological response to infection and surgery is designated an A-host. A compromised patient may exhibit either local (BL), systemic (BS), or combined (B-LS) deficiency in wound healing. Systemic factors affecting immune surveillance, metabolism, and local vascularity include malnutrition, renal failure, liver failure, alcohol abuse, immune deficiency disease (e.g., RA, SLE, HIV), drug- or radiation-induced immune deficiency states, chronic hypoxia, malignancy, diabetes mellitus, malnourishment, extremes of age, steroid therapy, and tobacco use. Similarly, adverse local factors include chronic lymphedema, venous stasis, major vessel compromise, arteritis, extensive scarring, and radiation fibrosis. Finally, a C-host requires either ablative, suppressive, or no treatment as the therapeutic interventions or the results of curative treatment for osteomyelitis/osteitis in these patients are more compromising than the therapeutic alternatives.

In the treatment of all musculoskeletal infections, Goris stresses the importance of identifying the causative organism(s), usually by aspiration, biopsy, and tissue culture. The common causative organisms are well described, with the caveat that foot infections from penetrating wounds (i.e., through shoes) are typically associated with *Pseudomonas* species infections. Similarly, in patients with recurrent urinary tract infections and pressure ulcers (e.g., spinal cord injuries), osteomyelitis caused by enteric Gram-negative organisms may occur by local spread or hematogenous dissemination. Patients with other chronic infections may seed osseous and nonosseous sites (e.g., subacute bacterial endocarditis) and should be evaluated for these diagnoses.

It is of paramount importance that antibiotic therapy be based on the results of culture and sensitivity data providing a quantitative measurement of minimum inhibitory concentration of the antimicrobial needed to inhibit the in vitro growth of the involved pathogen(s). Because of the frequency of polymicrobial infections and the emergence of resistant strains of bacteria, consultation with an infectious disease specialist is helpful, to guide the administration of multiple antibiotics with synergistic effects and to monitor effective tissue levels, side effects, and toxicities of the recommended therapy.

In addition to antibiotic administration, surgical debridement of necrotic, ischemic, and infected tissues is necessary when there is abscess formation or dead bone. Sinus tracks can be injected with a mixture of methylene blue and hydrogen peroxide immediately prior to operative debridement, to delineate the track and facilitate operative excision. Cierny and colleagues [3] have proposed an anatomical classification for osteomyelitis that is useful in directing surgical treatment. Four types are described: superficial, localized, medullary, and diffuse. Adequacy of surgical debridement may be assessed macroscopically by the presence of bleeding (the "paprika sign" seen in cortical bone), or mechanically with tools such as the laser Doppler. In addition to surgical debridement, adjunctive therapies to consider include:

- The use of various local antibiotic delivery systems such as impregnated PMMA beads, bioresorbable polymers, coated osseous conduction substrates and bead pouches
- The use, type, and timing of soft tissue coverage
- Hyperbaric oxygen when anaerobic organisms are present

The treatment algorithms presented in this chapter are thorough though they may be enhanced by general treatment principles and adjunctive therapies. General principles as related to source control in infections include:

- Complete resuscitation of trauma patients (e.g., to permit clotting, thereby preventing hematoma or seroma formation, which may provide a substrate for bacterial proliferation)
- Minimizing operating room foot traffic to eliminate other infectious sources
- Using ultraviolet light or other clean air technologies (e.g., laminar flow rooms)
- Optimizing the host by nutritional support to provide a healing and anabolic environment
- Management of host comorbidities (e.g., tight glucose control in diabetics, cessation of smoking, monitoring/supplementing low tissue oxygen saturation)

Omitted from this chapter is discussion of debated topics relating to bone and joint infections. These include:

- The timing, duration, and coverage of antibiotic treatment
- The best skin cleansing (prep) solutions

- The methods used to minimize external fixator contamination prior to staged surgical treatment
- The relative merits of different wound irrigation and cleansing solutions (i.e., saline, peroxide, Betadine, emulsifiers, etc.)
- The efficacy of pulsatile and nonpulsatile irrigation processes
- The decision on whether contaminated or infected wounds should be left open or closed (primarily or delayed)
- The relative merits of various wound drains as they relate to source control (i.e., suction, gravity, wick, no drain, etc.)
- The best wound dressings (sterile gauze, occlusive dressing, wick dressing, biological dressings, etc.)
- The optimal timing of soft tissue coverage in the author's treatment algorithm
- The physiological and biological effects of various implants and their influence on infection control (e.g., internal fixation, external fixation)

References

1. Morrissy RT, Haynes DW, Nelson CL (1980) Acute hematogenous osteomyelitis: the role of trauma in a reproducible model. Trans Orthop Res Soc 5:324
2. Whalen JL, Fitzgerald RH Jr, Morrissy RT (1988) A histological study of acute hematogenous osteomyelitis following physeal injuries in rabbits. J Bone Joint Surg 70A:1383–1392
3. Cierny G III, Mader JT, Penninck JJ (1985) A clinical staging system for adult osteomyelitis. Contemp Orthop 10:17–37

28 Incisional Surgical Site Infections

JAMES T. LEE

Key Principles

- Incisional infections develop because host defenses cannot eradicate contaminating pathogens. Intraoperative contamination of normally sterile tissues by pathogenic microbes is the most frequent antecedent of incisional infections.
- Detection of incisional infections relies on the fact that infection is one cause of wound healing failure. Infection must be ruled out when routine postoperative incision examination suggests that healing is not proceeding as expected. Therapy of incisional infections is based on a simple anatomic classification. Source control always includes an element of mechanically altering geometry and content of infected spaces.

General Approach

Nosocomial infections delay recovery from operations. Pneumonia, urinary tract infection, and blood stream infections collectively differ in two important respects from surgical site infections (SSI), which are infections of the tissues, organs, or spaces contacted by surgeons. Only SSI prevention tactics target a particular area in the hospital (the operating room), particular employees (surgeons and surgical nurses), and a particular temporal phase (immediately before and during operation). In addition, SSIs are diagnosed and treated by surgeons. By convention, SSIs are defined as those occurring within 30 days of index operations, excepting operations in which prosthetic devices are implanted, for which surveillance continues during at least 1 year [1, 2]. It is unusual for SSIs to present later than 4 weeks after index operations if standardized surveillance protocols and diagnostic definitions are utilized [3-7].

The term "surgical site infection" was formulated by the Centers for Disease Control and Prevention (CDC) in 1992 following a consensus meeting of surgical infection experts and infectious disease specialists [5]. The intent was to encourage comprehensive surgical infection surveillance. The CDC defines two SSI categories:

- Incisional SSI comprises all infections that surgeons have traditionally named "wound infections".
- Organ/space SSI are postoperative infections of body cavities or organs manipulated by surgeons.

Two incisional SSI types are superficial incisional SSI and deep incisional SSI. The former type is the most common incisional infection in modern practice and only the subcutaneous adipose layer is invaded by pathogens. Deep incisional SSIs develop much less frequently but have more serious consequences because these infections can spread quickly to invade the body wall fascia(e) and/or muscle(s) that define the subcutaneous wound's deep boundary (see Chap. 22, "Soft-Tissue Infections"). Multiple organisms, with presumed synergy of action, are often isolated from deep incisional SSI.

Primary skin closure is employed in the vast majority of operations. When substantial contamination occurs, the probability of incisional SSI is greatly reduced by simply leaving the skin open, followed by either delayed primary closure or healing by secondary intention (i.e., open wound care). For the purposes of this chapter, only primary skin closure is considered. By definition, superficial incisional SSI is impossible if the subcutaneous space is left unclosed and allowed to heal by second intention. Deep incisional SSI can potentially occur in a contaminated wound that is left open from the time of operation, but the author is unaware of credible reports of this phenomenon.

The development of SSI indicates that host defenses could not eradicate an initial pathogen burden. It has long been recognized that different types of operations entail different degrees of intrinsic intraoperative contamination and the most common SSI pathogens for differing procedures have been catalogued in authoritative reviews [1]. Consequently, the choice of antimicrobial agents for presumptive SSI therapy, when indicated, is straightforward [8]. The likelihood of SSI is shaped by the interplay of multiple variables besides the type of operation [2, 3, 6, 7]. Surgical patients present with variable degrees of host defense competence and the physiological effects of surgery and anesthesia have additional impacts on that competence. The species and initial wound density of contaminating microbes are usually the most powerful variables influencing the likelihood of SSI.

Primarily closed skin incisions are sealed from external contamination by a fibrin layer that bridges the apposed skin edges [2]. Within 24-36 h, this "caulking" supplied by the coagulation system has integrity and immediately beneath it, within a few hours of wound closure, are numerous activated neutrophils. It has been suggested that incisional infection may result from postoperative surface contamination of a primarily closed skin incision, based on reports describing isolation of organisms whose peculiar speciation prompted formal epidemiological investigations. Organism carriers were found to be healthcare professionals who had no opportunity to contact patients' incisions or dressings before patients entered the recovery room [1]. It is also plausible that SSI may develop secondary to bacteremia occurring at a vulnerable time in the early inflammatory phase of wound healing. This hypothesis has been supported by data gathered using animal models, but only occasionally finds support in clinical observations. However, most evidence indicates that intraoperative contamination is the source of nearly all SSI pathogens, regardless of the anatomic extent of infection.

With few exceptions, the pathogens isolated from SSI are bacteria. Organ transplant recipients occasionally develop the otherwise very rare fungal SSI [1].

Surgical breach of intact skin, a barrier to external contamination, is central to the pathogenesis of SSI, but no skin preparation method renders the skin sterile, so that normal skin flora are frequently incisional SSI pathogens [1, 3, 4, 6, 7]. Surgical entry into a hollow viscus and or surgical breach of established infection are other SSI precursor events. The duration of the operation and the premorbid health of the patient are other risk factors for incisional SSI. Authoritative epidemiology texts seldom mention that failure to correctly employ indicated SSI prevention measures is also an important predictive variable in SSI genesis [2].

Patients with superficial incisional SSI do not usually appear seriously ill, seeding of the bloodstream is rare, and the complication is rarely lethal. Superficial incisional SSI are functionally subcutaneous abscesses and resolution is usually achieved by simply opening primarily closed incisions (or incisions managed by delayed primary skin closure) to allow egress of inflammatory exudates and wound debris. Infrequently, sharp excision of necrotic fat or fibrin is warranted. Antibiotic therapy is indicated if cellulitis is present or a patient is systemically toxic [8]. Topical antiseptics or other chemicals add no benefit during open wound care (i.e., regular dressing changes). It is also irrational to administer antimicrobial drugs under the misguided inspiration that healing will be accelerated or that granulation tissue will somehow become sanitized.

Deep incisional SSIs are more serious complications than superficial incisional SSIs because there is ongoing enzymatic and/or ischemic destruction of the posterior adherence of subcutaneous fat to underlying body wall fascia, allowing unhindered spread of inflammatory fluids and bacteria. Indeed, this anatomic feature of fasciitis is pathognomonic of a necrotizing process in the interstitial space [8]. Myonecrosis may also occur. Patients with deep incisional SSI generally appear seriously ill. Empirical systemic antimicrobial therapy and immediate excision of involved tissues are absolutely necessary [8, 9]. Specimens for Gram's staining and cultures of fluid and tissue should be obtained in the operating room. Antimicrobial therapy continues after the reoperation and can be converted to directed therapy according to antimicrobial sensitivity reports. Details of operative and drug therapy for deep incisional SSI generally match those outlined by authorities on the de novo necrotizing soft tissue infections [8, 9] (see Chap. 22).

The present chapter concerns incisional SSIs, yet organ/space SSIs must be mentioned because they sometimes present with findings that mimic those of a typical incisional SSI. As described by other contributors to this text, organ/space SSIs are very serious complications, associated with appreciable morbidity and mortality risks. It is notable that these infections do not always present dramatically. For example, after abdominal operations, organ/space SSI may be occult when patients have resumed eating, are ambulatory, and have otherwise recovered in a seemingly uneventful fashion. An intact operative skin incision may conceal a sub-fascial abscess through the body wall. Source control for an organ/space SSI entails acquiring confirmatory diagnostic imaging information, initiating presumptive systemic antibiotic therapy, and externally draining an infected organ or space by reoperation or interventional radiology hardware placement. When an organ/space SSI exists, proper and prompt attack is essential to arrest the events that can trigger lethal multiple organ system failure. Superficial incisional SSIs almost never provoke this situation but deep incisional SSIs, especially if treated casually, late, or without attention to surgical details, must be considered dangerous systemic insults.

Decision-Making Algorithm

The CDC anatomic classification of SSI provides a foundation for an organized approach to therapy. Both superficial and deep incisional SSI represent closed space infections, and the necessary source control response for either includes mechanical conversion of a closed, infected three-dimensional space to an open, contaminated two-dimensional surface. Conscientious surgeons are alert in the postoperative period for answers to a sequence of yes/no questions displayed in algorithmic sequence:

- Is the incision suspicious? (e.g., drainage, inordinate erythema, incongruent pain or tenderness with unexplained fever).
- Open the skin incision to examine the wound space.
- Is SSI confirmed after the skin closure is taken down (i.e., pus or culture-positive hematoma present)? *SSI is confirmed.*
- Is there superficial incisional SSI? (i.e., involvement of only the subcutaneous fat layer and underlying fascia intact). Superficial incisional SSI is present.
- Start open wound care (regular dressing changes) with adjunctive antimicrobial therapy only for cellulitis or systemic toxicity.
- Is deep incisional SSI suspected? Is there evidence of deep incisional SSI (e.g., muscle or fascial necrosis, loss of intact plane between fat and fascia, etc.)?
- Deep incisional SSI is present. Schedule immediate emergency reoperation for wound examination and debridement of involved tissues, start broad spectrum antimicrobial therapy, obtain tissue cultures for both aerobic and anaerobic organisms.
- Is organ/space SSI masquerading as incisional SSI? Imaging studies to rule out subfascial collection and/or fistula from hollow organ.

Controversy

Staphylococcus is one of the most frequently isolated pathogens from superficial incisional SSI [1, 6, 7] and growing concern about the threat of methicillin-resistant *Staphylococcus aureus* (MRSA) suggests a simple rule that may be controversial: if a superficial SSI requires antibiotic therapy for the reasons described previously, culture effluent at the time of diagnosis and order antimicrobial sensitivity testing for the isolate(s). Adjunctive antibiotic therapy directed against the most likely pathogens has a limited period of utility in this setting and clinical resolution often will be obvious (perhaps because the incision was opened) before sensitivity testing is complete. There are no clinical features that mandate vancomycin therapy (or its alternatives) while awaiting culture results. In the author's view, when any type of incisional SSI develops in a patient known preoperatively to be an MRSA carrier, and adjunctive antimicrobial therapy is indicated, a surgeon should initially use an agent active against MRSA until definitive sensitivity test results are in hand. Unfortunately, isolation of MRSA from SSI has steadily increased in recent years at the few institutions where comprehensive SSI microbiology data are gathered [6, 7].

Summary

Superficial incisional SSI does not require reoperative therapy for source control. When deep incisional SSI is suggested by findings at the time of bedside incision reopening, formal operative exploration of the wound and tissue excision, as needed, are essential. The reoperation is an emergency and any delay in source control may increase lethality.

On occasion, after a suspicious incision is opened in anticipation of finding an incisional SSI, effluent characteristics or volume may suggest that an organ/space SSI or incipient viscerocutaneous fistula has drained through the fascial closure. Imaging information is then a high priority. In abdominal surgery, computerized tomography is often diagnostic and affords needle access to fluid collections for specimen culturing and drain placement by modified Seldinger techniques. If organ/space SSI collections or fistulae cannot be controlled by interventional radiology techniques, open operation is indicated [10]. Equivocation is inappropriate; the major principle of SSI source control, regardless of SSI category or type, is to transform an infected closed space to a contaminated, open surface that may be annoying, but will heal with safety. Source control is mechanical, not pharmacological.

References

1. Mangrum AJ, Horan TC, Pearson ML, Silver LC, et al (1999) Guideline for the prevention of surgical site infection, 1999. Infect Control Hosp Epidemiol 20:247–280
2. Lee J (1995) Wound infection surveillance for quality improvement. In: Fry D (ed) Surgical infections. Little-Brown, New York, pp 145–159
3. Lee J (1992) Wound infection surveillance. Surg Clin North Am 6:643–656
4. Garabaldi RA, Cushing D, Lerer T (1991) Risk factors for postoperative infection. Am J Med 91(Suppl 3B):158–163
5. Horan TC, Gaynes RP, Martone WJ, et al (1992) CDC definitions of nosocomial surgical site infections, 1992: a modification of CDC definitions of surgical wound infections. Infect Control Hosp Epidemiol 13:606–608
6. Lee J, Olson M (1999) Wound infection surveillance for 85,260 consecutive operations. J Surg Outcomes 2:27–42
7. Olson M, Lee J (1990) Continuous, ten-year wound infection surveillance: results, advantages, and unanswered questions. Arch Surg 125:794–803
8. Fry D (2001) Infection, inflammation, and antibiotics. In: Corson JD, Williamson RCN (eds) Surgery. Mosby, Philadelphia
9. Ahrenholz D, Simmons RL (1995) Infections of the skin and soft tissues. In: Howard RJ, Simmons RL (eds) Surgical infectious diseases, 3rd edn. Appleton & Lange, Norwalk
10. Lee J (1996) Reoperative care of postoperative external fistulas: stomach, pancreas, duodenum, and small intestine. In: McQuarrie D, Humphrey E, Lee J (eds) Reoperative general surgery: timing, tactics, and techniques, 2nd edn. Mosby Year Book, Saint Louis

Invited Commentary

ALLAN POLLOCK

Ask anyone who is not a surgeon to tell you about surgical site infection (SSI) and they will say that it is caused by doctors and nurses in the wards who do not wash their hands often enough. This may be half true. It is certainly true in the burns unit, where surgical site infection is unquestionably related to the transfer of bacteria to the wound by air and hands. This is what some people call secondary or ward-acquired infection as opposed to primary or operating-room-acquired infection. It is not, however, only burns that can become secondarily infected. A closed surgical wound is immune within a few hours even to the smearing on of feces, but let that wound discharge blood or serum or lymph or bile or pancreatic juice and it can, just like a burn, trap those airborne and hand-borne bacteria. For some reason these secondary invaders are much more likely to be *staphylococci* than enteric bacteria (which, of course, cause most primary SSIs because they have been planted in the wound during the incision of a contaminated viscus).

That is all very well, you will say, and you will agree that a contaminated operation is much more likely to result in a SSI. But you will recall in your practice the apparently inexplicable infection that arose in a surgical wound after a clean operation. You know that the patient's skin can never be completely sterilized and that the air in most operating rooms is not sterile (and the more people that are in the room and the more they move about the greater the bacterial contamination). A few bacteria will land on the surgical wound and be dealt with promptly by the host's humoral and cellular defenses.

Why is it then that from time to time, despite the utmost asepsis, the whole thing goes wrong, the patient gets a SSI (and the attorney a writ)? The answer would seem to lie in the ability of the host to mount this rapid defense. The problem is not only recognized states of immune suppression such as AIDS or cytotoxic chemotherapy, but also a matter of blood supply. Wounds on the head, neck, and arms are less likely to become infected than wounds on the abdomen or lower limbs, and there is evidence that a warm body is in a better position to throw off bacterial contamination than one whose temperature has been allowed to fall a couple of degrees as a result of being exposed on the operating table.

One of the tragedies in orthopedic surgery is for a hip or knee prosthesis to become infected. The infection often shows itself clinically months after the skin has healed. We used to think that a lot of these SSIs were blood-borne, but I think this is probably wishful thinking: there seems to be no doubt that ultra-clean operating conditions do result in lower rates of infection. The low-grade pathogens that were implanted at the time of operation have taken their time to cause symptoms from tissue destruction.

So far I have not even mentioned antibiotics. The consensus is that a single dose immediately before operation is enough and that there are dangers not only to the hospital ecology but also to the patient in prolonged courses of prophylactic antibiotics. Resistance to antibiotics is related closely to the prolixity with which antibiotics are prescribed.

Finally I want to mention a contentious issue and one that I doubt can ever be resolved by normal research methods. And that is that some surgeons get more SSIs than others. Is this because these surgeons operate on more patients with compromised immune systems? Or is it that some surgeons are more aggressive (one might say brutal) in their handling of tissues, so that they leave dead tissue to be a pabulum for contaminating bacteria? Nobody has come up with a good way of assessing surgeons, not for their competence (that is fairly easy), but for their performance. It is only the anesthesiologist who can offer an opinion about who is the gentle surgeon and who the butcher. Or is the answer, in the words of my friend Hiram C. Polk Jr., that surgeons who have extremely low rates of SSI suffer from "selective forgetfulness"?

Part III: Special Problems

29 Timing of Intervention

ULRICH SCHÖFFEL

Key Principles

- As a general principle, every established source of infection should be controlled as soon as possible.
- The urgency of intervention is determined by the rapidity of the progression of clinical symptoms.
- In complicated infections, any additional insult must be kept to a minimum. Thus, rapid, minimally invasive, temporizing, or palliative measures may be superior to definitive but lengthy and more traumatizing procedures.
- If the clinical signs of infection improve, the need for intervention must be reconsidered. At least there will be ample time for a thorough diagnostic work-up and careful planning of the therapeutic strategy.

General Approach

Source of Infection

Elimination of an infectious focus is the most decisive step in the treatment of surgical infections [1-3]. However, an infectious focus is not necessarily identical to the source of contamination. Many clinically apparent infections such as soft tissue infections, infections of parenchymatous organs, or intra-abdominal abscesses may present as a definable infectious focus without a determinable or accessible source of contamination. Thus, as described in detail elsewhere, attempts at source control may be directed at both the primary source of contamination and the primary site of infection (Table 1).

Ideally, the aims of all such interventions would be achieved by complete removal of the source of infection. However, in complicated infections, the primary goal is the control of the source of contamination by resection, exclusion, sealing,

Table 1. Aims of interventions for source control

Prevent further contamination
Reduce bacterial load at site of infection
Dampen local inflammation
Prevent spread of infection
Reestablish blood flow

or drainage. This will prevent further contamination and may help to reduce the bacterial load at the site of infection. At the same time, adjuvants such as necrotic tissue or hematoma are removed and every attempt is made to reestablish blood flow to the site of infection to deliver cellular and humoral mediators of host defense and anti-infective drugs.

Sequelae of Bacterial Contamination

The consequences of bacterial contamination of sterile tissues depend on two factors:
- The bacterial factor includes such considerations as bacterial load, composition of the inoculum, growth requirements, and microbial virulence factors such as wall components, invasive capacities, and specific toxins.
- The host defense factor is defined by local availability and function of cellular and humoral components of inflammation and also includes the general condition of a patient and therapeutic influences.

Both Factors and Their Balance Are Highly Time-Dependent

Both the transition of contamination to local infection and distant spread of invading bacteria, and the development of the local inflammatory response, its confinement to the primary site of infection, and its eventual insufficiency, exhaustion, or generalization are time-dependent phenomena.

The time from experimental contamination to bacterial peritoneal adhesion or invasion depends on the species involved, the number of bacteria, and the action of constitutive defense mechanisms present in the abdominal fluid and the peritoneal lining [4]. From experimental studies it is known that bacteria injected into the peritoneal cavity are rapidly cleared; approximately 90% of the total number are removed within 1-2 h [5]. Bacterial clearance is counteracted by sterile faeces, which inhibit local defenses and support growth by providing nutrients. In the cecal ligation and puncture model, the number of bacteria adhering to the peritoneum increases logarithmically from 10 organisms per milligram of tissue after 1 h to stable populations of 10-100 million aerobes and anaerobes beyond 12 h [6].

Clinically, the concentration of bacteria at the time of surgical intervention seems to be comparably high in intraabdominal infections and in soft tissue abscesses, averaging 200 million colony forming units (cfu) per milliliter [7]. It may be speculated that the degree of inflammation, and thus the indication to intervene, is correlated with the bacterial load at the source of infection. Additionally, it has been demonstrated that the severity of the inflammatory response and not the length of history is the major determinant of prognosis in intraabdominal infections [8].

Multiple, ill-defined mechanisms influence the time of the development of a generalized inflammatory response. A certain amount and duration of proinflammatory activation seems to be necessary, and occurs during the early stages

Table 2. Sequelae of infection

Local increase
Generalized response (sepsis)
Fulminant spread
Localization
Spontaneous resolution

of a septic response [9, 10]. However, *the time course of an infection can never be reliably predicted in the clinical setting.*

Moreover, depending on the efficacy of host defenses, and on general recuperative capacities, the bacterial challenge may sometimes be spontaneously controlled. It may then either become sealed off by abscess formation or may even resolve completely (Table 2). With some exceptions such as diffuse secondary peritonitis, catheter-related bacteremia, or gas-associated necrotizing soft tissue infections, the spontaneous outcome of an infection is also difficult to predict in the individual patient. Consequently, in the clinical situation, decisions must be made on the basis of a worst-case scenario.

Interventional Insult

Source control may be life-saving. However, the interventions per se may interfere with host defenses (Table 3). Not only are local defense mechanisms compromised by direct manipulation and sterile access sites contaminated, but invariably further activation of the inflammatory response to tissue trauma occurs. Whether this will result in local damage, early exhaustion, or overstimulation is difficult to predict. According to the second hit theory, such an additional insult may add to the existing inflammatory state and so induce a full-blown state of clinical sepsis with multiorgan dysfunction [11]. Because of this, a one-step approach to definitively eliminate the source of infection may sometimes prove inferior to temporizing, palliative procedures. In many situations, simple open or percutaneous drainage of an accumulation of infected fluid will be sufficient to reduce inflammation, so that any major attempt at focus elimination and repair can be postponed.

Diagnostic Delay

When clinical symptoms suggest the presence of severe inflammation and signs of deterioration are recognizable or to be expected, an urgent attempt must be

Table 3. Adverse effects of operative intervention

Impairment of local host defense
Additional trauma (second hit)
Contamination of access sites
Spillage of infectious material

made to define the source of infection. Localized pain or other clinical signs may reveal the anatomical site. However, often identification of the source requires further diagnostic evaluation. Once a suspected focus is defined, the question arises whether additional imaging procedures or measures such as guided fine-needle aspiration are necessary to prove the source of infection. This decision may be difficult. On the one hand, further investigations take time; on the other hand, a negative exploration may increase the morbidity.

The clinical picture, the availability and practicability of diagnostic modalities, and the respective findings will decide which and how many measures are deemed necessary before a decision is made to operate. Clinical experience and careful observation of the patient are invaluable in finding a path between the danger of time-consuming, extensive diagnostics and that of a nondirected approach.

The Improving Patient

Spontaneous sealing or even complete resolution of an infectious process may take place under conservative treatment and is suggested when objective clinical signs improve. Even when a defined source has been diagnosed and operative intervention is planned, this strategy may need reevaluation based on the clinical trajectory of the patient. Of course, some improvements are temporary only and operative measures will later be needed. However, clinical improvement indicates that there is no need to rush into the operating room. Instead, delaying intervention allows further diagnostic work-up with regard to local conditions – which may have changed – and the underlying etiology.

Controversies

The Length of Preoperative Optimization

A certain delay in operative intervention may be unavoidable if prior resuscitation and stabilization of homeostasis are necessary. With fulminant infection, however, such attempts have to be limited. There are often arguments between anesthesiologists and surgeons over how long a period of stabilization is appropriate in a severely ill and unstable patient. There are patients who are too ill to be operated upon. If, despite all attempts at resuscitation, the patient remains hemodynamically unstable, operative intervention is unlikely to be successful. On the other hand, if sepsis is the reason for severe organ dysfunction, stabilizing measures will never lead to normalization until the underlying mechanism is successfully addressed.

Two points must be clarified: first, how much stabilization must be achieved to meet the minimal requirements for a reasonably safe anesthetic? Corrections of metabolic derangements or secondary coagulopathies should not take too much time. Second, are there opportunities for temporizing or palliative measures, which might substitute for operative intervention? Ultrasound-guided percutaneous drainage, for example, can easily be performed as a bedside approach in the ICU. Even if such intervention does not always result in complete focus control, a form of focus reduction may also temporarily improve the situation.

Critical Factors and Decision Making: Summary

Time is a crucial factor in any event which leads to infection and sepsis. Untreated sources of contamination increase the bacterial load at a given site of infection. Both bacterial mechanisms such as growth, adhesion, and invasion and mechanisms of host defense are time-dependent. However, the number of bacteria released, their growth rate or virulence within a given environment, and the efficacy of host defenses are not predictable.

Thus the severity of clinical symptoms, rapidity of deterioration, degree of organ dysfunction, and the severity of the inflammatory response are the parameters which influence clinical decision making. Severity of disease and rapidity of clinical deterioration are the key factors in determining the urgency of source control (Table 4). However, the risk of additional trauma and of blind, nondirected exploration has to be considered. Whether prolonged attempts to stabilize homeostatic derangements may justify delayed intervention must be evaluated in the individual situation. Spontaneous clinical improvement requires reconsideration of the therapeutic concept of operative source control (Table 5).

Table 4. Urgency of source control

	Examples
Immediate	Diffuse secondary peritonitis
	Necrotizing soft tissue infections
Urgent	Loculated process (abscesses)
	Infected pancreatic necrosis
	Suspected focus in stable patient
	Infected devices (implants)
Delayed	Established focus, clinical improvement
	Palliatively controlled source

Table 5. Contraindications to (immediate) intervention

Hemodynamically unstable patient

Severe metabolic derangement

Secondary coagulopathy

Undefined source

Clinical improvement

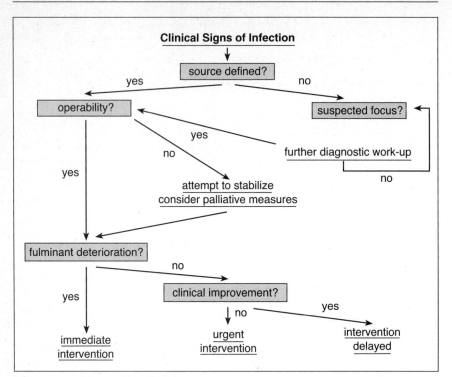

Clinical Signs of Infection

source defined?

yes   no

operability?   suspected focus?

yes

no   further diagnostic work-up

yes   no

attempt to stabilize
consider palliative measures

fulminant deterioration?

no

yes   clinical improvement?

yes

no

immediate   urgent   intervention
intervention   intervention   delayed

Diagram 1. Decision-making algorithm

References

1. Ohmann C, Yang Q, Hau T et al (1997) Prognostic modelling in peritonitis. Eur J Surg 163:53–60
    Critical evaluation of prognostic factors and scoring systems in peritonitis.
2. Hau T, Ohmann C, Wolmershäuser A et al (1995) Planned relaparotomy vs relaparotomy on
    demand in the treatment of intraabdominal infections. Arch Surg 130:1193–1197
    Case-control study on the role of planned relaparotomy.
3. Farthmann EH, Schöffel U (1990) Principles and limitations of operative management of in-
    traabdominal infections. World J Surg 14:210–217
    Reviews the basics of surgical therapy of peritonitis.
4. Farthmann EH, Schöffel U (1998) Epidemiology and pathophysiology of intraabdominal in-
    fections. Infection 26:329–334
    Concise summary of the current concept of the pathophysiology of peritonitis.
5. Nyström PO (1996) Transition from contamination to infection: implications in colonic sur-
    gery. Eur J Surg 576 (Suppl):42–46
    Reviews interesting experiments on the fate of intraperitoneal bacteria.
6. Edmiston CE, Goheen MP, Kornhall S, et al (1990) Fecal peritonitis: microbial adherence to
    serosal mesothelium and resistance to peritoneal lavage. World J Surg 14:176–183
    The classic study on bacterial adherence and the problems of lavage.
7. König C, Simmen HP, Blaser J (1998) Bacterial concentrations in pus and infected peritoneal
    fluid – implications for bactericidal activity of antibiotics. J Antimicrob Chemother 42: 227–232
    Interesting comparison of bacterial counts in different infections, questioning the value of
    results of routine sensitivity testing.

8. Schöffel U, Zeller T, Lausen M, et al (1989) Monitoring of the inflammatory response in early peritonitis. Am J Surg 157:567–572
   Early report showing that systemic parameters of inflammation best reflect the severity of secondary peritonitis, irrespective of the source of contamination.
9. Plank LD, Hill GL (2000) Sequential metabolic changes following induction of systemic inflammatory response in patients with severe sepsis or major blunt trauma. World J Surg 24:630–638
   Reviews several studies of this group on metabolic sequelae of SIRS.
10. Riché FC, Cholley BP, Panis YH, et al (2000) Inflammatory cytokine response in patients with septic shock secondary to generalized peritonitis. Crit Care Med 28:433–437
   Confirmatory prospective study on the early cytokine response in peritonitis.
11. Garrison RN, Spain DA, Wilson MA, et al (1998) Microvascular changes explain the "two-hit" theory of multiple organ failure. Ann Surg 227:851–860
   Experimental study demonstrating alterations in microvascular reactivity to systemic inflammation by prior pathophysiological stress.

Invited Commentary

Graham Ramsay

While I agree with the majority of the content I will take the opportunity to focus on important points and present an alternative view regarding some priorities in treatment.

One of the key principles stated is "generally, every established source of infection has to be brought under control as soon as possible." While it is difficult to argue with this as a general principle, I would prefer to add that this applies only to patients who have been adequately resuscitated. Later, Schöffel states that a certain delay in operative intervention may be unavoidable if prior resuscitation and stabilization of homeostasis are necessary. I would express this more strongly, stating that a delay in operative intervention is desirable until such time as resuscitation has been achieved. For an analogy, consider trauma care where resuscitation takes first priority. Intervention in a surgical sense takes place only when bleeding is so severe that the patient cannot be stabilized. Such a situation is virtually unknown in sepsis. A stable situation can almost always be achieved, although this may require invasive monitoring and the use of inotropic and vasopressor support. Old surgical literature taught us that a patient who is passing urine prior to undergoing surgery is less likely to suffer renal failure or other organ failure postoperatively. In any event, resuscitation in an intensive care unit allows further monitoring of the patient during the operative procedure to be carried out in a more thorough and safe manner. In addition, there is good evidence from studies that the admission of patients to an intensive care unit for resuscitation prior to high-risk surgery (including surgery for surgical infection) results in a significant reduction in mortality [1, 2]. The time taken to achieve complete or relative hemodynamic stability can be used to perform needle puncture or other techniques to obtain culture results. The provision of adequate antibiotic cover prior to the start of surgery has been shown to influence outcome [3].

Dr. Schöffel makes an interesting point in the section headed "The Improving Patient". He states that even if an infectious source has been identified the planned surgical intervention should be canceled if the patient shows significant and sustained clinical improvement. I support this view. An area of controversy which will be dealt with in Chap. 42, is the role of planned relaparotomy. The finding of severe peritoneal contamination during an initial laparotomy often leads to a request by the operator for a planned second look. The clinical signs of sepsis or organ disfunction should reinforce the need for a relaparotomy. On the other hand, it is my opinion that a planned relaparotomy should be canceled if the patient shows significant clinical improvement. This is particularly important since there is some evidence that the strategy of planned relaparotomy can lead to an increase in complications, including development of intestinal fistula [4].

The section entitled "Interventional Insult" underlines the importance of the second hit theory in determining organ dysfunction and poor outcome. The concept that a prolonged one-step approach to definitively eliminate the source of infection may sometimes prove inferior to temporizing, palliative procedures is interesting. Again, by analogy to trauma surgery, it fits in well with the concept of damage control. In other words, it may be wise to drain an infective focus, carry out further resuscitation of the patient, and, at a later stage, carry out definitive source control. While it is easy to agree with the apparent common sense of such a statement, it would be interesting to examine whether the view can be supported by references from the literature.

In the section entitled "Diagnostic Delay," a view is expressed that, where diagnostic certainty is difficult to achieve, patients should be subjected to further diagnostic procedures prior to intervention. This is a particularly important principle in the intensive care situation where sedated, ventilated patients are more difficult to assess clinically. My view is that signs of deterioration in organ function within 2 or 3 days of a laparotomy for intraabdominal infection should lead, in the absence of other causes, to a relaparotomy. However, when clinical deterioration occurs 4 or more days after a previous laparotomy, it is almost always better to carry out CT scanning prior to a surgical intervention, since at that stage localization of infection is more likely and percutaneous drainage may be an option.

In the section entitled "Controversies", the author states that "there are patients who are too ill to be operated upon." An alternative view is that patients who are so ill must be operated upon, since allowing a patient to die of infection without an attempt at surgical source control is usually inappropriate. Moribund patients should not be operated upon when it is virtually certain that they will die during the surgical procedure. On the other hand, an intensive care patient who is ventilated with full invasive monitoring, in whom a degree of hemodynamic stability can be achieved, should not be denied a surgical intervention.

References

1. Boyd O, Ground RM, Bennett ED (1993) A randomized clinical trial of the effect of deliberate perioperative increase of oxygen delivery on mortality in high-risk surgical patients. JAMA 270:2699–2707

2. Boyd O (1999) The high risk surgical patient – where are we now? Clin Inten Care 10:161–167
3. McCabe WR, Olans RN (1981) Shock in Gram-negative bacteremia: predisposing factors, pathophysiology, and treatment. Cur Clin Top Infect Dis 2:121–150
4. Van Goor H, Hulsebos RG, Bleichrodt RP (1997) Complications of planned relaparotomy in patients with severe general peritonitis. Eur J Surg 163:61–66

Editorial Comment

When confronted with any surgical infection, the surgeon has a very limited menu of strategic options to choose from:

- Surgery now: run to the OR. As both Drs. Schöffel and Ramsay emphasize, this situation, when a patient is too sick to be adequately resuscitated for at least 1-2 h, almost never exists in the settings of surgical infection.
- Surgery tonight: this the commonest scenario, when the patient with clinical peritonitis and free air on X-ray is operated on a few hours after admission.
- Surgery tomorrow: well-localized conditions such as acute appendicitis or cholecystitis, in the absence of severe local and systemic manifestations, can be safely added to the day operative list.
- Surgery maybe in a few days: the patient with a contained leak after anterior resection – let us try to cool him down and see.
- No surgery: most patients with acute diverticulitis.

That the time factor is crucial but notoriously unpredictable may be exemplified with a patient sustaining a perforation of his colon during colonoscopy. Based on the mechanisms of perforation and the clinical, local, and systemic, manifestations this patient may be treated with no surgery or surgery tonight. When the no surgery approach fails, it is substituted with surgery tomorrow. On the other hand, we have seen such patients rapidly deteriorate within a few hours and die in intractable septic shock. In court the plaintiff's lawyer will always claim that the negligent delay in operation was the cause of death. And usually the jury will accept such a claim!

Two of Dr. Schöffel's statements are sufficiently important that they bear repeating: that the time course of an infection can never be reliably predicted in the clinical setting and that in the clinical situation decisions must be made through consideration of a worst-case scenario.

30 Complications of Source Control

MARK A. MALANGONI

Key Principles

- Complications of source control often result from technical errors or local factors that impair healing.
- Diagnosis and drainage of local infection and correction of fluid and electrolyte disorders are important for successful treatment.
- Control of fistulous drainage and provision of appropriate nutritional support are important secondary goals of management.

General Comments

In spite of optimal efforts to obtain appropriate control of the source of intraperitoneal infection, complications will occasionally develop. Two of the most frustrating and difficult problems encountered are anastomotic leaks and fistulas. At best, the development of these complications substantially increases the complexities of patient management and hospital length of stay. At worst, the associated mortality for these events is high.

Whenever a leak from an anastomosis or suture line occurs, it is important to critically review the circumstances of the original operation. Sometimes errors in technique or judgment that may have contributed to these complications can be identified. This exercise is an important one and can help target areas where quality improvement is necessary.

Vague, nondescript symptoms and signs such as abdominal pain and distension, ileus, a low-grade fever, and leukocytosis often precede the appearance of anastomotic leaks and fistulas. Whenever an incisional infection develops after an operation for intra-abdominal infection, a suture line leak should be suspected, since this is often the initial manifestation of this complication and is followed later by drainage of intestinal contents through the incision.

There are a variety of causes for failure of suture line healing (Table 1). Experience suggests that impairment of venous drainage due to improper mesenteric dissection near the anastomotic area is an important cause for anastomotic failure. Impaired healing of a suture line or anastomosis can be a result of other circumstances (Table 2). The same factors that contribute to the development of a leak also will prevent a fistula from closing spontaneously [1]. It is imperative to avoid these problems either by not performing an anastomosis or repair, constructing the suture line at an area that is not involved by these abnormalities, or physically moving the anastomosis to a remote area.

Table 1. Technical causes of anastomotic leaks and fistulas

Tension on the suture line or anastomosis
Impairment of blood supply due to:
  Arterial compromise
  Occlusion of venous drainage
  Overlapping suture lines
Improper placement of sutures resulting in:
  Defect in the closure
  Eversion of mucosa
Entrapment of intestine during fascial closure
Unintentional injury due to:
  Electrocautery
  Lysis of adhesions

Table 2. Additional factors contributing to anastomotic leaks and fistulas

Persistent infection
Distal intestinal obstruction
Cancer
Acute inflammatory bowel disease
Radiation enteritis
Improper placement of a drain
Intestinal tuberculosis (rare)

The major causes of death from an anastomotic leak or fistula are uncontrolled sepsis, fluid and electrolyte imbalances, and malnutrition. The surgeon should make an immediate effort to identify whether these complications are present and, if so, they should be treated rapidly. First and foremost, any fluid and electrolyte abnormalities should be corrected, by adequate resuscitation using crystalloid and/or colloid solutions to increase intravascular volume. Renal function should be assessed before intravenous potassium is given, unless the patient has profound hypokalemia. Parenteral antibiotics should be started and agents effective against intra-abdominal infections should be selected. It is extremely important to assess whether the draining enteric content is or can be controlled, since failure to control infection is the leading cause of death due to intestinal leaks.

The gut should be put "at rest" by stopping enteral intake and placing a gastric drainage tube until the amount of drainage can be quantified and the impact of these maneuvers can be assessed. Abdominal computed tomography will help identify any fluid collections or abscesses that need to be drained either by operation or by percutaneous methods. Drainage from a fistula often can be controlled with a continuous suction or sump drain. If these measures do not control the drainage adequately, then operation is needed. Operation also is indicated when there is a large area of anastomotic disruption (>1 cm^2), a short, epithelialized fistulous tract (<2 cm), or for any of the other reasons contributing to a persistent fistula as listed above.

Once these immediate priorities have been addressed, a fistulogram should be done to guide treatment decisions and better define the likelihood of spontaneous closure. The fistulous drainage should be controlled to minimize skin irritation. An enterostomal therapist can often help to construct an appropriate skin barrier in this situation. In addition, the patient's nutritional requirements will need to be satisfied [2]. Enteral nutritional support is preferred since enteral feeding results in a reduced incidence of multiple organ failure and superior outcomes compared to parenteral nutritional support. There are times when it may not be appropriate to use enteral feeding unless it can be directed distal to the leak. Conversely, some fistulas of the large intestine and pancreas will not be adversely affected by enteral feeding. When enteral nutritional support is not feasible, total parenteral nutrition should be started after fluid and electrolyte disorders have been corrected. The goal of management of anastomotic leaks and fistulas is closure. Adequate nutritional support helps reduce the risk of developing other complications such as pneumonia, which also can increase mortality.

Patients who develop significant anastomotic disruption or who have obvious peritonitis should be resuscitated and readied for an emergency operation; broad-spectrum antimicrobial agents should be started immediately. The choices for source control at this operation are generally similar to those at the previous operation for source control; however, it is more likely that a stoma or other diversionary procedure will be needed at reoperation.

The primary goal of the management of anastomotic leaks and fistulas is closure [3-5]. It is very important to determine whether spontaneous closure is likely or whether the patient will be better treated by operation (Table 3). Once it has been determined that an operation is needed, the procedure should be performed without delay. Fistulas that recur following spontaneous closure almost always require operation. The operative treatment of anastomotic leaks and fistulas should not be viewed as competitive with nonoperative management; rather, these methods both can result in successful resolution of the problem. What is important is to select the most appropriate treatment based on safety, experience, and the circumstances at hand.

Table 3. Factors that prevent spontaneous closure of an intestinal fistula

Disruption of intestinal continuity
Distal intestinal obstruction
Presence of a foreign body (e.g., prosthetic mesh, drain)
Fusion of the intestinal mucosa and skin
Active peritonitis or abscess

The Operation

When operation is needed, it may be beneficial to choose an incision away from the previous one. This allows for easier and more rapid entry into the abdominal cavity and can help avoid unintentional injury to the surrounding intestine, a factor that can result in fistula recurrence. In general, the fistula should be excised completely to include a margin of bowel and a primary anastomosis or suture performed at an area of normal intestine. Attempts at so-called local repair usually are unsuccessful. The fistulous track should be excised or curetted to destroy any residual mucosa. Failure to do so often results in delayed healing or a persistent sinus. The skin generally is left to heal by secondary intention or is managed by delayed primary closure. Diversion of proximal enteric contents from the site of closure is another important component of treatment and can usually be accomplished by sump tube decompression. A feeding jejunostomy or post-pyloric feeding tube should be placed when operating on fistulas of the upper gastrointestinal tract. One should avoid placing drains in the area of repair and suture lines should be remote from any abscess cavity.

Specific Considerations

Esophagus

Because of a strong tendency for recurrence, these leaks should be reinforced with other tissues [6]. The stomach can be used to reinforce suture lines of the distal esophagus. Otherwise, an intercostal muscle flap placed over the suture line has been demonstrated to result in superior healing. Pleural patches usually do not work as well as intercostal muscle (see Chap. 20).

Stomach

Gastric resection and conversion to a gastrojejunostomy should be used to treat gastroduodenal anastomotic leaks. Leaks or fistulas from a gastrojejunal anastomosis are best treated by drainage since resection is associated with a high incidence of recurrence. Distal gastric fistulas should be managed with gastric resection and gastrojejunostomy (see Chap. 11).

Duodenum

Lateral duodenal fistulas have a very low rate of spontaneous closure. Early operation to divert gastric secretions from the area of involvement is strongly recommended. A tube duodenostomy and sufficient drainage are essential components of management.

Small Intestine

Patients with recurrent or multiple fistulas should have a proximal enterostomy to divert enteric contents in order to optimize chances for healing. Fistulas of the distal ileum are more likely to close spontaneously than proximal fistulas. Appendiceal fistulas are rare; their occurrence suggests distal obstruction from colon cancer.

Large Intestine

These fistulas are most likely to close spontaneously. When operation is needed, creation of a colostomy is often needed for success.

Pancreas

Pancreatic fistulas will usually close within 30-60 days. Distal pancreatectomy is commonly necessary for fistulas of the body or tail. External drainage is preferred for fistulas of the proximal pancreas. There also has been recent success with endoscopic stents for proximal fistulas.

Critical Issues and Summary

The development of an anastomotic leak or fistula following operations for source control often results from technical and judgmental errors at the initial operation. When a leak or fistula occurs, the essential principles of management are:
- Gain control of any associated infection and begin antimicrobial treatment.
- Correct fluid and electrolyte abnormalities immediately.
- Control any fistulous drainage and provide nutritional support.

Remember that the goals of management are patient survival and fistula closure.

References

1. Schrock TR, Deveney CW, Dunphy JE (1973) Factors contributing to leakage of colonic ana-stomoses. Ann Surg 177:513–518
2. Soeters PB, Ebeid AM, Fischer JE (1979) Review of 404 patients with gastrointestinal fistulas: impact of parenteral nutrition. Ann Surg 190:189–202
3. Edmunds LH Jr, Williams GM, Welch CE (1960) External fistulas arising from the gastroin-testinal tract. Ann Surg 152:445–471
4. Reber HA, Roberts C, Way LW, Dunphy JE (1978) Management of external gastrointestinal fistulas. Ann Surg 188:460–467
5. Malangoni MA, Madura JA, Jesseph JE (1981) Management of lateral duodenal fistulas: a study of fourteen cases. Surgery 90:645–651
6. Richardson JD, Tobin GR (1994) Closure of esophageal defects with muscle flaps. Arch Surg 129:541–549

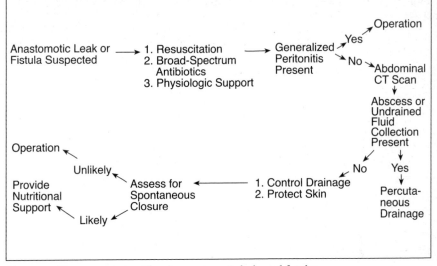

Diagram 1. Management algorithm for anastomotic leaks and fistulas

Invited Commentary

Hannes Wacha

Anastomotic leaks and fistulas are among the most frustrating and difficult problems of source control. Other complications of source control include wound infections and abscesses, wound dehiscence and hernia, and systemic infectious complications such as sepsis and pneumonia.

Fistula

Postoperative abscesses and peritonitis and delayed postoperative bowel function may be early signs of fistula formation. Fistulas following perforation of the upper GI tract are the exception. The incidence of fistulas varies according to the type of operation, ranging from 2% after perforated appendicitis to 6% after large and small bowel surgery and 11% in postoperative peritonitis [1].

Common causes of fistula formation include repeated operations and technical complications after radical debridement [2]. While proponents of planned reoperation believe this technique has the advantage of early detection of anastomotic leaks and fistulas, radical debridement and planned reoperations do not improve survival; why do more than necessary in the management of source control?

It is generally accepted that a stoma or a diversionary procedure is necessary for patients with an anastomotic dehiscence. This philosophy has not changed despite new suture techniques and planned relaparotomy. In some cases, however, a reanastomosis done in infected area may be successful if protected by absorbable mesh (personal experience). The time of reintervention should be chosen carefully. In cases of fistula in the upper GI tract, this may be difficult because of high fluid loss leading to metabolic and nutritional problems. The definitive operation should not be attempted before the 3rd week and in the colon before 6-8 weeks. I do not agree that wounds should always be left to heal by secondary intention. In my experience, primary closure is reasonable when excision of the fistula or dehiscence can be accomplished and an anastomosis created. Wound excision, primary closure, and appropriate antibiotics will result in primary healing in most cases.

Wound Infection and Abscesses

Even following diffuse peritonitis, major wound complications are uncommon. Their frequency varies from 8% in patients with perforated ulcers of the stomach and duodenum, to 20% in patients with perforated appendicitis [1]. These results were achieved with primary wound closure and appropriate antibiotics. The diagnosis of wound infection may be delayed because of prolonged antibiotic administration. This is one reason to limit antibiotic therapy for 3-5 days.

In my experience, adequate reopening of an infected wound does not require opening up the incision completely. Foreign material must be removed, because of delayed resorption in the presence of pus. Intraabdominal or retroperitoneal abscesses require drainage. Depending on the duration, contents, and localization, open drainage is not always required. When there is a single abscess and minimal necrotic tissue, percutaneous puncture using ultrasound or radiological guidance is possible. Relapse is to be expected when drainage procedures are incomplete or when surrounding organs do not allow shrinking of the abscess. Subphrenic abscesses can be drained transcostally, pelvic abscesses transrectally or transvaginally.

Dehiscence and Hernia

Wound dehiscence and hernias may develop following operations for diffuse secondary peritonitis. The incidence varies from 3% following perforation of the stomach or colon to 13% in small bowel perforation, and up to 25% in postoperative peritonitis. The more operations that are performed, the higher the likelihood is of developing a hernia. Whenever tension-free closure of the abdomen is not possible, absorbable mesh can be used to protect the bowel. Mesh is well tolerated in infected wounds, but for definitive wound closure, autologous fascial grafts should be used [3].

Sepsis and Pneumonia

Certain extraperitoneal infective complications seem to be typically related to the site of origin of peritonitis [1, 4]. There is a high incidence of pneumonia in patients with a perforated stomach or postoperative peritonitis (32%). The sepsis rate was highest in postoperative peritonitis (34%) and significantly higher in patients with inadequate antibiotic coverage (39%) or in patients undergoing planned reoperations (45%). Are these typical complications of source control?

Enterococci and Source Control

The influence of microbiological findings including enterococci and the impact of an appropriate antibiotic regime on the prognosis of peritonitis is controversial. Enterococci are markers for patients at increased risk of developing complications. Patients with intra-abdominal infections who did not receive appropriate antibiotics had a significantly higher postoperative infective complication rate than those treated with antibiotics effective against enterococci. There was, however, no significant difference in mortality in this group of patients. Both bacterial complication rates (38% vs 70%) and mortality (14% vs 47%) have been shown to differ in patients having or not having source control [1]. Most complications occur in patients having more than one operation and particularly in those patients having planned reoperations [5].

Conclusion

In my opinion, complication rates correlate with overtreatment. These complications are the result of a surgical technique performed too vigorously or of prolonged parenteral nutrition or antibiotics.

I would include as a key principle in the prevention and treatment of complications of source control early enteral feeding and the normalizing of the bowel function [6], because failure of the gut often precedes further complications. Delayed recovery of GI motility is a characteristic response to abdominal surgery. There is no single measure that can reduce postoperative ileus. Early oral feeding stimulates secretion of intestinal hormones that exert a stimulatory effect on gastrointestinal motility. Early feeding and limited antibiotic treatment normalizes the intestinal flora; conversely, immobilization of the patient, anesthesia, inadequate pain management, and nasogastric tubes favor the development of pneumonia and depress gastrointestinal motility [7]. In addition to adequate surgery, a comprehensive approach in the surgical ICU may reduce and treat complications of source control.

References

1. Wacha H, Hau T, Dittmer R, Ohmann C and the Peritonitis Study Group (1999) Risk factors associated with intraabdominal infections: a prospective multicenter study. Langenbeck's Arch Surg 384:24–32
2. Kriwanek S, Gschwantler M, Beckerhinn P, Armbruster C, Roka R (2000) Reconstructive intestinal surgery after open management of severe intraabdominal infection. World J Surg 24:999–1003
3. Disa JJ, Goldberg NH, Carlton JM, Robertson BC, Slezak S (1998) Restoring abdominal wall integrity in contaminated tissue-deficient wounds using autologous fascia grafts. Plast Reconstr Surg. 101:979–986
4. Teichmann W, Herbig B (2000) Therapie-Prinzipien bei der diffusen Peritonitis. Chirurg 71:120–128
5. Mustard RA, Bohnen JMA, Rosati C (1991) Pneumonia complicating abdominal sepsis: an independent risk factor for mortality. Arch Surg 126:170–175
6. Hau T, Ohmann C, Wolmershäuser A, Wacha H, Yang Q, for the Peritonitis Study Group of the Surgical Infection Society – Europe (1995) Planned relaparotomy vs relaparotomy on demand in the treatment of intra-abdominal infections. Arch Surg 130:1193–1197
7. Minard G, Kudsk K (1998) Nutritional support and infection: does the route matter? World J Surg 22:213–219

Editorial Comment

In this chapter, Dr. Malangoni provides an overview of an often lethal complication of source control: anastomotic dehiscence. Commentator Wacha stresses the contribution of overtreatment to the genesis of postoperative intestinal leaks and underlines the importance of the overall care in the salvage of these patients.

There are two common clinical scenarios of postoperative intestinal leak:

- The leak is obvious: intestinal contents are draining from the operative wound or from the drain site.
- One suspects a leak but does not see one.

There is little controversy that an established postoperative external enterocutaneous fistula should initially be treated *conservatively*. But what about early postoperative intestinal leakage, presenting a day or two after the initial operation for source control? Should it be managed with an immediate reoperation as we would do for any simple gastrointestinal perforation, or should we treat it conservatively as we would treat an established fistula?

The Role of Nonoperative Management

As Dr. Malangoni writes, with adequate conservative-supportive management, and in the absence of distal obstruction or loss of bowel continuity, the majority of postoperative fistulas will close spontaneously. Those that fail to close within 6 weeks will require an elective reoperation. Surgery performed on an anabolic patient, in a less hostile peritoneal environment, will restore the gastrointestinal tract with a minimal rate of complication. A crucial issue when deciding on a trial of conservative management is the absence or presence of peritonitis and/or sepsis: *clinical peritonitis is an indication for an immediate operation*. Even when clinical peritonitis is not present, clinical evidence of sepsis should promote an aggressive search for drainable intraabdominal pus. This search is best accomplished with a CT scan: abscesses should be drained percutaneously or by laparotomy. Notably, in contemporary unselected series of postoperative enterocutaneous fistulas one-third of patients still die – usually from neglected intraabdominal infection [1].

The Role of Operative Management

There is a great temptation to attempt reanastomosis in patients with an anastomotic leak; however, attempts at primary closure of a leaking intestinal suture line in the presence of postoperative peritonitis are doomed to fail. Although such an attempt may occasionally be successful, saving the patient a prolonged hospitalization and morbidity, when a leak redevelops, it represents a tremendous "second hit" – in an already primed, susceptible and compromised host – and death or significant morbidity is common.

We believe that a trial of conservative management of anastomotic dehiscence is warranted when:

- There is no clinical peritonitis.
- There are no associated abscesses on CT that cannot be drained percutaneously.
- The surgeon knows the underlying cause of the leak, had performed the first operation, and knows with a reasonable certainty where the leakage is originating from (an anastomosis or an enterotomy). Obviously these conditions may not be met in a patient transferred from another institution.

An immediate relaparotomy is warranted when:

- There is clinical evidence of peritonitis.
- Abdominal compartment syndrome is present.
- The surgeon does not have adequate information about the index operation.

What to Do During an Emergency Relaparotomy?

The decision is based on several factors, including the condition of the bowel, the condition of the peritoneal cavity, and the condition of the patient. *Very rarely*, in a stable, minimally compromised patient, when peritonitis is macroscopically minimal, the bowel appears to be of good quality and the serum albumin is normal, we will resect the involved segment and reanastomose. Such a decision is made when a leak presents within a day or two of operation, typically as a result of a technical mishap. The less heroic but logical and life-saving option of exteriorization of the leak as an enterostomy should be performed if there is any question about the safety of primary repair.

Conservative Management

- Protection of the skin around a fistula from the corrosive intestinal juice can often be accomplished using a well-fitting colostomy bag. Alternatively, drainage from a fistula can be controlled with a tube connected to continuous suction; stomadhesive sheaths are positioned around the defect and the entire field is then covered with an adhesive transparent dressing [2].
- Providing nutrition. Proximal gastrointestinal fistulas often require TPN, whereas distal small bowel and colonic fistulas will close spontaneously whether the patient is fed orally or not. When at all possible, the intestine should be used as the preferred route of nutritional support. For patients with high fistulas, it is often possible, and probably beneficial, to collect the fistulous output, reinfusing it with the enteral diet into the bowel below the fistula.
- Delineate anatomy. This is best done with a sinogram, injecting water-soluble contrast medium into the fistulous tract to document the level of the defect and the presence or absence of distal obstruction or loss of continuity, prerequisites for successful conservative management.

Colonic anastomotic leaks are best visualized with a Gastrografin enema. For upper gastrointestinal and small bowel anastomoses Gastrografin can be given from above, combining the contrast study with a CT scan to look for free intraperitoneal contrast or abscesses.

The initial output of a fistula is of little prognostic significance. A fistula which drains 1,000 ml/day during the first week has the same chance of spontaneous closure as one with an output of 500 ml/day. While attempts to decrease the fistulous output by starvation and administration of a somatostatin analogue are cosmetically appealing; these strategies have not proven to be beneficial.

Fistula Associated with a Large Abdominal Wall Defect

Commonly, the result of intestinal leaks and reoperative surgery is an abdominal wall defect with multiple intestinal fistulas in its base. *This so-called complex or type IV fistula represents a catastrophe, which carries a very high mortality rate* [3] (according to our classification, type A are foregut fistulas; type B small bowel; type C colonic [1]). The distance of the fistulous opening in the intestine from the surface of the defect and the condition of the peritoneal cavity influence the treatment of this condition. It is practical to distinguish between two situations.

- Type IV-A fistula. When the fistula is located in the depth of the infected abdominal defect, the prolonged contact of large peritoneal surfaces with gastrointestinal contents allows increased absorption of toxic products, perpetuating a local and systemic inflammatory response and organ dysfunction. In such instances, reoperation is necessary to exteriorize or divert the intestinal leak away from the defect.
- Type IV-B fistulas are exposed fistulas near the surface of the defect. Also called bud fistulas, they result from damage to intestine exposed at the base of the

defect. Because the peritoneal cavity is usually clean and sealed away from intestinal contents, an expectant approach is indicated. A simple rule of thumb is that the condition of the abdominal wall defect reflects the condition of the peritoneal cavity. A well-contracted abdominal wall defect in which the fistula looks like a surgical stoma suggests that an elective intervention is possible and safe. An exposed-bud fistula can be managed temporarily (until definitive reconstruction) by defining the mucosal and submucosal layer of the pouting intestinal hole and closing it with a fine monofilament suture. The repaired bowel and surrounding abdominal wall defect are then covered with a split-thickness skin graft.

Anastomotic leaks comprise a spectrum of conditions requiring a variety of therapeutic approaches. To minimize morbidity, treatment must be tailored to the specific leak, its degree, and the affected patient.

References

1. Schein M, Decker G (1991) Postoperative external alimentary tract fistulas. Am J Surg 161: 435–438
2. Schein M, Saadia R, Jamieson JR, Decker GAG (1986) The "Sandwich" technique in the management of the open abdomen. Br J Surg 73:369–370
3. Schein M, Decker GA (1990) Gastrointestinal fistulas associated with large abdominal wall defects: experience with 43 patients. Br J Surg 77:97–100

31 Reoperation After Source Control Surgery for Intra-abdominal Infection

Ori D. Rotstein

Key Principles

- In general, reoperation should be delayed for several months following resolution of all complications arising from the source control operation. It seems prudent to delay surgery for at least 6 months.
- The sensitive nature of reoperation for prior complications requires a strong physician-patient relationship to minimize patient anxiety prior to the procedure.
- In all reoperative cases, it is critically important for the operating surgeon to fully understand the nature of prior surgeries.
- It is preferable to enter the peritoneal cavity through a "virgin area" of the abdominal wall.

Introduction

Several general principles underlie the surgical management of patients with intra-abdominal infection. These include drainage and debridement of infection or infected tissues in the abdominal cavity, management of the underlying pathological process, and appropriate wound management. For the purpose of this manuscript, the model of colonic anastomotic dehiscence following elective colon resection will be used as the template for considering approaches to reoperation following initial source control surgery for diffuse postoperative peritoneal infection. At the initial reoperation, the patient would likely have had a repeat laparotomy through the initial midline abdominal wall incision. Fecal material as well as purulent exudates are aspirated from the peritoneal cavity complemented by irrigation with warmed crystalloid solution to facilitate removal of particulate debris. Depending on the location of the dehiscence, the degree of breakdown of the anastomosis and the amount of peritoneal soiling, the anastomosis will have been taken down entirely with formation of an end stoma and mucus fistula/closed stump or alternatively have been defunctioned with a proximal stoma and drained externally at the site of the anastomotic breakdown. If possible, the abdominal wall fascia is closed primarily but otherwise an absorbable mesh is secured to fascia or skin to maintain the intestines in situ and hence right of domain. Finally, the skin is left open to minimize postoperative wound infection in a markedly contaminated field. In the postoperative period, the patient may require insertion of a percutaneous drain to treat recurrent or residual intra-abdominal infection. The wound is allowed to epithelialize with or without the help of split thickness skin grafts. The stage is now set: after a complicated initial hospital course, the patient is discharged facing the prospect of reoperation to return him to his preoperative state.

Preparing for the Reoperation

Timing

In general, reoperation should be delayed for several months following resolution of all complications arising from the source control operation. The most compelling reason relates to the general nutritional and metabolic status of the patient. Patients who have had repeat interventions for intra-abdominal infection lose weight and muscle mass as a result of reduced caloric intake in a setting of hypermetabolism. Once infection has resolved, wounds have healed and adequate caloric intake has been reinitiated, the stimuli for hypermetabolism are removed, permitting full restoration of the premorbid state, including nutritional, metabolic, and immunological parameters. These will impact on wound healing, coagulation, and ability to resist infection following restorative surgery. The optimal route of nutritional support during the period prior to reoperation will depend on the patient's underlying anatomy. A patient with an intact upper gastrointestinal tract and distal stomas will usually tolerate enteral nutrition. Often tube feeding is necessary initially until the patient regains appetite and the ability to consume sufficient calories by oral diet. Even patients with GI fistulas should be offered a trial of enteral nutrition since this frequently has little impact on fistula output and is well tolerated. Patients requiring total parenteral nutrition (TPN), particularly in the home setting, require considerably more care and are subject to the risks of TPN including line complications, line infection and metabolic imbalance.

The second major reason for delaying reoperative intervention relates to the ease of surgery. One of the major technical obstacles during reoperative peritoneal surgery is the presence of dense vascularized adhesions. These make entry into the peritoneal cavity and mobilization of structures both difficult and precarious. Even mobilization of stomas from the abdominal wall is rendered difficult by dense adhesions between the subcutaneous tissues and the segment of bowel as it passes through the abdominal wall. While the presence of these vascularized adhesions is a normal component of the acute proliferative phase of healing, studies by Ellis have shown that ischemic and necrotic tissues present in the peritoneal cavity at the initial reoperation augment the vascularity of subsequent adhesions [1, 2].

Few studies have evaluated the effect of timing on outcome following closure of stomas. One report assessed the effect of timing of closure of Hartmann's procedure on complications related to the operation. In this retrospective study, a multivariate analysis showed that a prolonged interval (>6 months) between the initial Hartmann's procedure and its closure was associated with a lower incidence of anastomotic complications and a shorter hospital stay [3]. In another study examining outcome of colostomy closure, the authors reported that all wound, small bowel, and anastomotic complications related to stoma closure for Hartmann's procedure or other colostomy types occurred when the closure was performed less than 6 months after the initial procedure [4]. Overall, it seems prudent to delay surgery for at least 6 months following surgery for source control.

Preoperative Preparation

Consent

As for all operations, the patient should be fully apprised of the nature of the procedure and its potential for complications. Frank discussion with the patient is particularly important for reoperative surgery since the patient will invariably have significant anxieties related to his/her prior surgery and the fact that it was complicated by postoperative infection. In my discussions with patients, I regularly raise the issue of the potential difficulty of the procedure, pointing out the potential for adhesions and therefore inadvertent injury and excessive bleeding. The patient and the family should know that the procedure may be prolonged and may require an ICU stay in the postoperative period. Some of the anxiety of the patient may be related to mistrust of physicians in general following a previously complicated operation. The patient may request information about the previous operation and the reasons for its failure. Whether the surgeon for the reoperative procedure is the same as for the original procedure or a different surgeon, it would seem most appropriate to attempt to focus most of the discussion on the upcoming procedure, its nature, and the potential for problems. Clearly, the sensitive nature of reoperation for prior complications requires a strong physician-patient relationship to minimize patient anxiety prior to the procedure.

Patient Preparation

Definition of the Anatomy

In all reoperative cases, it is critically important for the operating surgeon to fully understand the nature of the prior surgeries. Reviewing the previous operative notes as well as speaking with the original surgeon will consolidate one's knowledge of the initial pathological process and the precise anatomy to be corrected in the reoperative setting. In the absence of clear information, one should be very liberal about using preoperative contrast imaging or endoscopy to define the anatomy. In the hypothetical case of reoperation after a colonic anastomotic dehiscence, the need for definition of the anatomy varies according to the initial source control procedure. A prior operation consisting of exteriorization of an end colostomy with nearby mucus fistula or exteriorization of the disrupted anastomosis are circumstances where investigation is probably unnecessary. In preparation for closure of a Hartmann's procedure, the rectal stump should be routinely investigated by endoscopy. This may help with planning of the operation as well as locating the stump at surgery. Closure of a defunctioning ileostomy or colostomy should also be preceded by investigation of the original anastomosis. This is intended to rule out the presence of a stricture or persistent defect at that site. This approach should be contrasted to studies examining closure of stomas created to manage intestinal trauma closure following prior trauma patients. In this patient group, investigation of the distal colon prior to colostomy closure has been shown to yield little useful information and does not alter morbidity of the procedure [5]. In one study, the defunctioning stoma was performed following penetrating trauma in a generally young patient population. Ninety-eight percent of contrast studies were negative and the complication rate following stoma closure did not differ between patients with or without preoperative barium enema. These results may similarly apply to nontrauma patients such as those following anastomotic dehiscence, although the possibility of stricture due to initial anastomotic ischemia would seem to be increased. Finally, contrast studies are essential when complex fistulas exist and are to be treated by reoperative surgery.

Perioperative Preparation

The general principles related to preparation for any surgery should be applied to reoperation. These would include optimization of the general medical status of the patient, administration of subcutaneous heparin and/or other antithrombotic strategies, and initiation of measures aimed at reducing postoperative infectious complications. Orthograde intestinal lavage by mouth as well as distally via the defunctioned limb has been recommended for mechanical preparation of the bowel and should be supplemented by the use of perioperative intravenous antibiotics [6]. The latter should include broad spectrum coverage of both facultative Gram-negative enterics as well as anaerobic bacteria.

Operative Intervention

Patient Positioning

Patients should be positioned to permit optimal exposure to the field of surgery, to take into account potential requirements for extension of the operative field, and to facilitate optimal reconstruction of the gastrointestinal tract and/or drainage of the operative field. In the majority of situations, the supine position is adequate. Concomitant lithotomy positioning is often helpful, particularly when reconstruction involves the left colon or rectum, where transanal access for endoscopy or stapling may be useful. When reoperation involves the upper GI tract, left lateral decubitus positioning will allow an initial thoracoabdominal incision or extension of an abdominal incision into the chest. If flank drainage is anticipated, supine positioning with placement of a sandbag under the flank may facilitate dependent drainage of the field.

The Incision and Entering the Abdominal Cavity

Stoma Closure

Most stomas where both proximal and distal limbs are positioned together in a single stoma site can be closed by using the stoma site itself as the access point to mobilize the bowel as it passes through the abdominal wall. The skin is opened 2-3 mm from the mucocutaneous junction of the stoma, providing tissue to grasp during mobilization. Occasionally this will have to be lengthened to facilitate dissection down to the level of the fascia. The limbs are then dissected from the subcutaneous tissues and released from attachments to the abdominal fascia. This mobilization will provide length for closure of the bowel and also permit repair of the abdominal wall defect after the bowel is returned to the abdominal cavity. Injury to mesenteric vessels or to the seromuscular layer of the bowel during mobilization will predispose to dehiscence of the closure or the development of a parastomal fistula in the postoperative period. These injuries are minimized by using meticulous dissection and by avoiding excessive traction on the limbs. Parastomal hernias complicate stoma formation in 1%-2% of patients and the surgeon should be mindful of their possible presence during stoma mobilization [7]. In order to return the reconstructed bowel to the peritoneal cavity, it is necessary to free the bowel from its fascial attachments and to gain some mobilization of intraperitoneal structures away from the surrounding abdominal wall for a few centimeters in all directions. The extent of peritoneal adhesions will influence the ease of accomplishing this. Care should be taken to avoid injury to adherent loops of intestines as well as to control bleeding from vascularized adhesion and omentum. This occasionally requires some extension of the fascial incision. It also underscores the importance of delaying reconstructive surgery, since this will minimize the extent and vascularity of these adhesions.

Entering the Peritoneal Cavity

When the abdominal cavity must be entered for stoma closure or reconstruction of bowel following fistula excision, careful planning of the location and type of incision is mandatory. It is preferable to enter the peritoneal cavity through a "virgin area" of the abdominal wall. This facilitates entry into the abdominal cavity by avoiding the areas where the most intense adhesions would be expected, i.e., beneath the previous abdominal wall incision and in the region of the abdomen where the inflammation might have been the most severe. Inadvertent enterotomy is relatively common during reoperation, occurring in approximately 20% of patients, and is associated with a higher rate of postoperative complication and a longer postoperative hospital stay [8]. In addition, it is a frustrating beginning to a potentially long and tedious operation.

The use of the previous midline incision, beginning with entry either cephalad or caudad to this initial incision through an unoperated field is the most common approach to reentering the abdomen. This approach provides broad access to the peritoneal cavity with opportunity for extension and is also readily closed.

Other approaches may include unilateral or bilateral subcostal incisions, transverse incisions, flank incisions or thoracoabdominal incisions. In general, these should be considered when a specific area of the abdomen is operated on, since they generally afford less access to the overall peritoneal cavity. For example, a subcostal incision may provide excellent exposure for reoperation in the biliary tree but would be a poor choice for rectosigmoid surgery. When placing new incisions, care should be taken not to render intervening tissue bridges ischemic. This might occur when a midline incision is placed adjacent to a previous paramedian incision. It is preferable to use the previous paramedian incision with extension into the midline above or below. Similarly, placement of a midline incision crossing a subcostal incision may leave a triangle of ischemic tissue where the incisions intersect. Placement of the incisions such that they do not intersect may prevent this complication.

Upon entering the peritoneal cavity, adhesions between the anterior abdominal wall and the underlying omentum and bowel must be released. By 6 months following the initial surgery, adhesions are generally relatively filmy and readily divided using scissor or cautery dissection. Gentle traction on the bowel with counter-traction on the abdominal wall will facilitate exposure of the appropriate tissue plane for division. A similar approach is appropriate for dense adhesions, with some surgeons preferring knife dissection. During this dissection, it may be necessary to leave patches of abdominal wall (peritoneum with or without fascia) adherent to bowel to avoid enterotomy. During operations such as these, one of my mentors was known to caution, "It is better to leave abdominal wall on bowel than bowel on abdominal wall." It is also noteworthy that enterotomies are not invariably due to injury by surgical instruments during dissection. Rather, they may be due to traction on the bowel due to overexuberant traction on the abdominal wall by an enthusiastic resident. Clearance of the fascial edges along both sides of the entire incision is necessary to achieve adequate and safe closure of the abdominal wall.

Surgical Correction

Managing Intra-abdominal Adhesions

Having successfully entered the abdominal cavity, one faces varying degrees of interloop adhesions. The degree to which these must be lysed depends upon the particular operation to be performed. When one is operating on the colon for the purpose of stoma closure or reestablishment of colonic continuity, there is generally little need to exhaustively take down small bowel adhesions. The fact that the patient has been tolerating a normal diet preoperatively provides ample evidence that the small bowel adhesions are not of physiological significance. While not having to lyse all adhesions, it is necessary, however, to free small bowel loops from their attachments to the colon so that the latter might be adequately mobilized to permit easy closure or anastomosis. When operating to close a small bowel stoma or to correct an enterocutaneous fistula, I am much more fastidious about lysis of interloop adhesions, particularly distal small bowel ones. The presence of a stoma or fistula may serve to defunction a distal small bowel adhesive obstruction prior to surgery and may therefore preclude its recognition. The presence of a distal obstruction following upstream anastomosis could prove catastrophic in the postoperative period.

Adhesiolysis varies considerably in its degree of difficulty. Even when the re-operation is delayed more than 6 months since the initial operation and vascula-rized adhesions are no longer present, the number and density of residual fi-brous adhesions may still be significant and represent a significant technical challenge. As described for opening the peritoneal cavity, good lighting of the operative field, excellent surgical assistance and a dose of patience are absolute requirements for this part of the operation. Two experienced surgeons working together seems to facilitate adhesiolysis. One surgeon can splay the adhesions so that the other can use scissor dissection to divide them. Occasionally, cautery dissection is appropriate when bowel loops are widely separated but should be considered contraindicated when loops of bowel are closely adjacent. I frequent-ly use Lauer dissection to demonstrate particularly fibrous adhesive bands for di-vision by my assistant. During lysis of adhesions, one should also be wary of en-countering previous anastomoses. Adhesions may be particularly tenacious in these areas, particularly when the anastomosis was performed using a stapled technique. For stapled side-to-side functional end-to-end stapled anastomoses, the crotch of the anastomosis may be mistaken for intense adhesions. Failure to recognize this may result in inadvertent enterotomy and the attendant increased morbidity.

Closure of Ostomies and Bowel Anastomosis

Several reviews have addressed various issues related to stoma closure, where the initial stoma was performed during either elective surgery or as part of a source control procedure under emergency circumstances. Closure rates are lower than one might anticipate when performing them at the initial source control proce-dure. One review followed 73 patients who underwent emergency colostomy for-mation after colorectal surgery [9]. Only 60% of patients ultimately had colo-stomy closure, with the rate of closure higher in patients with diverticular disease (84.6%) compared to patients presenting initially with colorectal cancer (48.3%). Another study reported the rate of closure of stomas following source control surgery for anastomotic leakage following an anterior resection [10]. For "high" anastomoses, defined as being above the pouch of Douglas, the rate of closure of Hartmann's procedure was 91% (11/12 patients), whereas Hartmann's closure af-ter "low" anastomoses was 0% (0/7 patients). Further, another nine patients trea-ted with a defunctioning stoma following low anastomotic dehiscence had suc-cessful restoration of gastrointestinal continuity with closure of the stoma. These findings are relevant to preparing the patient as to the potential success of their restorative procedure as well as the decision-making process that should occur at the initial source control operation.

Several options are available for closure of defunctioning loop ileostomies. These include:

- Simple closure of the enterotomy by suturing
- Stapled side-to-side closure
- Limited resection with hand-sewn or stapled anastomosis.

The overall complication rate varies from approximately 10% to 30%, with the majority of complications being wound infection, fever, small-bowel obstruction, and anastomotic leak [6, 11, 12]. In one study, postreversal bowel obstruction was highest for limited resection with anastomosis, lowest for simple closure by suturing, and intermediate for stapled side-to-side anastomosis. Other complications did not differ. This study was retrospective in nature and therefore subject to bias related to patient selection [11]. Hull and colleagues compared takedown of loop ileostomies using either simple closure or stapled technique assigned by random allocation [12]. These authors had a remarkably low morbidity rate and showed no difference between the two techniques, except that the hand-sewn operation was marginally faster.

For colostomy closure, both hand-sewn and stapled techniques appear to be commonly used. For loop colostomies, mobilization without formal laparotomy is usual and closure is frequently performed using a hand-sewn technique. For closure of stomas via a transperitoneal approach, it is critically important to achieve adequate mobilization of the colon and/or small intestine to ensure a tension-free anastomosis. This invariably requires mobilization of the left or right colon (or both) from their retroperitoneal attachments. Whether continuity is reestablished using the hand-sewn or stapled technique is somewhat controversial, but is likely relatively unimportant. A recent Cochrane Review compared hand-sewn to stapled methods for colorectal anastomoses [13]. No difference was found for overall mortality, anastomotic dehiscence rate, wound infection, or hospital stay. Hand-sewn anastomoses appeared to have a slight reduction in stricture formation and reoperation rate, while stapled anastomoses were slightly faster. The authors concluded that the evidence did not support the superiority of one technique over the other.

Hartmann's procedure is a frequently performed source control procedure for the management of perforation of the sigmoid and rectum. Both hand-sewn and stapled approaches have been described for Hartmann's closure, although the modern circular stapling device seems to have made this approach preferable. At surgery, the patient is positioned in a lithotomy position for insertion of the stapling device. After dissecting the small bowel out of the pelvis, the residual stump is identified. Identification is obviously easier when the distal stump is long and protrudes into the peritoneal cavity. Insertion of a "sizing instrument" transanally can help identify the rectal stump. Needless to say, it is essential that the sizer is passed transanally in women and not transvaginally since this would result in a colovaginal anastomosis if not recognized. Some surgeons actually pack the vagina preoperatively to prevent this complication and more importantly, to identify the apex of the vagina to prevent injury. The rectum need only be cleared for a length of 4-6 cm prior to performing either a hand-sewn or stapled anastomosis. Some studies have suggested a higher stricture rate for stapled anastomoses. For Hartmann's closure, it is preferable to use the largest stapler diameter possible in order to minimize this complication. For both hand-sewn and stapled anastomoses, tension-free anastomosis of well-vascularized bowel will help minimize this complication. Recent reports have suggested that reversal of a Hartmann's procedure may be successfully accomplished laparoscopically [14]. Indeed, this colonic procedure seems ideally suited to a laparoscopic approach since the mobilized stoma is readily available for insertion of the stapler anvil, while the stapler itself is passed transanally to achieve an intracorporeal anastomosis. While this approach appears promising, it remains in the realm of the expert laparoscopist with skill at lysis of adhesions, division of mesenteric vessels, and performance of intracorporeal suturing and stapling.

Summary

Success after reoperative surgery requires comprehensive preoperative preparation of the patient plus skill and patience in the operating room. Together, these hold the greatest promise for achieving an optimal outcome.

References

1. McQuarrie DG (1997) The pathophysiology of wound healing and its relationship to reoperative surgery. In: McQuarrie DG, Humphrey EW, Lee JT (eds) Reoperative general surgery, 2nd edn. Mosby, St. Louis, pp 144–161
2. Ellis H (1971) The cause and prevention of post-operative intraperitoneal adhesions. Surg Gynecol Obstet 133:497–511
3. Pearce NW, Scott SD, Karran SJ (1992) Timing and method of reversal of Hartmann's procedure. Br J Surg 839–841
4. Mosdell DM, Doberneck RC (1991) Morbidity and mortality of ostomy closure. Am J Surg 162:633–637
5. Sola JE, Buchman TG, Bender JS (1994) Limited role of barium enema examination preceding colostomy closure in trauma patients. J Trauma 36: 245–246
6. Riesener JP, Lehnen W, Hofer M, Kasperk R, Braun JC, Schumpelick V (1997) Morbidity of ileostomy and colostomy closure: impact of surgical technique and perioperative treatment. World J Surg 21:103–108
7. Park JJ, Del Pino A, Orsay CP, Nelson RL, Pearl RK, Cintron JR, Abcarian H (1999) Stoma complications: the Cook County Hospital experience. Dis Colon Rectum 42:1575–1580
8. Van Der Krabben AA, Dijkstra FR, Nieuwenhuijzen M, Reijnen MM, Schaapveld M, Van Goor H (2000) Morbidity and mortality of inadvertent enterotomy during adhesiotomy. Br J Surg 87:467–71
9. Mealy K, O'Broin E, Donohue J, Tanner A, Keane FBV (1996) Reversible colostomy. What is the outcome? Dis Colon Rectum 39:1227–1231
10. Parc Y, Frileux P, Schmitt G, Dehni N, Ollivier JM, Parc R (2000) Management of postoperative peritonitis after anterior resection: experience from a referral intensive care unit. Dis Colon Rectum 43:579–589
11. Phang PT, Hain JM, Perez-Ramirez JJ, Madof RD, Gemlo BT (1999) Techniques and complications of ileostomy takedown. Am J Surg 177:463–466
12. Hull TL, Kobe I, Fazio VW (1996) Comparison of hand-sewn with stapled loop ileostomy closures. Dis Colon Rectum 39:1086–1089
13. Lutosa SAS, Matos D, Atallah AN, Castro AA (2001) Stapled versus hand-sewn methods for colorectal anastomosis surgery (Cochrane Review). In: The Cochrane Library, 4, Oxford, Update Software
14. Wexner SD, Reissman P, Pfeifer J, Bernstein M, Geron N (1996) Laparoscopic colorectal surgery: analysis of 140 cases. Surg Endosc 10:133-136

Invited Commentary

Timothy C. Fabian

Dr. Rotstein has written a fine manuscript concerning late reoperation after source control surgery. Salient principles including patient and surgeon preparation, timing for the reoperative procedure, and technical details concerning the conduct of the operative procedure were addressed. I will begin by stating that I am in agreement with essentially all of the principles which are outlined. After a few introductory comments, this commentary will address the issue of abdominal wall reconstruction in those cases where large ventral hernia defects result from initial wound management in some of these complex cases. As can be said for many issues in life, "timing is everything" in operative management of these patients. The general recommendation in this article is that there be an interval of at least 6 months between the initial procedure and reoperation. We have a fairly large experience with these cases at our institution and it is rare that we would reoperate before 6 months with 80% of our cases being done in the 6- to 9-month interval. We have a biological measurement which we rely on heavily for decisions for reoperation and I will return to a discussion of that measurement in a bit.

An excellent recommendation for reviewing the previous operative notes has been made by the author and I heartily concur. This seems like an obvious principle in management, but one that is often overlooked. God, indeed, rewards those who enter the operating room with a prepared mind. That preparation is best for the outcome of the patient and the confidence of the surgeon. These two issues are, of course, intimately intertwined.

There are several practical points made concerning surgical dissection. It is clearly better to enter the peritoneal cavity at a point above or below the previous incision, as there are minimal adhesions to the peritoneal surface in that location. I use a variety of techniques for adhesiolysis and settle with the one in each case that seems to be working best. These involve scalpel dissection, use of electrocautery, or, frequently, the suction tip works very nicely as a vacuum, which amazingly lyses dense adhesions from the peritoneal wall with minimal blood loss. At times it seems as though there is a brain in the suction tip that allows it to find the perfectly appropriate adhesion plane between bowel wall and parietal peritoneum. Additionally, I would certainly agree that lysis of all small-bowel adhesions is not required because I believe that the bowel is locked in the open position by these chronic adhesions. Further dissection generally causes unnecessary blood oozing and lost time. Relative to the technique of anastomosis, I do not believe it makes any difference whether it is hand-sewn or stapled, as long as the chosen technique is meticulously performed. I have always thought that one of the commonest reasons for anastomotic failure in colon surgery revolves around a simple point of dissecting the fat from the bowel, including the mesenteric border as well as the appendices epiploicae so that the seromuscular layer involves indeed seromuscular tissue and not fat. I believe incorporation of fat in the anastomosis cannot be a good thing. Like most things in surgical technique, it is the importance of meticulous attention to simple surgical technique, including tissue handling, dissecting in appropriate planes, and avoidance of strangulation of tissues that contribute to optimal outcomes.

Abdominal Wall Reconstruction in Complex Hernias Following Source Control

Attention will now be turned to abdominal wall reconstruction in complex hernias resulting from either prior severe abdominal sepsis as outlined by Dr. Rotstein or in the management of the abdominal cavity that has been left open for either damage control and/or abdominal compartment syndrome. Our institutional approach has been to routinely use absorbable mesh following reexploration in the overwhelming majority of these cases. If this is not performed, the fascia is often closed with undue tension resulting in strangulation of tissues leading to necrotizing fasciitis with severe sepsis and the patient ultimately having multiple fistulas through an open wound. Since turning to nearly routine use of absorbable mesh, we see almost no necrotizing fascial infections and enteric fistulas are far less common than was the case a decade or so ago. Application of this technique allows cinching up of the mesh either in the ICU or in the operating room over the ensuing 3-7 days in those patients who are resolving their systemic inflammatory response with diuresis and a decrease in bowel edema and intra-abdominal tension. Approximately half of our patients can be closed over the course of the first week by gradual cinching on a daily basis. However, the other half do not resolve their inflammatory response and/or septic state and their abdomens cannot be closed. In that circumstance, we routinely let the wound granulate and cover the wound with split-thickness skin graft. Occasionally, woven absorbable mesh will be totally absorbed but, in our hands, well over 90% of the mesh is not absorbed but begins separating from the bowel at 2-3 weeks in those patients who are doing well; we remove the mesh at the time of split thickness skin grafting, which is quite easily done. I believe a skin graft improves the nutritional status by eliminating what I consider to be a catabolic drain for the patient. I believe it helps in improving the protein and fluid losses associated with any large wound not dissimilar to the important principle of covering third-degree burns. Equally important regarding the split thickness skin grafting, is that once the graft is placed, it essentially eliminates the risk of fistula formation. Furthermore, if a granulating wound is allowed to chronically granulate, it substantially increases the rate of enterocutaneous fistula development. Therefore, we make every effort to get the wound grafted within 2-3 weeks.

I would like to now return to the issue of reconstruction and what I alluded to as a biological timepiece for that reconstruction. For several months, the skin graft is densely adherent to the underlying intestines. However, at around 6 months, when the patient is examined, one can pinch the skin graft away from the bowel and there are mainly loose, filmy adhesions at that time. So this approach demonstrates the important principle that Dr. Rotstein has alluded to of waiting 6 months before reconstruction. This is a very real and practical measure. It is rare to find dense and vascular adhesions when the graft is soft, pliable, and can easily be pinched from the bowel. At the time of reoperation and reconstruction, the skin graft is incised with a knife and using hemostat dissection, the graft is eventually opened in its mid-portion from top to bottom and the adhesions are dissected from the skin graft. These adhesions are generally quite filmy. The only part that is consistently more dense is at the musculofascial aponeuroses at the lateral aspect of the graft. It is routinely a more tedious dissection in that area. It generally takes approximately 45 minutes to remove the skin graft from the wound. Following removal of the graft, our approach to abdominal wall reconstruction has been use of a modified component separation technique. This technique was originally reported by Ramirez et al. [1]. We subsequently developed a modification of that approach and have used it extensively in several hundred cases over the last decade [2]. It is a method of tissue advancement that eliminates the requirement for prosthetic mesh reconstruction in these moderate-to-large hernias. This is especially important in dealing with cases as depicted in the current article where an ostomy is in place. The component separation technique avoids the risk associated with bacterial contamination of a foreign body. I would refer the reader to the aforementioned references for a full description of technique but will briefly describe it here. The skin and subcutaneous fat are mobilized from the fascia as with any ventral hernia. Dissection usually occurs to the anterior axillary line bilaterally. The tissue advancement occurs by performing long relaxing incisions of the external oblique component of the anterior rectus fascia (divided approximately 0.5-1 cm lateral to the lateral rectus), extending from the costal margins of the approximately 9th through 12th ribs down to near the pubis. Performed bilaterally, this form of relaxation allows tissue advancement and will permit closure of some of these smaller defects. However, in our experience, some of the defects will require more extensive tissue advancement and, therefore, we have modified the originally described procedure. This entails division of the internal oblique component of the anterior rectus sheath down to the arcuate line. It is important not to divide the internal oblique component below further because there is no posterior rectus fascia below that point on the abdominal wall. Following this division, there is marked mobilization bilaterally, allowing as much as 6-7 cm of mobilization of each side in the upper abdomen and as much as 12 cm in the midabdomen. This allows for closure of nearly all of these defects. The reconstruction continues by mobilizing the rectus muscle free from the posterior rectus fascia from top to bottom. Final reconstruction entails suturing of the medial portion of the posterior rectus fascia to the lateral portion of the anterior rectus fascia (that which has been divided). Then we routinely use four closed suction drains in these wounds. This technique has provided good long-term results with only occasional small hernia recurrences.

References

1. Ramirez OM, Ruas E, Dellon AL (1990) "Components separation" method for closure of abdominal-wall defects: an anatomic and clinical study. Plast Reconstr Surg 86:519–526
2. Fabian TC, Croce MA, Pritchard FE, Minard G, Hickerson WL, et al (1994) Planned ventral hernia: staged management for acute abdominal wall defects. Ann Surg 219:643–653

32 Trauma

Lillian S. Kao, Avery B. Nathens

Key Principles

- Management of blunt and penetrating abdominal trauma depends upon early diagnosis of injuries, prompt control of active hemorrhage, and control of peritoneal contamination.
- An early assessment of the extent of anatomic injury, the degree of physiologic derangement, and the ability of the patient to tolerate a prolonged operative procedure are critical in the decision-making process.
- Primary restoration of gastrointestinal continuity may be safely achieved for most injuries.

General Approach

Improvements in prehospital care in concert with aggressive resuscitation and management of hemorrhagic shock have reduced the early mortality associated with severe intra-abdominal injuries. Patients who in the past would not have survived their initial insult now survive only to experience a prolonged ICU course complicated by intra-abdominal sepsis, multiple organ failure, and late mortality.

Successful management of the trauma patient requires balancing the competing priorities of prompt hemorrhage control with control of peritoneal contamination. In the absence of severe derangements in physiology, both hemostasis and source control with definitive reconstruction of the gastrointestinal tract may be performed at the time of initial laparotomy. However, in selected patients in whom the vicious cycle of coagulopathy, hypothermia, and acidosis threatens survival, definitive restoration of intestinal continuity may best be deferred to a subsequent operation. The operative strategy is therefore dependent on the location and extent of the injury, taking into consideration the physiologic status of the patient.

The general principles of source control for peritoneal contamination following trauma are no different than those that guide the management of non-traumatic perforations and include excluding, resecting, or closing the involved segment(s) of bowel. Thorough lavage of the peritoneal cavity to remove particulate debris and blood may lessen the risk of subsequent infection. Antimicrobial therapy must be administered as soon as possible following injury. In cases without established peritonitis, prolonged antimicrobial therapy is unwarranted as there is no difference in the rate of intra-abdominal infections in patients receiving 24 h versus 5 days of antimicrobial coverage [1].

Gastric and Small-Bowel Injury

Gastric injuries are most common in patients suffering penetrating injury. In patients with an anterior gastric injury, it is critical to evaluate the posterior gastric wall through the lesser sac to avoid missing a second injury. Additionally, injuries in the region of the gastroesophageal junction may be difficult to identify and typically require mobilization of the left triangular ligament. Most gastric injuries can be simply repaired in one or two layers. Lacerations in the region of the pylorus may be managed by incorporating a pyloroplasty in the repair. More extensive disruptions of the distal stomach and/or gastroduodenal junction may require resection with either a Billroth I or II reconstruction.

The management of traumatic small bowel perforations depends on both the mechanism and extent of injury. In general, wounds that involve less than 50% of the circumference of the bowel wall can be repaired primarily using a single or two-layer closure. Wounds involving more of the bowel wall generally require resection and anastomosis. This approach may be altered to some extent by the mechanism of injury. For example, wounds without significant tissue injury (e.g., stab wounds) can be readily repaired even if greater than 50% of the circumference is involved, as long as luminal compromise is unlikely. By contrast, there is typically more tissue injury following blunt trauma or firearm injury. In these settings resection and anastomosis is preferred. Additionally, the presence of several wounds in close proximity typically warrants a resection rather than repair.

Duodenal Injury

Duodenal injuries may be problematic because of the propensity for repairs to leak and their frequent coexistence with pancreatic and major vascular injuries. Any evidence of duodenal injury, including periduodenal hematoma, bile staining, or crepitus of the retroperitoneum mandates a thorough exploration of the duodenum. The entire duodenum can be exposed with a combination of an extensive Kocher maneuver and a Cattell-Braasch maneuver, or right medial visceral rotation. Not infrequently, it is necessary to mobilize the ligament of Treitz to access the distal third and proximal fourth part of the duodenum to allow a reliable assessment of the extent of injury. This extensive mobilization also limits tension on any subsequent duodenal repair.

The type of repair is governed largely by the mechanism and extent of injury and the interval between wounding and repair [2, 3] (Table 1). Most duodenal in-

Table 1. Classification scheme for duodenal injuries

	Mild	Severe
Mechanism	Stab wound	Gunshot wound or blunt
Extent	<75% of duodenal wall	≥75% of duodenal wall
Site	3rd, 4th part of duodenum	1st, 2nd part of duodenum
Interval to repair	<24 h	≥24 h
Associated injury	No CBD or pancreatic injury	Pancreatic or CBD injury

CBD, common bile duct.

juries may be managed using relatively straightforward surgical techniques. Simple injuries may be repaired primarily in two layers. These repairs are best buttressed using an omental patch. More complex injuries require considerable judgment and experience, particularly in the relatively immobile second portion of the duodenum. Extensive lateral defects can be managed using a side-to-end Roux-Y duodenojejunostomy or, if the defect is more extensive, an end-to-end duodenojejunostomy with oversewing of the distal duodenal stump. These and other severe injuries mandate exclusion of the duodenum from the passage of gastric secretions to protect the duodenal suture line and allow the repair to heal. The most frequently employed technique, referred to as pyloric exclusion, calls for closure of the pylorus through a gastrotomy using an absorbable suture, along with creation of a gastrojejunostomy. Pyloric patency is reestablished once the sutures resorb, thus accomplishing a method of temporary diversion that allows for subsequent restoration of normal gastrointestinal physiology. Pancreatico-duodenectomy for source control is rarely required and should only be considered in cases where the ampulla is involved or in the face of unreconstructable injuries to the duodenum and the head of the pancreas.

Duodenal fistulae are not uncommon following duodenal repairs, particularly when the injury is complex. For this reason most surgeons routinely place closed-suction drains. Similarly, a feeding jejunostomy may simplify management in the later postoperative setting.

In critically injured patients with multiple coexisting injuries or in the face of hypothermia, coagulopathy or acidosis, complex reconstructions should not be attempted at the initial laparotomy. In these settings, temporary source control by oversewing, stapling, or draining the injury may be lifesaving. Definitive repairs may then be accomplished over the next 24-72 h.

Colonic Injuries

Source control for colonic injuries has changed dramatically over the past decade, particularly for penetrating trauma. There is now clear evidence that primary repair without colostomy is the preferred course of management for patients with nondestructive intraperitoneal penetrating colon injuries [4]. In this subset of patients, the lower morbidity, low incidence of intra-abdominal septic complications and the lower cost, coupled with avoidance of the stigma of a colostomy have set a new standard of care for these injuries (Table 2). By contrast, the management of patients with destructive colonic injuries requiring resection is less clear. Many trauma surgeons elect to perform resection with primary anastomosis in very select clinical settings. Our practice is to limit this approach to patients who would require an ileocolonic anastomosis to restore continuity. Patients with injuries to the left of the middle colic vessels who would require a colocolonic anastomosis might be better served with a resection and colostomy.

Table 2. Evidence-based guidelines for the management of penetrating intraperitoneal colon injuries (from [4])

Clinical setting	Guidelines for method of source control	Level of recommendation[a]
Nondestructive colon wound (< 50% circumference of colon without devascularization) and no peritonitis	Primary repair	Level 1

Destructive colon wounds (> 50% circumference of colon or devascularization of a segment) if:
  No history of shock
  No significant underlying disease
  Minimal or no associated injuries
  No peritonitis
	Colon resection and primary anastomoses	Level 2

Destructive colon wounds with any of above factors present	Colon resection and colostomy	Level 2

[a] Level 1 recommendations are based on prospective randomized trials. Level 2 recommendations are based on a combination of prospective and retrospective data along with expert opinion.

Rectal Injury

Traditionally, rectal injuries have been treated with repair, proximal diversion, irrigation of the rectal stump, and in the case of extraperitoneal injuries, presacral drainage. Recently, all of these tenets have been challenged. Wounds of the intraperitoneal rectum with little loss of the rectal wall may be managed with primary repair in a similar fashion to intraperitoneal colon injuries. More extensive injuries typically require rectal resection in the form of a Hartmann procedure. Extraperitoneal injuries typically require a diverting colostomy for source control. Direct repair of these injuries may not be possible and attempts should not be made to do so if extensive dissection is necessary. Routine adjunctive maneuvers to control ongoing contamination, including distal rectal washout and presacral drainage remain controversial and may be of value only in select circumstances (see "Controversies") [5].

Source Control in the Context of Damage Control

Over the past decade, the concept of abbreviated laparotomy for damage control has evolved. In patients who arrive in extremis, it is now recognized that prolonged attempts at achieving definitive management of major vascular, solid organ, or hollow viscus injuries may be detrimental and potentially lethal. In this critically ill subset of patients, the goals of initial laparotomy should be limited to achieving hemostasis, controlling ongoing peritoneal contamination, and providing a mechanism of temporary abdominal closure. Definitive management of injuries may be attempted at staged, repeat laparotomies once the profound phy-siologic derangements have been corrected in the intensive care unit. There are no established criteria for the determination of the need to "bail-out" of the in-itial laparotomy, but suggested parameters include early significant blood loss, systolic blood pressure under 70 mmHg, arterial pH less than 7.25, core tempe-rature lower than 34°C and severe, multisystem injury [6,7]. Regardless of the cri-teria used to determine the need to perform an abbreviated laparotomy, it is clear that the decision to terminate the laparotomy must be made early in order to optimize the chance for survival.

In these patients, simply oversewing the bowel injury or ligating the bowel proximal and distal to the injury using an umbilical tape or stapling device [6,8] should achieve initial control of peritoneal contamination. Resection may or may not be carried out at the initial laparotomy, depending on the anticipated time required for its completion and the physiologic status of the patient. Blind loops of bowel are generally not left more than 72 h before definitive diversion or re-storation of gastrointestinal continuity. While exteriorization of the intestine at the original laparotomy may appear to be a reasonable option, this approach should be avoided to allow for early termination of the laparotomy and to avoid retraction of the ostomy with increased abdominal wall edema. For biliary tract and pancreatic injuries, external tube drainage may be performed. Reconstruc-tion should not be attempted until the patient has undergone resuscitation in the intensive care unit and all metabolic derangements have reversed.

Controversies

Scheduled Relaparotomy in Circumstances Other Than Damage Control

There is a subset of patients with massive peritoneal contamination following multiple gunshot wounds or close-range abdominal shotgun wounds in whom the probability of a missed hollow viscus injury or subsequent intra-abdominal infection is significant. In these circumstances there may be some merit in per-forming a planned relaparotomy at 48-72 h following injury. In addition to pro-viding a second opportunity to evaluate for missed injuries and to remove any particulate debris and/or hematoma, this second-look laparotomy allows the surgeon to limit the development of loculated fluid collections and deal with ear-ly abscess formation. The advantages of this approach have never been evaluated in a prospective fashion and probably will never be assessed formally because of the rare circumstances in which it may offer benefit. However, many feel the mor-bidity of early relaparotomy is low and the potential for benefit is great.

Stapled Versus Hand-Sewn Anastomoses

In elective general surgery, there appears to be no difference in the risk of ana-stomotic dehiscence or abscess formation in patients undergoing stapled vs hand-sewn anastomoses. Whether these two techniques are similar in the trauma patient is unclear. The extensive visceral edema seen at laparotomy in trauma patients may increase the risk of anastomotic failure in patients undergoing stapled anastomoses as the staples and the stapling techniques were designed for relatively normal bowel. One retrospective cohort study in which the risk of anastomotic complications was compared in patients undergoing stapled vs hand-sewn anastomoses suggested a greater risk of postoperative intra-abdominal septic complications in the former group [9]. However, this analysis did not differentiate between small and large bowel injuries, nor did it control for the surgeon or the specific technique utilized for hand-sewn anastomoses. A subsequent retrospective analysis limited to small bowel injuries demonstrated no difference in outcome in either cohort of patients [10]. Similar to the first report, this analysis did not control for potential confounders that may place a patient at risk for subsequent infection. Specifically, hollow viscus injuries tend to be repaired using a hand-sewn technique when there are few associated injuries and the element of time is not critical. Obviously, these patients are at particularly low risk for anastomotic failure, thus biasing any retrospective analysis.

Distal Rectal Irrigation and Presacral Drainage Following Penetrating Rectal Injury

There are four main management considerations following rectal injuries, including:
a) Fecal diversion
b) Repair of the rectal injury when possible
c) Presacral drainage
d) Distal rectal irrigation

Although there is no consensus on the routine application of any of these adjunctive procedures, presacral drainage and distal rectal irrigation remain the most controversial. Enthusiasm for routine presacral drainage and rectal irrigation originated from the morbidity associated with high-velocity missile injuries during military conflict. The lower velocity injuries and consequent lesser degrees of tissue injury associated with civilian trauma have led to a reevaluation of this dogma.

The principal underlying distal rectal washout is that by reducing the fecal (and thus bacterial) load in the rectal stump, the incidence of infectious complications would be reduced. One potential disadvantage to this approach is that forced irrigation of luminal contents into the perirectal tissues may increase the risk of pelvic sepsis. There are no prospective data evaluating the merits of routine distal rectal washout for penetrating rectal injuries. In recent retrospective studies limited by small sample size, there appears to be no significant benefit to routine irrigation [11]. As a result, many trauma surgeons have abandoned this practice [12].

The value of routine presacral drainage for extraperitoneal rectal injuries remains even more controversial. A single, small (48 patients) prospective randomized study evaluating presacral drainage demonstrated no difference in the rate of infectious complications in patients undergoing presacral drainage [13]. However, others suggest that presacral drainage may offer benefit in select clinical circumstances, including patients with high velocity missile injuries, significant rectal wall loss (or situations where repair cannot be accomplished), and associated genitourinary injuries [5].

Critical Factors and Decision Making

Although it is quite straightforward to present an algorithm for the management of source control based on purely anatomic criteria, it is now clear that the intra-

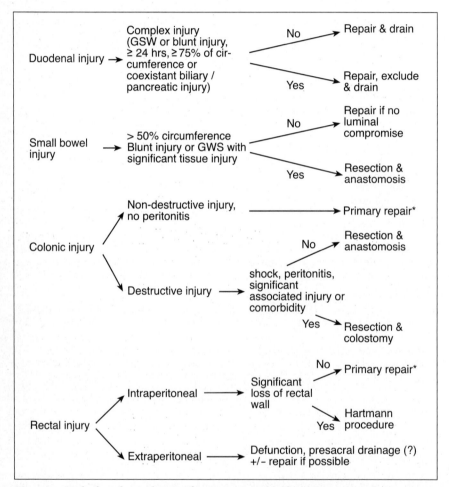

Diagram 1. Methods and consideration for source control in the trauma patient. An assessment of the physiologic status of the patient is critical to intraoperative decision making (see "Critical Factors and Decision Making"). *A colostomy is preferred in the face of peritonitis

operative decision-making and the sequelae of these decisions are based on factors other than the anatomic pattern of injury (Diagram 1). For example, it is evident that for patients with the same degree of anatomic injury, one may be at greater risk of suture-line dehiscence and subsequent intra-abdominal infection if there is greater physiologic derangement at the time of repair. It is also clear that early source control is of secondary importance to hemorrhage control. There is no point in completing a definitive repair of a duodenal injury in a patient succumbing from acidosis and hypothermia following repair of a complex caval injury. There are always solutions available for early source control in this context and these should be applied liberally to maximize early survival.

References

1. Luchette FA, Borzotta AP, Croce MA, O'Neill PA (2000) Practice management guidelines for prophylactic antibiotic use in penetrating abdominal trauma. J Trauma 48:508–518
   Evidence-based review of antimicrobial therapy in patients with penetrating abdominal trauma.
2. Velmahos GC, Kamel E, Chan LS, Hanpeter D, Asensio JA, Murray JA, et al (1999) Complex repair for the management of duodenal injuries. Am Surg 65:972–975
   A retrospective case series of contemporary management of duodenal injuries in a level I trauma center.
3. Degiannis E, Boffard K (2000) Duodenal injuries. Br J Surg 87:1473–1479
   An excellent review of the classification and management options for duodenal injuries.
4. Pasquale M, Fabian TC (1998) Practice management guidelines for trauma from the Eastern Association for the Surgery of Trauma. J Trauma 144:941–957
   Evidence-based guidelines for the management of penetrating colon injuries. Updated at www.east.org.
5. Morken JJ, Kraatz JJ, Balcos EG, Hill MJ, Ney AL, West MA, et al (1999) Civilian rectal trauma: a changing perspective. Surgery 126:693–700
   Retrospective review of rectal injuries, concluding that management should be tailored based on the severity and pattern of injury.
6. Carillo C, Fogler RJ, Shaftan GW (1993) Delayed gastrointestinal reconstruction following massive abdominal trauma. J Trauma 34:233–235
   Summarizes management of gastrointestinal injuries in the context of damage control.
7. Eddy VA, Morris JA Jr, Cullinane DC (2000) Hypothermia, coagulopathy, and acidosis. Surg Clin North Am 80:845–854
   A review of the underlying concepts behind damage control in the trauma patient.
8. Hirshberg A, Walden R (1997) Damage control for abdominal trauma. Surg Clin North Am 77:813–820
   Description of damage control as applied to abdominal trauma; specifically describes methods of controlling abdominal spillage and peritoneal contamination.
9. Brundage SI, Jurkovich GJ, Grossman DC, Tong WC, Mack CD, Maier RV (1999) Stapled versus sutured gastrointestinal anastomoses in the trauma patient. J Trauma 47:500–507
   A retrospective review of stapled versus hand-sewn anastomoses in the trauma setting. Demonstrates an increased leakage rate in patients undergoing stapled anastomoses.
10. Witzke JD, Kraatz JJ, Morken JM, Ney AL, West MA, Van Camp JM, et al (2000) Stapled versus hand sewn anastomoses in patients with small bowel injury: a changing perspective. J Trauma 49:660–665
    Retrospective review of small bowel injuries requiring resection demonstrated no significant difference in the rate of complications between hand-sewn and stapled techniques.
11. McGrath V, Fabian TC, Croce MA, Minard G, Pritchard FE (1998) Rectal trauma: management based on anatomic distinctions. Am Surg 64:1136–1141
    Contemporary case series of the management of rectal trauma. Addresses issues of presacral drainage and distal washout.

12. Velmahos GC, Gomez H, Falabella A, Demetriades D (2000) Operative management of civi-
    lian rectal gunshot wounds: simpler is better. World J Surg 24:114–118
    A retrospective case series of the contemporary management of rectal injuries.
13. Gonzales RP, Falimirski ME, Holevar MR (1998) The role of presacral drainage in the mana-
    gement of penetrating rectal injuries. J Trauma 45:656–661
    A small, randomized controlled trial of presacral drainage in patients with penetrating extra-
    peritoneal rectal injuries. Demonstrates that presacral drainage offers no benefit.

Invited Commentary

ERIC R. FRYKBERG

Source control in trauma is a very important issue, because infection remains a
major cause of postinjury morbidity and mortality [1]. All of the issues discussed in this chapter are appropriate considerations in controlling infection in this
setting. Several deserve emphasis and further clarification, and other issues merit mention.

Damage Control

As asserted by Dr. Kao and Dr. Nathens, prompt control of hemorrhage and
wound contamination remains the most basic and important factor in source
control following trauma. This must be accomplished by rapid diagnosis of
injury so as to remove contamination before infection becomes established.
Minimizing surgery in severely injured patients through damage control is critical.
This is true not only in the abdomen, but in any open wound of the body, especially
those associated with fractures and open body cavities, (i.e., extremity fractures,
open skull wounds with dural penetration, open chest wounds).

Source Control and "Toilet"

Spillage of enteric contents into the abdomen should be controlled immediately
by clamping proximal and distal to bowel injuries, especially in the colon. Prompt
resection of devitalized tissue also reduces bacterial contamination, thus reducing the risk of intra-abdominal infections. Many advocate large-volume peritoneal irrigation as a means of reducing the bacterial load. However, this strategy
is not supported by any degree of evidence. In fact, there is reason to suspect that
excessive irrigation, beyond that necessary to facilitate removal of gross debris,
may actually be harmful, by impairing the host defenses of the peritoneum.

Avoid Immunosuppression

The control of hemorrhage is important not only as a life-saving maneuver, but also because of the immunosuppressive effects of hemorrhage, transfusions, and shock, all of which directly increase the risk of infection. Splenectomy exacerbates this risk, suggesting that splenic salvage also may be an important method of source control [2, 3]. Antibiotics alone cannot reduce this immunosuppressive risk to any significant degree. However, immune enhancers, such as granulocyte colony stimulating factor and interferon gamma, have shown experimental promise and may contribute to source control in clinical settings in the near future.

Foreign Bodies

It is important to find and remove foreign bodies and exogenous debris from all wounds, as they serve as a potent nidus of infection. Examples include dirt, bits of clothing tracked in by a bullet, and shotgun shell wadding. Studies have shown that bullets which have traversed an obviously contaminated area, such as the unprepped colon, significantly increase the risk of an abscess if not removed [5].

Drains

Drains have been used extensively in past years with the belief that they reduce infection by evacuating fluid collections. However, recent data show that drains generally at best make no difference, and may actually increase infection risk. There are select indications for the use of drains, but they should be used sparingly and should only be of the closed-suction type [6].

Colostomy for Pelvic-Perineal Injury?

Another controversial issue is the use of routine fecal diversion for open pelvic fractures. The need for diverting colostomy for severe extraperitoneal rectal injuries is not disputed. Several small retrospective studies in the past indicated that routine colostomy is necessary as well in open pelvic fractures even in the absence of rectal injury. However, more recent data indicate this is not true [7]. As long as these open wounds are accessible for aggressive debridement and cleansing, routine fecal diversion does not appear necessary. This allows avoidance of an otherwise unnecessary open operation on the abdomen, which may actually extend contamination and increase the risk of infection.

Antibiotics

The role and dosing of prophylactic antibiotics is plagued by misperceptions and wide variations in practice. The data are clear that only a short course of antibiotics, of less than 24 h, is necessary for maximal infection prophylaxis in abdominal trauma, as well as in open fractures [8, 9]. This is true regardless of the degree of contamination, as long as contamination has not been present for more than 12 h (after which time it is generally agreed that infection should be assumed and a therapeutic rather than a prophylactic regimen of antibiotics should be initiated). In fact, there is little credible evidence that antibiotics have any role at all in preventing intra-abdominal infection, as most efficacy has been shown only for wound infection [9]. Antibiotics cannot substitute for proper wound management by the surgeon. Attention should be paid to proper antibiotic dosing in trauma patients. A single perioperative dose may not suffice in cases of severe hemorrhage or shock, as blood levels may wash out more quickly than normal and bioavailability is altered. Increased doses and frequency of antibiotics should be considered in this setting [9].

We must realize that there is no magic potion for source control following trauma. Antibiotics, drains, massive irrigation, and colostomy all play limited and secondary roles.

References

1. Dellinger EP, Oreskovich MR, Wertz MJ, Hamaski V, Lenard ES (1984) Risk of infection following laparotomy for penetrating abdominal injury. Arch Surg 9:20–27
2. Blackwood JM, Hurd T, Suval W, Machiedo GW (1988) Intra-abdominal infection following combined spleen-colon trauma. Am Surg 54:212–216
3. Duke BJ, Modin GW, Schechter WP, Horn JK (1993) Transfusion significantly increases the risk for infection after splenic injury. Arch Surg 128:1125–1132
4. Croce MA, Fagian TC, Patton JH et al (1998) Impact of stomach and colon injuries on intra-abdominal abscess and the synergistic effect of hemorrhage and associated injury. J Trauma 45:649–655
5. Poret HA, Fabian TC, Croce MA, Bynoe RP, Kusk KA (1991) Analysis of septic morbidity following gunshot wounds to the colon: the missile is an adjuvant for abscess. J Trauma 31:1088–1095
6. Fabian TC (1992) Prevention of infections following penetrating abdominal trauma. Am J Surg 165 (Suppl):14S–19S
7. Woods RK, O'Keefe G, Rhee P, Routt ML, Maier RV (1998) Open pelvic fracture and fecal diversion. Arch Surg 133:281–286
8. Dellinger EP, Caplan ES, Weaver LD et al (1988) Duration of preventive antibiotic administration for open extremity fractures. Arch Surg 123:333–339
9. Luchette FA, Borzotta AP, Croce MA et al (2000) Practice management guidelines for prophylactic antibiotic use in penetrating abdominal trauma: the EAST practice management guidelines work group. J Trauma 48:508–518

Editorial Comment

The commandments of source control in trauma are elegantly articulated here by Drs. Kao and Nathens and commentator Frykberg:

- Achieve hemostasis before source control.
- Do the minimum in the unstable patient and come back later.
- Avoid fancy reconstructions.
- Ostomies are rarely indicated but should be performed when indicated.
- Drains are usually useless foreign bodies.
- Intestinal injury represents contamination rather than infection: a course of antibiotics longer than 24 h is seldom indicated.
- Avoid missed injuries: the number of holes in the GI tract must be paired, because an unpaired number raises the probability of a missed injury. Although it is possible to have a "tangential" penetration or to have the missile lodge inside the bowel, this is less common then a missed injury. The trajectory of the wounding missile (e.g., sequence of injured organs) should make sense. One must be able to construct a logical mental picture of the bullet trajectory; if the trajectory is noncontinuous or nonlinear a missed injury must be suspected.

33 The Burn Wound

Annmarie L. Dunican, William G. Cioffi

Key Principles

- Important risk factors for the development of burn wound infection include patient age, comorbidities, and extent of the burn.
- Burn wound sepsis is prevented through use of topical antimicrobials, early excision of the burn eschar and barrier isolation precautions.
- Differentiation between wound colonization and invasive infection can be made by biopsy of the burn wound.
- Treatment of burn wound infection entails use of subeschar clysis and excision of the burn wound.
- Nosocomial infections in burn patients include pneumonia, urinary tract infections, and suppurative thrombophlebitis.

Management of the burn wound poses a unique challenge for the surgeon. The skin serves an important function as a mechanical barrier to microbial invasion. Disruption by burn injury results in loss of this barrier function. The burn eschar, which consists predominantly of coagulated proteins, does not provide sufficient barrier to microbial colonization, invasion and infection. Rather it may serve as a medium for bacterial growth [1]. The local release of inflammatory mediators coupled with protein accumulation in the burn wound, local tissue hypoxia, and ischemia all contribute to the propensity for the development of local infection. As a consequence of the effects of local mediator release, burn wound infection was a common occurrence as recently as the 1960's and was associated with significant morbidity and mortality.

While burn wound specific factors increase the risk of an infection in the thermally injured patient, defects in systemic immunity also play a role in lowering resistance to infection. The alterations in host immunity include altered cell mediated immunity as well as decreased responsiveness of circulating neutrophils [2, 3]. The changes in the burn wound coupled with systemic immunosuppression predispose the burn patient to infection-related complications. Understanding the factors that lead to burn wound infection and taking appropriate steps to prevent it are critical to the successful management of these patients.

Risk Factors for Burn Wound Infection

Patient age is an important factor in the development of burn wound infection. Invasive infection occurs most commonly in children and the elderly; it occurs least commonly in young adults. The propensity to develop burn wound infection at the extremes of age is related to patient comorbidities, depth of burn injury, and the likelihood of more severe systemic immunosuppression [4]. Burn wound depth tends to be greater at the extremes of age as a consequence of skin thickness: skin is thinnest in children, and becomes progressively thicker until approximately the fourth decade of life. While partial thickness burn wounds rarely develop invasive infection, the likelihood of invasive infection increases as burn wound depth increases. One of the most important risk factors in the development of burn wound infection is the extent of burn. Simply stated, larger burns are more likely to develop invasive infection. Factors responsible for this include delayed closure of large burns due to the unavailability of autograft skin, increased immunosuppression, and the increased likelihood that mechanical ventilatory support is required [5-7]. In addition, delay in burn wound excision results in an increased likelihood of colonization of the burn wound by resistant organisms and opportunistic pathogens. The development of biologic dressings and the increased use of allograft allows for early excision of the burn wound and protection of the excised area.

Prevention of Burn Wound Sepsis

The three most critical advances leading to a decrease in the incidence of burn wound infection are improved local wound care, the employment of rigid infection control policies, and the early surgical removal of the burned tissue. Topical application of antimicrobials has helped to reduce the incidence of burn wound sepsis by reducing burn wound microbial colonization. Prior to the development of adequate topical therapy, systemic sepsis was a cause of death in approximately 60% of burn patients who succumbed to their injury [8]. The development and liberal use of topical agents such as mafenide acetate, 0.5% silver nitrate, and silver sulfadiazine resulted in a significant reduction of burn wound sepsis as a cause of death in thermally injured patients. In addition, early surgical excision and closure of the burn wound further reduced the incidence of burn wound infection and subsequent mortality so that in the year 2000, burn wound sepsis was responsible for only 6% of deaths from thermal injury [9].

The development of strict infection control policies centered around burn patient isolation resulted in delayed colonization of the burn wound and represents another important factor in the declining incidence of burn wound infection. Exposure to exogenous bacteria and prevention of cross-contamination of burn wounds with virulent bacteria is easily accomplished by enforcement of hand washing and barrier precautions. The use of isolation techniques has contributed to a decrease in the incidence of Gram-negative bacteremia from 31% to 12% and to an associated reduction in mortality [10]. Such techniques obviously will not prevent colonization by endogenous flora. Although the use of individual isolation rooms for severely burned patients is now common, shared areas such as burn showers and treatment rooms require thorough cleansing between patient use.

The flora which colonizes the burn wound, follows a fairly predictable pattern. Early in the postinjury period, the flora of the wound consists predominantly of

Gram-positive organisms. These organisms typically originate from the thermally injured skin or from hair follicles or sweat glands from the adjacent uninvolved skin. *Staphylococcus* is the most common Gram-positive organism recovered from burn wounds in this period and is typically sensitive to methicillin. By the end of the first postburn week, Gram-negative organisms are more commonly recovered from the wound. Gram-negative organisms have unique properties that contribute to their increased virulence compared to Gram-positive organisms. These include the elaboration of exotoxins and extracellular polysaccharides, the elaboration of endotoxin, and organism motility. *Pseudomonas*, a typical Gram-negative organism causing burn wound infection, is the offending organism in up to 25% of burn wound infections [11]. The incidence of invasive bacterial wound infections has dropped to less than 4% and occurs less frequently than invasive fungal wound infections [12]. While *Candida albicans* is the most common nonbacterial organism recovered from burn wounds, it has little invasive potential and is not a common cause of burn wound infection [13]. True fungi such as *Aspergillus* are more likely to be responsible for invasive burn wound infection. In some series, invasive infections caused by these fungi are responsible for mortality rates up to 74%, likely related to extensive burn size; they are found in 47% of patients with associated inhalation injury [12].

Differentiation Between Wound Colonization and Invasive Infection

Burn wound infection may be classified into three categories: cellulitis, impetigo, and invasive infection. Pain, tenderness, and erythema characterize cellulitis, which may be the result of burn wound infection or simply of the release of inflammatory cytokines within the wound. Progressive erythema with associated lymphangitis should prompt treatment with antibiotics directed at Gram-positive organisms. Impetigo is an infection that occurs in a re-epithelialized surface such as the previously grafted burn wound, a healed donor site, or a partial thickness burn wound which has healed primarily. It typically begins as a small ulceration or a superficial abscess and is not usually associated with systemic signs of infection such as fever and leukocytosis. Gram-positive organisms such as *Staphylococcus* are the common causative bacteria and treatment consists of local wound care and topical antimicrobial application. Invasive burn wound infection must be differentiated from burn wound colonization. The presence of bacteria within the burn wound is not indicative of burn invasive infection. Invasive infection is defined as bacteria within viable tissue beneath the burn wound eschar. Typical clinical changes signifying potential burn wound infection include burn wound appearance changes outlined in Table 1. Since these changes can occur very rapidly, twice-daily assessment of the burn wound by the burn team is essential. Although the diagnosis of burn wound infection is more likely when the bacterial density exceeds 10^5 colony-forming units, quantitative cultures of the burn wound do not always correlate with histologic findings of a burn wound biopsy [14]. Although surface cultures of the burn wound may aid in the selection of systemic antibiotics, they are not useful in making the diagnosis of

Table 1. Local signs of invasive burn wound infection

Dark brown, black, or purple discoloration of the wound
Conversion of partial thickness injury to full thickness necrosis
Subcutaneous tissue with hemorrhagic discoloration
Edema and dark discoloration of unburned skin at wound margin
Rapid sloughing/separation of the eschar
Pyocyanotic appearance of subeschar tissue
Black or purple discoloration in unburned tissue (ecthyma gangrenosum)

invasive burn wound infection. The most reliable mechanism to diagnose invasive burn wound infection is a biopsy of the wound with subsequent histologic evaluation. The definitive histologic findings of an invasive burn wound infection include the presence of bacteria or fungi at the interface between viable and nonviable tissue or within the viable tissue beneath the burn wound eschar. Other characteristics include small vessel thrombosis, marked inflammatory changes, and ischemic necrosis of unburned tissue. A negative burn wound biopsy in a patient with systemic signs of sepsis should lead to prompt evaluation for other sources of infection. Although false-negative biopsies are rare, reasons for failure include sampling from an area that is not infected, improper preparation of the tissue, or misinterpretation of the histologic findings. Strong clinical suspicion in the face of a negative histologic evaluation should prompt repeat biopsy.

Treatment of Burn Wound Infection

When invasive burn wound infection is diagnosed, systemic antibiotics should be started immediately. Broad-spectrum antibiotics that provide suitable coverage against Gram-negative organisms to include *Pseudomonas* should be initiated. Antibiotic choice can be tailored based on culture results but one should not wait for culture results to initiate treatment.

Surgical excision of the infected wound is the mainstay of therapy and should follow subeschar antibiotic clysis of the infected burn tissue [15]. Suitable antibiotics for clysis include semisynthetic penicillins that have broad Gram-negative activity. After debridement of the infected tissue, topical wound care with either 0.5% silver nitrate or 5% mafenide acetate soaks should be performed and the patient returned to the operating room at 24-48 h for further debridement. When all infected tissue has been removed, the patient's excised area should be covered with either a biologic dressing or a skin graft.

Nosocomial Infections in Burn Patients

Despite a significant decrease in mortality from burn wound sepsis, infection-related complications remain the most common cause of morbidity and mortality in thermally injured patients. Pneumonia has replaced burn wound infection as

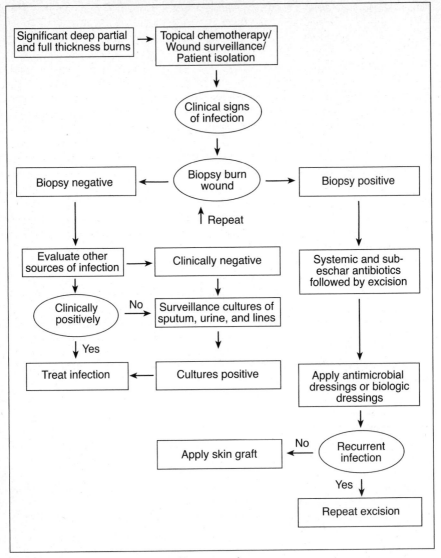

Diagram 1. Algorithm for treatment of burn wounds

the most frequently diagnosed infection following thermal injury. Prior to the development of adequate topical chemotherapy, the broad use of burn wound excision and the initiation of strict infection-control policies, pneumonia typically resulted from hematogenous spread of infection from the burn wound. Today, hematogenous pneumonia is uncommon and most affected patients develop bronchopneumonia from airborne bacteria [16]. With this shift from hematogenous to bronchopneumonia, the causative organisms have also changed. Gram-positive organisms such as *Staphylococcus* have replaced Gram-negative organisms such as *Pseudomonas* as the most commonly isolated bacteria from the airway of burn patients with pneumonia. Age, burn size, and the presence of inhalation injury are the most common predisposing factors for the development of pneumonia [17]. Clinical suspicion of respiratory infection should lead the clinician to obtain a chest X-ray and a sputum sample for Gram stain and culture. The presence of white cells in the sputum in combination with a predominant single organism, in a clinical setting which includes bronchorrhea, fever, and an elevated white blood cell count, and an infiltrate on the chest roentgenogram should lead to the initiation of empiric antibiotics that cover the predominant organisms found in the burn unit. Suppurative thrombophlebitis has become an uncommon infection in burn patients as control of burn wound colonization has occurred. In addition, a policy mandating frequent catheter changes has resulted in a decrease in the incidence of suppurative thrombophlebitis from 6.9% in 1970 to less than 1% in burn patients in 1990 [16]. Urinary tract infections occur frequently in these patients because of a need for long-term indwelling catheter use. Patients with obvious clinical signs of infection should have urine cultures obtained and treatment tailored appropriately.

The decrease of burn wound infection as a cause of morbidity and mortality in thermally injured patients is a true success story in infection source control. The factors responsible for the decreased incidence of burn wound infection include a delay in burn wound colonization following the use of topical antimicrobial agents, the initiation and strict adherence to infection control techniques, and most importantly, the use of surgical excision to promptly remove the burn wound.

References

1. Pruitt BA Jr, Moncrief JA (1967) Current trends in burn research. J Surg Res 7:280–293
2. Winkelstein AU (1984) What are the immunologic alterations induced by burn wound injury? J Trauma 24:S72–S83
3. Stein MD, Stevens JM, Herdon DN (1983) Defective neutrophil chemotaxis resulting from thermal injury. Clin Immunol Immunopathol 27:234–239
4. Pruitt BA Jr (1984) The diagnosis and treatment of infection in the burn patient. Burns 11:79–91
5. Pruitt BA Jr, Cioffi WG Jr (1995) Diagnosis and treatment of smoke inhalation. J Intens Care Med 10:117–127
6. Pruitt BA Jr, Mason AD Jr (1996) Epidemiological, demographic and outcome characteristics of burn injury. In: Herndon DN (ed) Total burn care. London, WB Saunders, pp 5–15
7. Munster AM (1984) Immunologic response of trauma and burns: an overview. Am J Med 76 (Suppl. 3A):142–145
8. Pruitt BA Jr, O'Neill JA Jr, Moncrief JA, Lindberg RB (1968) Successful control of burn wound sepsis. JAMA 203:1054–1056
9. Pruitt BA Jr (1999) The development of the international society for burn injuries and progress in burn care: the whole is greater than the sum of its parts. Burns 25:683–696
10. McManus AT, Mason AD, McManus WF, Pruitt BA (1994) A decade of reduced Gram-negative infections and mortality associated with improved isolation of burned patients. Arch Surg 129:1306–1309

11. Lesseva MI, Hadjiiski OG (1996) Staphylococcal infections in the Safia Burn Centre, Bulgaria. Burns 22:279–282
12. Becker WK, Cioffi WG Jr, McManus AT, Kim SH, McManus WF, Mason AD Jr, Pruitt BA Jr (1991) Fungal burn wound infection: a 10-year experience. Arch Surg 126:44–48
13. Bruck HS, Nash G, Stein JM, Lindberg RB (1972) Studies on the occurrence and significance of yeast and fungi in the burn wound. Ann Surg 176:108–110
14. McManus AT, Kim SH, McManus WF, Mason AD Jr, Pruitt BA Jr (1987) Comparison of quantitative microbiology and histopathology in divided burn wound biopsy specimens. Arch Surg 122:74–76
15. McManus WF, Goodwin CW Jr, Pruitt BA Jr (1983) Subeschar treatment of burn wound infection. Arch Surg 118:291–294
16. Pruitt BA Jr, McManus AT (1992) The changing epidemiology of infection in burn patients. World J Surg 16:57–67
17. Shirani KZ, Pruitt BA Jr, Mason AD Jr (1987) The influence of inhalation and pneumonia on burn mortality. Ann Surg 205:82–87

Invited Commentary

BASIL A. PRUITT JR.

The authors have provided a concise review of the current management of burn wound infections with special emphasis on the interaction between microorganisms and the patient. They have properly highlighted the central importance of prompt excision and closure of the burn wound to limit the duration of risk for development of invasive infections. A few points deserve expansion and emphasis.

Effective topical antimicrobial chemotherapy not only decreased the incidence of invasive burn wound sepsis, but also reduced the bacterial density of the burn wound to such an extent that wound manipulation-related bacteremia is uncommon in patients with burns of less than 40% of the body surface. Even in those patients with extensive burns, wound manipulation seldom evokes bacteremia before the 10th postburn day, which provides an expanded window of opportunity for burn wound excision unassociated with bacteremia.

The authors note that the histologic examination of a burn wound biopsy is the most accurate means of differentiating burn wound colonization from invasive burn wound infection and call attention to the unreliability of even quantitative cultures in making that differentiation. However, quantitative cultures yielding low bacterial counts, i.e., 10^4 or fewer organisms per gram of tissue, are consistent with the absence of invasive burn wound infection. If the histologic examination of successive wound biopsies reveals a progressive increase in bacterial density within the eschar and proliferation of organisms at the viable/nonviable tissue interface without evidence of invasive infection, the topical agent being used should be changed to mafenide acetate, which can penetrate the eschar and limit bacterial proliferation. Additionally, following excision of an infected burn wound, other areas of unexcised burn wounds should be treated with mafenide acetate burn cream to limit intraeschar bacterial proliferation. In the case of intraeschar fungal proliferation, clotrimazole cream should be applied twice daily as topical therapy.

The authors identify *Aspergillus* sp. as the most common cause of invasive fungal burn wound infection, but those organisms are slow to traverse fascial planes. The *Phycomycetes*, however, are aggressive invaders, which rapidly traverse fascial planes and readily invade the microvasculature of the affected tissue to cause thrombosis and necrosis. Acidosis predisposes burn patients to the development of phycomycotic infections and the rapid centrifugal extension of ischemic necrosis in the burn wound of an acidotic patient mandates immediate biopsy. Confirmation of phycomycotic invasion necessitates prompt institution of amphotericin B therapy, and a "wide-margin" excision of the infected tissue, which may require whole limb amputation if muscle compartments are involved.

A particular strength of the chapter is the algorithm developed by the authors, which serves as a road map for the diagnosis and treatment of burn wound infections. The current prevalence of nonbacterial invasive burn wound infections speaks for adding a recommendation for systemic administration of an antifungal agent prior to excision of such an infection. Additionally, systemic antibiotic or antifungal therapy should be continued following excision until one is certain that all infected tissue has been excised.

The authors cite the usefulness of the burn center microbial surveillance program in the selection of initial empiric antibiotic therapy for infections in burn patients. It should be noted, however, that the surveillance program also permits one to assess the effectiveness of infection control procedures, the emergence of resistant organisms, and temporal changes in the prevalence of infecting organisms. The authors report a prevalence of Gram-positive organisms as the causative agents of airborne pneumonia, but surveillance data in the past 2 years are consistent with a recrudescence of Gram-negative organisms as the cause of pulmonary infections. Although hematogenous pneumonia has been superseded by airborne pneumonia as the prevalent form of pneumonia, hematogenous pneumonia can still arise from an intravenous infection and infected burn wounds. The sudden appearance of the solitary rounded pulmonary infiltrate pathognomonic of hematogenous pneumonia should prompt a meticulous search for an area of burn wound infection or a focus of suppurative thrombophlebitis in previously cannulated veins.

The authors properly emphasize that infection remains the most common cause of death in extensively burned patients even though invasive burn wound sepsis has been "controlled" by current techniques of burn wound care. The frequency of life-threatening infections justifies a program of scheduled microbial surveillance for each burn center as well as a program of infection surveillance for each burn patient. Such programs facilitate identification of infections in their earliest stages and optimize initial therapy to achieve prompt control of the infections and thereby minimize infection-related morbidity and mortality.

34 Organ Transplant Patients

Tim Pruett

Key Principles

- Transplant recipients frequently have surgical infections, requiring prompt control of the graft/host interface. The decision to invoke an operative, interventional radiological or endoscopic approach is dependent upon patient factors. Control of the source of the infection is key to successful resolution.
- Superinfection or concomitant systemic viral or fungal infection is common.
- The patient's underlying comorbid diseases and nutrition are significant determinants of the successful management of surgical infection.
- Removal of the allograft and the cessation of immunosuppressive agents is rarely required, but remains an option which needs to be contemplated.

General Approach

Infections in organ transplant recipients are typically thought to be an amalgam of problems caused by uncommon viral, fungal, or poorly classified infectious agents. Although this patient population does have a disproportionate number of exotic infectious agents, the transplant recipient population has its share of typical surgical infections.

Each of the commonly transplanted organs has a peculiar predilection for infection. It will be the purpose of this review to summarize the clinical presentation and the options for therapy. As with most surgical infections, the key to management is decompression and control of the site proximal to the problem. A common theme in the etiology of many, but not all, posttransplant infections is that the source of the infection is often technical or ischemic in origin. Successful management therefore includes not only the control of the infected fluid, but also control of the leak (urine, bile, exocrine pancreas or air). In addition, if possible, management should be consistent with a long-term functioning allograft. As with most types of surgical infections, the use of appropriate antimicrobial therapy is desirable but rarely sufficient to treat the complication. Widespread use of broad spectrum antibacterial agents, in combination with steroids, the concomitant presence of diabetes, significant malnutrition, and the common use of invasive lines in this patient population predispose the transplant patient to fungal or yeast infections.

Significant decreases in immunosuppressive agents are typically not necessary. The development of clinical rejection can be problematic, however. Administration of bolus doses of steroids or antilymphocyte antibodies should be avoided in the face of serious infection. As the majority of the immunosuppressive agents do not significantly affect the innate immune system, significant adjustment of drugs is not felt to be necessary; however, leukopenia will necessitate modifications.

Clinical Signs and Symptoms

Although it is commonly taught that immunosuppression will mask deep infection, the transplant recipient with deep space infections typically presents with complaints of pain, nausea, fever, and wound drainage [1]. Leukocytosis is common. The typical transplant recipient has many comorbid diseases and is receiving numerous medications, all of which can confuse the diagnosis. Abdominal pain can be a consequence of mycophenolate mofetil ingestion, cytomegalovirus infection, or constipation associated with diabetic enteropathy after kidney or pancreas transplantation. It is important to gain an accurate, prompt diagnosis. Combinations of blood testing and imaging techniques can quickly identify the majority of deep infections in the transplant population. Radiographic sampling of fluid collections has become routine, with samples being assayed for the products of the transplanted organ (creatinine, bilirubin, amylase) as well as for cell count and culture for pathogens. Abnormally elevated levels of products from the allograft in intra-abdominal fluid collections demands a more precise evaluation regarding the source of the disruption.

Kidney Transplantation

Deep space infections directly related to the transplanted kidney are rare. The two most common causes of deep space fluid collections are lymphoceles and ureteral leaks. Infection of the former is uncommon in the absence of persistent or repetitive instrumentation. Lymphoceles usually are not clinically evident during the first 2 postoperative weeks. Definitive treatment of an uninfected lymphocele is intraperitoneal drainage [2], but when the lymphocele is infected, an extraserous catheter drainage system should be employed to evacuate the cavity: the inflammatory response to infection is effective in closing the lymphatic leak. Urine leaks from ureteral disruptions are especially problematic. The optimal approach is not the same for each patient. Operative intervention often yields the best long-term *functional* outcome, but for some patients, the price of wound complications, nutritional insult, and risk of death outweighs the potential benefits of operative control [3, 4]. In many instances, placement of a percutaneous nephrostomy across the anastomosis into the bladder provides effective control of the leak. Extraserous drainage of a urinoma is commonly necessary for resolution of the deep space infection. Late correction of strictures through operative, interventional radiographic or endourologic techniques all have their proponents.

Liver Transplantation

Intra-abdominal infections are relatively common after liver transplantation [5]. Sources for infection include biliary leaks or strictures, and gastrointestinal disruption from leakage of an intestinal anastomosis (Roux-en-Y) or damage to the bowel in the removal of the native liver. Occasionally bowel contamination at the time of operation or hematogenous spread of microorganisms to intraperitoneal fluid collections give rise to infection and result in an abscess without an obvious ongoing source. In the more common event of an ongoing source for postoperative infection, prompt identification and control of the contaminating focus is essential for successful resolution. Delayed diagnosis is associated with an increased likelihood of multiorgan dysfunction in a patient population with reduced physiologic reserve. *Candida* infections are common in the liver transplant population and the use of antifungal agents in reoperative or urgent transplant patients is a routine practice [6].

Intestinal sources typically require operative control in the form of suture closure, exteriorization, serosal patch, or rarely, in the severely adhesed abdomen, tube drainage. Biliary leakage is amenable to nonoperative control by either endoscopic retrograde cholangiopancreatography (ERCP) biliary stent placement or transhepatic biliary catheter placement [7-9]. It is often necessary to drain infected collections of fluid contiguous to the leak. Long-term management of biliary leaks or strictures is often a coordinated effort involving endoscopic or interventional radiographic stent placement and surgical control [10].

Pancreas Transplantation

Perioperative surgical site infection has been a significant problem for the pancreas recipient [11]. The pancreas has a proclivity for infection [12] from the associated duodenal stump closure, the duodenal anastomoses to the bladder or bowel, or from persistent graft pancreatitis and infection of the surrounding fat necrosis. Enteric drainage of the pancreas has received a renewed interest. In contrast to early experience that suggested a high likelihood of infection, it now appears that intra-abdominal infection and duodenal leaks are less frequent than with bladder drainage [13] Closure of the duodenal leaks either by direct suture or with a serosal patch, in combination with distal decompression, will usually control the leak and preserve function of the graft. Bacterial or fungal infection in association with significant early graft pancreatitis usually requires removal of the allograft in order to save the patient. Delaying graft pancreatectomy in the setting of suppurative peritonitis and pancreatitis is usually fatal for the patient [14].

Thoracic Transplantation

Sternal wound infection is a significant cause of morbidity for the heart transplant recipient. Infection is typically the consequence of contamination at the time of the procedure, in association with an underlying perfusion abnormality.

Prompt recognition, debridement, and the use of vascularized muscle flaps has reduced the associated mortality. In the early days of pulmonary transplantation, bronchial disruption with associated bronchopleural fistula was common. Surgical techniques have improved and its occurrence is now infrequent [15]. Management includes split bronchial ventilation, stenting, muscle flaps, and drainage.

Control of transplant infections is a race against time. The longer the complication exists, the greater the morbidity for the patient and the higher the risk of death. Because many transplant-associated infections arise at the operative site, persistence of infection can jeopardize the vascular anastomoses. Hemorrhage from anastomotic disruption or thrombosis of the graft may be the consequence of protracted infection and infection of vascular anastomoses [16, 17]. Evacuation of infected material and prevention of its reaccumulation by control of the source is crucial for successful resolution. Both contamination at the time of surgery and superinfection with either nosocomial pathogens (multidrug-resistant Gram-positive or Gram-negative organisms) pose difficult problems. Because of the potential range of infecting organisms, the use of broad-spectrum antimicrobial agents is commonplace. The use of these agents predisposes to the evolution of multiresistant bacterial flora and/or the development of yeast or fungal overgrowth. Early treatment with either amphotericin or the imidazole antifungals is warranted in this setting. Observation for secondary infection by imidazole-resistant yeast (*T. glabrata or C. crusei*) will allow for the prompt, effective use of amphotericin B [18, 19].

Controversies

The objective of therapy in transplant recipients is a live patient with a functioning allograft. Methods to achieve this goal are numerous and not standardized. A technique that works in one institution will not have equal applicability at another. Fortunately, the frequency of technical complications after organ transplantation has decreased over the past decade. Yet the risk of loss of graft is increased in patients who experience an operative site or intra-abdominal infection. As many infections in transplant patients arise from the graft/host interface, mechanisms to control the flow of urine, bile, or pancreatic exocrine secretions are key to long-term success. In the early days of transplantation, surgery was the only approach. Today endoscopic or percutaneous placement of nephrostomy or biliary drainage tubes will clarify anatomy and decompress and sometimes control the ureter or bile duct. Additional percutaneously placed catheters are necessary to drain intra-abdominal collections of fluid which are associated with a leak. Transient control, however, does not translate into good long-term results. Early operative intervention, if feasible, should be performed to minimize the risk of stricture, erosion of tubes into vessels, and infection from plugged catheters, in appropriate candidates. Unfortunately, not all patients are candidates for operative repair and if subjected to a major surgical procedure will suffer significant wound complications, bleeding, and superinfection, with an unforgiving debility.

Differentiation of the patient who would benefit from early operative intervention from the one who is best served by catheter drainage and percutaneous control is not clear. The literature suggests that the elderly, malnourished, and obese do less well than the young, lean recipient; but this is consistent with intuition. Better predictors of outcomes are needed.

Whether antifungal agents should be routinely employed following liver transplantation has been controversial [20]. Because the liver patient population has to wait longer for an allograft, they become more debilitated, increasing the likelihood of fungal infection. In recipients of other allografts, the isolation of fungal pathogens is uncommon. Awaiting culture confirmation of yeast infection prior to treatment is common practice. Imidazole agents such as fluconazole have few significant side effects and their use has increased dramatically. There is concern that extended administration will result in an increasing prevalence of resistant yeast forms. Amphotericin B is an agent to be used with caution in the transplant patient population, because of the ubiquitous impairment of renal function.

Critical Factors and Decision Making

Prompt, precise diagnosis is key to successful management of deep space infections in transplant patients. The integration of contrast and interventional radiographic techniques and endoscopic evaluation is the most commonly employed approach to complications of the biliary tree and ureter. To avoid protracted use of stents and drainage bags, one can make the case for operative correction when leaks occur within the first 2 weeks of transplantation in the young, otherwise healthy patient. When catheters are used for control of infected fluid and the flow of urine or bile, repetitive radiographic assessment is necessary until the leak and intra-abdominal fluid has been shown to be controlled. Whenever gastrointestinal disruption is seriously entertained, operative evaluation should be promptly employed.

As a general rule, samples from all deep space fluid collections should be sent for culture. These patients have typically been ill for some time and will often grow nosocomial pathogens in the first infectious event. The need for tailored antimicrobial therapy is great, because of the probability of multiresistant organisms.

References

1. Sawyer RG, Crabtree TD, Gleason TG, Antevil JL, Pruett TL (1999) Impact of solid organ transplantation and immunosuppression on fever, leukocytosis, and physiologic response during bacterial and fungal infections. Clin Transplant 13:260–265
2. Meyers A, Salant D, Rabkin R, Milne J, Botha R, Myburgh J (1976) Lymphocoeles in renal homograft recipients. Proc Eur Dial Transplant Assoc 112:452–60
3. Matalon TA, Thompson MJ, Patel SK, Ramos MV, Jensik SC, Merkel FK (1990) Percutaneous treatment of urine leaks in renal transplantation patients. Radiology 174:1049–1051

4. Smith TP, Hunter DW, Letourneau JG, Cragg AH, Darcy MD, Gastaneda-Zuniga WR, Amplatz K (1988) Urine leaks after renal transplantation: value of percutaneous pyelography and drainage for diagnosis and treatment. AJR 151:511–513

5. Busuttil RW, Shaked A, Millis JM, Jurim O, et al (1994) One thousand liver transplants. The lessons learned. Ann Surg 219:490–497; discussion 498–499

6. Patel R, Portela D, Bradley AD, Harmsen WS, Larson-Keller JJ, et al (1996) Risk factors of invasive Candida and non-Candida fungal infections after liver transplantation. Transplantation 62:926–934

7. Saab S, Martin P, Soliman GY, Machicado GA, Roth BE, Kunder G, et al (2000) Endoscopic management of biliary leaks after T-tube removal in liver transplant recipients: nasobiliary drainage versus biliary stenting. Liver Transpl 6:627–632

8. Pfau PR, Kochman ML, Lewis JD, Long WB, Lucey MR, Olthoff K, et al (2000) Endoscopic management of postoperative biliary complications in orthotopic liver transplantation. Gastrointest Endosc 52:55–63

9. Born P, Rosch T, Bruhl K, Sandschin W, Allescher HD, Frimberger E, Classen M (1999) Long-term results of endoscopic and percutaneous transhepatic treatment of benign biliary strictures. Endoscopy 31:725–731

10. Davidson BR, Rai R, Nandy A, Doctor N, Burrough A, Rolles K (2000) Results of choledochojejunostomy in the treatment of biliary complications after liver transplantation in the era of nonsurgical therapies. Liver Transpl 6:201–206

11. Ozaki CF, Stratta RJ, Taylor RJ, Langnas AN, Bynon JS, Shaw BW Jr (1992) Surgical complications in solitary pancreas and combined pancreas–kidney transplantations. Am J Surg 164:546–551

12. Humar A, Kandaswamy R, Drangstveit MB, Parr E, Gruessner AG, Sutherland DE (2000) Prolonged preservation increases surgical complications after pancreas transplants. Surgery 127:545–551

13. Firsch JD, Odorico JS, D'Allessandro AM, Knechtle SJ, Becker BN, Sollinger HW (1998) Post-transplant infection in enteric versus bladder-drained simultaneous pancreas-kidney transplant recipients. Transplantation 66:1746–1750

14. Humar A, Kandaswamy R, Granger D, Gruessner RW, Gruessner AC, Sutherland DE (2000) Decreased surgical risks of pancreas transplantation in the modern era. Ann Surg 231:269–275

15. Nunley DR, Grgurich WF, Keenan RJ, Dauber JH (1999) Empyema complicating successful lung transplantation. Chest 115:1312–1315.

16. Walsh TJ, Zachary JB, Hutchins GM, Sterioff S (1977) Mycotic aneurysm with recurrent sepsis complicating post-transplant nephrectomy. Johns Hopkins Med J 141:85–90

17. Calvino J, Romero R, Pintos E, Novoa D, Mardaras J, et al (1999) Renal artery rupture secondary to pretransplantation Candida contamination of the graft in two different recipients. Am J Kidney Dis 33:E3

18. Fortun J, Lopez-San Roman A, Velasco JJ, Sanchez-Sousa A, de Vicente E, et al (1997) Selection of Candida glabrata strains with reduced susceptibility to azoles in four liver transplant patients with invasive candidiasis. Eur J Clin Microbiol Infect Dis 16:314–318

19. Gleason TG, May AK, Caparelli D, Farr BM, Sawyer RG (1997) Emerging evidence of selection of fluconazole-tolerant fungi in surgical intensive care units. Arch Surg 132:1197–1202

20. Winston DJ, Pakrasi A, Busuttil RW (1999) Prophylactic fluconazole in liver transplant recipients. A randomized, double-blind, placebo-controlled trial. Ann Intern Med 131:729–737

Invited Commentary

Zakiyah Kadry, Pierre-Alain Clavien

Dr. Pruett provides a good general approach to the problem of infectious complications following transplantation. Key principles applicable to any solid organ transplant, including early aggressive investigation and treatment of infection, reduction of immunosuppressive therapy, correction of comorbid conditions and nutrition, along with early interventional or operative management of technical problems are emphasized early in the chapter.

The first 3 months following solid organ transplantation are a particularly critical period, because of the immunosuppressive regimen and the fact that technical problems relating to the transplant procedure are most likely to become manifest. The balance between acute rejection and overimmunosuppression is a particularly tenuous equilibrium and this is particularly evident when one examines the increased incidence of infectious complications in organ transplant patients requiring higher levels of immunosuppression such as recipients of intestinal allografts [1]. In the latter group of patients, bacterial translocation with loss of the intestinal barrier function during episodes of acute rejection is an additional predisposing factor to an infectious risk.

Dr. Pruett's chapter concentrates on typical surgical infections. However, the solid organ transplant recipient is more susceptible to certain forms of infection. Bacterial infections such as those associated with urinary tract infections, wound infections, technical complications such as biliary leaks or hepatic artery thrombosis, or sepsis caused by intravascular catheters tend to occur in the *first month*. Opportunistic infections such as cytomegalovirus occur most frequently after the first month following transplantation and often before 6 months have elapsed: a time period during which the patient is usually maximally immunosuppressed [2, 3]. After the first 6 months, patients are still at risk for opportunistic infections, as well as for infections caused by community-acquired bacterial pathogens [2,3]. *Viral infections* are an important cause of infection, both in the first 6 months and later following transplantation [2, 3].

The impact of fungal infections in solid organ transplant recipients is relatively underestimated in the chapter by Dr. Pruett. The incidence of fungal infection has been reported to be up to 5% in kidney allograft recipients, 10-35% in heart/lung recipients, 38% in pancreas recipients, 42% in liver recipients, and 33%-53% in small-bowel transplant recipients [4-6]. The high incidence in liver allograft recipients may reflect more than the longer waiting time and the state of debility of the patient. *Candida* is the predominant infectious agent [3] and colonization of the gastrointestinal tract by *Candida* has been reported to occur in up to 100% of potential liver allograft recipients [3-7], probably because of chronic liver disease necessitating multiple prior hospitalizations and antibiotic treatment for a variety of infections including spontaneous bacterial peritonitis. In 1994, Kusne et al. analyzed endoscopic samples at 7 alimentary tract locations in 30 randomly selected patients with advanced chronic liver disease undergoing a liver transplant evaluation [8]. Results of the analysis showed that 100% of the patients grew *Candida* in at least one site of the gastrointestinal tract, 50% in the duodenum. Most fungal infections in the liver transplant recipient tend to occur in the first 2 months after liver transplantation. Predisposing factors include disruption of the integrity of the biliary tract and intestine during the creation of a choledochojejunal anastomosis; however, additional risk for a clinically evident infection is associated with difficult or prolonged surgery, poor allograft function, retransplantation, and biliary leaks [6, 9, 10].

Dr. Pruett also does not touch on the subject of prophylaxis against prevalent infections that are not clinically significant before transplantation, for example, cytomegalovirus or bacterial colonization in lung transplantation for cystic fibrosis – which can become manifest in the postoperative period. The management principles of acute infection are, however, well emphasized. Although the therapeutic methods used to achieve the endpoint of a live patient and functioning allograft are not standardized between centers, the importance of early control of infection with antimicrobial therapy, aggressive radiological investigations and fluid/tissue sampling, and early correction of predisposing technical complications are clearly outlined.

References

1. The Intestinal Transplant Registry: http://www.lhsc.on.ca/itr/registry.htm
2. Flye WM (1989) Principles of organ transplantation: history of transplantation. WB Saunders Company, Philadelphia
3. Winston DI, Emmanouilides C, Busuttil RW (1995) Infections in liver transplant recipients. State of the art clinical article. Clin Infect Dis 21:1077–1091
4. Paya CV (1993) Fungal infections in solid organ transplantation. Clin Infect Dis 16:677–688
5. Hadley S, Karchmer AW (1995) Fungal infections in solid organ transplant recipients. Inf Dis Clin North Am 9:1045–1073
6. Tollemar JG (1998) Fungal infections in solid organ transplant recipients. In: Bowden RA, Ljungman P, Paya CV (eds) Transplant infections. Lippincott-Raven Publishers, Baltimore, pp 339–350
7. Collins LA, Samore MH, Roberts MS, Luzzati R, Jenkins RL, Lewis WD, Karchmer AW (1994) Risk factors for invasive fungal infections complicating orthotopic liver transplantation. J Infect Dis 170:644–652
8. Kusne S, Tobin D, Pasculle AW, Van Thiele DH, Ho M, Starzl TE (1994) Candida carriage in the alimentary tract of liver transplant candidates. Transplantation 57:398–402
9. Castaldo P, Stratta RJ, Wood RP, Markin RS, Patil KD, Schaefer Ms, Langnas AN, Reed EC, Li S, Pillen TJ, Shaw BW (1991) Fungal infections in liver transplant recipients: a multivariate analysis of risk factors. Transplant Proc23:1517–1519
10. Nieto-Rodriguez JA, Kusne S, Manez R, Irish W, Linden P, Magnone M, Wing EJ, Fung JJ, Starzl TE (1996) Factors associated with the development of candidemia and candidemia-related death among liver transplant recipients. Ann Surg 223:70–76

Editorial Comment

Although the transplant patient is at increased risk of infectious complications following transplantation, as emphasized by Dr. Pruett, these complications arise from the technical challenges of surgery more than from the effects of immunosuppression to prevent graft rejection. The typical infecting organisms are those that are isolated in critically ill patients and result from invasive monitoring devices and indiscriminate antibiotic use, rather than from systemic immunosuppression. Indeed, bacterial infection is largely controlled by innate immune mechanisms, including neutrophils and macrophages, and the integrity of these is not altered by antirejection medications that target the adaptive immune response.

35 Tertiary Peritonitis

ROBERT G. SAWYER

Key Principles

- The treatment of tertiary peritonitis involves a multidisciplinary approach requiring knowledge of gastrointestinal surgery, infectious diseases, critical care, nutrition, and radiology.
- As tertiary peritonitis progresses, the opportunity for aggressive open surgical intervention decreases and minimally invasive procedures are favored.
- The organisms associated with tertiary peritonitis are nosocomial in origin, often difficult to treat, but sometimes of unclear pathological relevance.
- Tertiary peritonitis is rarely cured rapidly and frequently requires long rehabilitation and secondary procedures weeks to months after initial presentation.

General Approach

The term tertiary peritonitis has been applied to describe recurrent infection of the peritoneal cavity after a prior episode of secondary peritonitis [1]. This entity encompasses a broad range of presentations, ranging from a pelvic abscess in an otherwise stable patient previously treated for a perforated appendix, to a desperately ill patient with ongoing infected necrotizing pancreatitis. Morbidity and mortality also vary based on the severity of the underlying pathology [2, 3]. Despite this, unifying themes in the diagnosis and management of tertiary peritonitis can be applied to all of these scenarios.

The diagnosis of tertiary peritonitis must be entertained in any patient previously treated for secondary peritonitis [4] whose recovery deviates from its expected course. The adequacy of the initial source control procedure must be kept in mind [5]. Although it is easy to identify recurrent infection in a patient with new onset fever, leukocytosis, hypotension, abdominal pain, and tenderness, most patients with tertiary peritonitis do not present with all of these signs and when they do, they are relatively late in their course. Any of these symptoms should make the surgeon think about further diagnostic testing, as should less obvious evidence of recurrent abdominal infection such as the new onset of food or tube feeding intolerance, ileus, or nausea and vomiting. In critically ill patients, other subtle signs include the need for increased ventilatory support, tachycardia, decreased urine output, hyperbilirubinemia, reduced tolerance of dialysis, hypothermia, or arrhythmias. Any of these conditions under the appropriate circumstances should trigger further diagnostic efforts.

Table 1. Characteristics of the last 129 cases of tertiary peritonitis at the University of Virginia (1996–2000)

Basic demography	Source	Initial source control procedure[a]	Treatment for tertiary peritonitis	Organisms	Mortality
Age	Esophagus, 0%	Drainage only, 30%	Drainage only, 67%	Gram (+): 77	All patients
50±1 years	Stomach/duodenum 16%	Repair/ patch, 20%	Repair/ patch, 8%	Gram (–): 40	25/129 (19%)
Gender	Pancreas, 21%	Diversion only, 2%	Diversion only, 5%	Fungi: 42	APACHE II ≤1(
70 M, 59 F	Small bowel, 22%	Resection, 38%	Resection, 15%		1/36 (3%)
APACHE II	Large bowel, 19%	Resect and divert, 7%	Resect and divert, 15%	C. albicans: 23	APACHE II 11–2
14.9±0.7< 3	Appendix, 2%	Antibiotics only, 3%	Antibiotics only, 4%	E. faecium: 21	4/65 (22%)
	Liver/biliary, 16%			E. faecalis: 19	APACHE II >2
	Kidney, 2%			E. coli: 11	10/28 (36%)
	Other, 3%			S. aureus: 9	

[a] Performed for presenting episode of tertiary peritonitis.

Tertiary peritonitis occurs in patients afflicted by secondary peritonitis (Table 1). Patients tend to present with a relatively high severity of illness (mean APACHE II score of 15). The most common original sites of infection are evenly distributed between stomach/duodenum, pancreas, liver and biliary tree, and small and large bowel, and tertiary peritonitis can develop after all methods of initial source control procedures for secondary peritonitis.

Abdominal Imaging

Computer tomographic (CT) scanning can reliably rule in or rule out a significant ongoing intra-abdominal infection. Blind re-exploration of the abdomen despite a negative CT scan is only rarely indicated. The CT scan provides several pieces of useful information:
- Free air more than 1 week after a prior intra-abdominal procedure frequently represents ongoing or new leakage from a hollow viscus.
- Abscesses of significant size are generally seen as rim-enhanced lesions.
- Fluid collections without the typical characteristics of an abscess can still be infected or indicate a leak; repositioning the patient may be necessary to determine whether or not the fluid is free-flowing and more likely benign.
- Visualization of extraluminal contrast material occasionally allows the localization of gastrointestinal (GI) leaks.
- The condition of the bowel itself, whether obstructed, edematous, ischemic, or normal can also be assessed.

Occasionally, ultrasound can substitute for CT scanning; although less sensitive and specific, it can be easily performed at the bedside in unstable patients. More specific localizing procedures such as an upper gastrointestinal series or fistulogram are helpful in certain cases.

Percutaneous Sampling

After a suspicious fluid collection is isolated, sampling should be performed under radiological guidance [6]. This procedure allows one to determine whether or not the fluid is infected and can provide information about the origin of any ongoing GI leaks. Fluid will routinely be sent for cell count, Gram stain and culture, and total bilirubin, amylase, and creatinine if biliary, pancreatic, or urinary fistulae are suspected. When patients are receiving, or recently have received antibiotics, care must be taken in interpreting negative culture results; significant numbers of bacteria on Gram stain or an elevated fluid white blood cell count may be sufficient to diagnose infection in the absence of viable pathogens.

Management Options

Once an active infection is diagnosed (frequently by immediate visual examination of aspirated fluid), several treatment options are possible. The first consideration is whether or not there is ongoing contamination from a hollow viscus. Operative management of a visceral leak includes repair, diversion, or resection combined with drainage of infected fluid. Not all leaks, however, require operation, and the placement of a drain to create a controlled fistula can often serve as successful temporizing therapy. The majority of patients can first be treated with a percutaneously placed drain (Table 1). In cases where a source control procedure is needed but a safe percutaneous route is not possible, surgical approaches that avoid contamination of the peritoneum, such as through the flank, should be considered.

Microbiology and Antibiotics

Culture data should be evaluated carefully, given the unpredictable nature of the pathogens involved (Table 1). Nosocomial organisms such as *C. albicans* and *Enterococcus* species are common, yet community-acquired organisms such as *E. coli* and *S. aureus* are also isolated [7]. We will frequently start broad-spectrum empiric therapy, for example, imipenem or piperacillin/tazobactam, and adjust the regimen on the basis of cultures. Although fungi are common isolates, we reserve empiric therapy with antifungal agents for cases involving the upper GI tract, and otherwise withhold treatment until after Gram stain and culture results return. The optimal duration of antibiotic therapy is unclear [8], since the infected space frequently cannot be sterilized. If physiologic improvement is noted, a 7- to 14-day course is reasonable. Even if the patient still remains febrile or demonstrates a leukocytosis at the end of a predetermined course of antibiotics, we still favor stopping therapy and repeating both cultures and radiological investigations, searching for cryptic sites of infection.

General Support

The role of physiologic support of the patient with tertiary peritonitis cannot be overstated. Nutrition must be provided, with increasing evidence that enteral tube feedings, possibly with immunologically enhanced formulas, are superior to parenteral nutrition. Other techniques to avoid further complications such as maneuvers to decrease the risk of pneumonia in intubated patients should be rigorously applied. Finally, the early involvement of physical therapists and rehabilitation specialists in the care of severely debilitated patients is mandatory.

One of the most difficult aspects of the management of this disease is how to determine when a course of treatment has failed and another round of diagnostic investigation is required [9, 10]. Many patients will have an exaggerated septic response for 1 or 2 days after an initial intervention, particularly after the stress of an open procedure. After this period, unequivocal improvement, even if slow, should be seen. If the patient worsens or stops improving, a renewed effort to diagnose infection, in the abdomen and at other sites, should be pursued [11, 12].

Controversies

There are many controversies regarding the pathogenesis and treatment of tertiary peritonitis.

- First, it is now clear that sterile inflammation such as pancreatitis can produce the clinical signs and symptoms characteristic of infection and sepsis. This population does not benefit from antibiotics.
- Second, the techniques of open surgical and percutaneous radiological management of intra-abdominal infection are complementary, rather than competing, modalities. It is much less important to determine which method is superior in cases when both could be used than to understand where one or the other is relatively contraindicated.
- Third, the role of repeated laparotomy, the open abdomen, or *etappenlavage* remains unknown [13-15]. Many small studies support or refute its use, implying that the exact patient population which might benefit from this technique has yet to be precisely defined.
- Fourth, many patients with persistent open or draining anatomic spaces will become colonized with nosocomial organisms which are not actively causing invasive infection, yet many commensal organisms such as *C. albicans* or *S. epidermidis* are quite capable of causing lethal infections. The necessity, type, and duration of antibiotic treatment under these circumstances, therefore, remain open to debate.
- Finally, opinions regarding the survivability of any episode of peritonitis have become more optimistic. For example, in the past an APACHE II score of 15 was

felt to predict a mortality of 50% among patients with intra-abdominal infections; among our most recent 86 patients treated for peritonitis with scores of 14-16, the mortality was only 11%. Although one must continue to remain circumspect, the prognosis for critically ill patients continues to improve and should be taken into account when withdrawal of support is considered.

Critical Factors and Decision Making

The management of tertiary peritonitis has evolved over time. The diagnosis must first be established, usually radiologically, to avoid procedures on patients who do not have active infection yet still look septic. The anatomic focus of infection should be localized as accurately as possible. An ongoing source of leakage must be sought and the necessity for further source control procedures considered. Percutaneous drainage is often the best first option. Drained material should be cultured for nosocomial pathogens, including fungi, and a course of antibiotics administered, guided by clinical response. Careful attention must be paid to physiologic support, particularly nutrition, volume management, and physical therapy, since these patients frequently are just beginning a long and complicated hospital course.

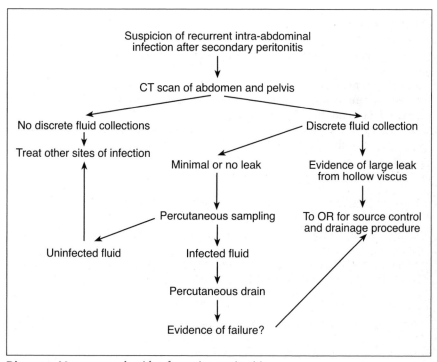

Diagram 1. Management algorithm for tertiary peritonitis

References

1. Malangoni MA (2000) Evaluation and management of tertiary peritonitis. Am Surg 66:157–161
   An excellent review of tertiary peritonitis.
2. Bohnen JM, Mustard RA, Oxholm SE, Schouten BD (1988) APACHE II score and abdominal sepsis. A prospective study. Arch Surg 123:225–229
   Prospectively validates the use of APACHE II scoring in 100 patients with generalized peritonitis or intra-abdominal abscess.
3. Reemst PH, van Goor H, Goris RJ (1996) SIRS, MODS and tertiary peritonitis. Eur J Surg Suppl 576:47–48
   Emphasizes the importance of the immune response in tertiary peritonitis.
4. Bosscha K, van Vroonhoven TJ, van der Werken C (1999) Surgical management of severe secondary peritonitis. Br J Surg 86:1371–1377
   Presents a fair review of the options for the management of severe secondary peritonitis.
5. Wilson SE, Faulkner K (1998) Impact an anatomical site on bacteriological and clinical outcome in the management of intra-abdominal infections. Am Surg 64:402–407
   In a study of 429 patients with intra-abdominal infections, mortality was associated with failure of an initial primary operation.
6. Butler JA, Huang J, Wilson SE (1987) Repeated laparotomy for postoperative intra-abdominal sepsis. An analysis of outcome predictors. Arch Surg 122:702–706
   Early paper studying 47 patients requiring reoperation for intra-abdominal infection, emphasizing the role for radiological localization and sampling.
7. Nathens AB, Rotstein OD, Marshall JC (1998) Tertiary peritonitis: clinical features of a complex nosocomial infection. World J Surg 22:158–163
   Of 59 patients admitted to an ICU, 74% developed tertiary peritonitis. The microbial ecology is also well described.
8. Visser MR, Bosscha K, Olsman J, et al (1998) Predictors of recurrence of fulminant bacterial peritonitis after discontinuation of antibiotics in open management of the abdomen. Eur J Surg 164:825–829
   Proposes a new scoring system to determine whether or not antibiotics can be stopped in patients undergoing open management of severe peritonitis.
9. Pusajo JF, Bumaschny E, Doglio GR, et al (1993) Postoperative intra-abdominal sepsis requiring reoperation. Value of a predictive index. Arch Surg 128:218–222
   This study presents an Abdominal Reoperation Predictive Index and continues to show that its application to patients possibly in need of a second procedure for peritonitis reduced mortality when compared to clinical judgment alone.
10. Seiler CA, Brugger L, Forssmann U, et al (2000) Conservative surgical treatment of diffuse peritonitis. Surgery 127:178–184
    A prospective analysis of 258 patients with diffuse peritonitis. Only 9% of patients with an adequate initial source control procedure required reoperation, while 71% of those with inadequate initial source controlled required reoperation.
11. Stone HH, Bourneuf AA, Stinson LD (1985) Reliability of criteria for predicting persistent or recurrent sepsis. Arch Surg 120:17–20
    A review of 2567 patients with peritonitis, none with a normal temperature, white blood cell count, and differential at the time of cessation of antibiotics required further procedures.
12. Lennard ES, Dellinger EP, Wertz MJ, Minshew BH (1982) Implications of leukocytosis and fever at conclusion of antibiotic therapy for intra-abdominal sepsis. Ann Surg 195:19–24
    A study of 65 patients with intra-abdominal infection, leukocytosis, and fever at the time of cessation of antibiotics were significantly associated with relapse.
13. Bosscha K, Hulstaert PF, Visser MR, et al (2000) Open management of the abdomen and planned reoperations in severe bacterial peritonitis. Eur J Surg 166:44–49
    Reviews the outcomes of 67 patients treated using the open abdomen technique; in hospital mortality was still 42%.

14. Christou NV, Barie PS, Dellinger EP, et al (1993) Surgical Infection Society intra-abdominal infection study. Prospective evaluation of management techniques and outcome. Arch Surg 128:193–198
    A non-randomized study of 239 patients undergoing operation for severe peritonitis, sponsored by the Surgical Infection Society. There was no difference in outcome between open and closed management of peritonitis.
15. Teichmann W, Wittmann DH, Andreone PA (1986) Scheduled reoperations (etappenlavage) for diffuse peritonitis. Arch Surg 121:147–152
    Early study of 61 patients proposing the utility of the open abdomen or *etappenlavage*.

Invited Commentary

JONATHAN L. MEAKINS

The introduction of a new term often engenders confusion about definition; to paraphrase Lewis Carroll, the word means what I mean it to mean. The concept of "persistent peritonitis" was first published in 1986 by Rotstein [1]. In this article, patients who had continuing nonresolving infection of the peritoneal cavity were found to have a different spectrum of organisms from those found in classic secondary peritonitis. Contrary to expectations, the flora was not the typical mixed anaerobic and aerobic bacteria of GI origin, but rather a flora whose growth is associated with antibiotic use or a commensal flora of uncertain pathogenicity. Characteristically *S. epidermidis*, enterococci, *P. aeruginosa* and *Candida* were found along with a wide spectrum of aerobes, but few anaerobes. Marshall et al. [2] subsequently found identical flora in the proximal GI tract of ICU patients at risk for nosocomial infection. In those patients with persistent peritonitis, the GI and peritoneal cultures were identical. The presence of persistent diffuse peritonitis and a dramatically different flora from that characteristically found in primary or secondary peritonitis led Rotstein and Meakins to coin the term "tertiary peritonitis," and use it at Grand Rounds, an American College of Surgeons Plenary Session [3]. The concept mirrored tertiary hyperparathyroidism, where following secondary hyperparathyroidism, the enlarged parathyroid glands take on a life of their own when the initiating event (renal failure) is managed by transplantation. Peritonitis in this setting takes on a life of its own with a different microflora, the inability to localize and no primary source.

What factors allow this entity to become established and to persist in the absence of an ongoing source of contamination? While there are no specific data, it is clear that patients with major infections having had surgery, with ongoing major systemic medical illness and major (multiple) organ dysfunction, have an acquired immunodeficiency [4]. Don Fry was heard saying in a discussion of the management of intra-abdominal abscess that the formation of the abscess was the first signal of the healing process; it was the failure or inability to form the abscess that was the problem. These patients could not localize or contain the infection and were therefore likely to be sicker and at greater risk of a poor outcome. Tertiary peritonitis is the extreme expression of the host's inability to contain and localize an intraperitoneal infectious process, which has no source. The peritoneal cavity is completely involved usually with watery, brackish-looking pus.

Dr. Sawyers' algorithm points out the importance of ensuring via imaging that there are *no* collections and *no* holes in the GI tract, as both require interventional solutions before infection can be resolved, i.e., source control. In the absence of a specific defect or source, another approach to management is required. We must think outside the box as it is common, perhaps the rule, that the state arises because of the quality of initial and subsequent surgical management. I have frequently thought that apart from tertiary peritonitis, there was not very much more we needed to study about the management of intraperitoneal infection.

Our own approach was to use the open abdomen, something we felt made a major difference to outcome. It has been impossible to prove. The microbial source seems to be the GI tract: is decontamination the solution? With the passage of time, better source control, earlier reoperation when initial treatment goes poorly, cleverer use of antibiotics, and generally better ICU and comprehensive care, the incidence of tertiary peritonitis in our center is now low, and usually a result of major trauma. Biotechnologic support of the immune system might also be the answer! However, when all is said and done, correct application of initial therapy, proper application of algorithms such as that presented and optimal clinical care will make tertiary peritonitis a rare entity.

References

1. Rotstein OD, Pruett TL, Simmons RL (1986) Microbiologic features and treatment of persistent peritonitis in patients in the intensive care unit. Can J Surg 29:247–250
2. Marshall JC, Christou NV, Horn R, et al (1988) The microbiology of multiple organ failure: the proximal gastrointestinal tract as an occult reservoir of pathogens. Arch Surg 123:309–315
3. Rotstein OD, Meakins JL (1990) Diagnostic and therapeutic challenges of intraabdominal infections. World J Surg 4:159–166
4. Meakins JL, Pietsch JB, Bubenik O, Kelly R, Gordon J, MacLean LD (1977) Delayed hypersensitivity: indicator of acquired failure of host defenses in sepsis and trauma. Ann Surg 86:241–250

Editorial Comment

What is tertiary peritonitis? Should any form of postoperative intra-abdominal infection be so defined? Dr. Sawyer thinks so and would include in this entity even a pelvic abscess after appendectomy for acute appendicitis. This is perhaps why his series of tertiary peritonitis has such a low mortality, while in most contemporary series around one-third of patients treated for severe postoperative peritonitis still die (see Chap. 42).

Our definition of tertiary peritonitis mirrors that of Dr. Meakins: "Peritonitis in this setting takes on a life of its own with different microflora, the inability to localize and no primary source." Thus, diffuse peritonitis resulting from a leaking colorectal anastomosis will become tertiary only after the leak has been controlled (colostomy) and following 5-7 days of antibiotic treatment, the patient is septic with peritoneal fluid collections containing peculiar organisms.

We should remember, however, that a new source or a drainable abscess might still develop in these patients. Careful bedside examination of all open wounds and connecting spaces, supplemented with serial CT scans, is crucial to discover treatable sources or collections in the otherwise surgically untreatable tertiary peritonitis. As Dr. Sawyer suggests, the key to patients' survival is a multidisciplinary approach, orchestrated, however, by the operating surgeon. If all sources are mechanically controlled, pus is evacuated, unnecessary invasive procedures reduced to minimum, enteral nutrition provided, courses of antibiotics limited, and maximal organ support provided the patient suffering from tertiary peritonitis may survive. But this usually takes many weeks and is expensive: prevention is simpler and cheaper. In our experience, most cases of nontraumatic tertiary peritonitis follow faulty initial management of secondary and postoperative peritonitis.

36 The Role of Laparoscopy

PIOTR GORECKI

Key Principles

- Laparoscopic evaluation of the peritoneal cavity permits magnified visualization of peritoneum and intra-abdominal organs with less tissue trauma than laparotomy.
- Laparoscopy can detect pus, feces, bile or blood – facilitating the identification of the source of intra-abdominal pathology and estimating its severity.
- Whether the therapeutic procedure is laparoscopic or conventional depends on the findings, the patient's condition, and the complexity of the planned procedure.
- Advantages of laparoscopy over laparotomy include reduced perioperative pain, shorter hospital stay, quicker recovery, and decreased wound complications, particularly wound infection and incisional hernias. In addition, laparoscopic procedures result in improved cosmesis and greater patient satisfaction.

General Approach

Gynecologists have used laparoscopy as a diagnostic tool for many decades. Rapid spread and acceptance of laparoscopic cholecystectomy in the early nineties and recent advances in laparoscopic instrumentation dramatically expanded the therapeutic application of laparoscopic techniques. Improved endoscopic stapling devices and laparoscopic suturing techniques have made it possible to perform most complex procedures. Over the past few years, laparoscopy has been used in the management of a wide variety of elective and emergent intra-abdominal problems.

Laparoscopy has been shown to be sensitive and organ-specific in determining the presence and nature of acute intra-abdominal disorders. In a group of 121 patients with acute abdominal pain, a definitive diagnosis was made in 98% of cases and therapeutic laparoscopic procedures were performed in 44% of patients [1]. Diagnostic laparoscopy has been associated with lower morbidity (3% vs 22%) and a shorter hospital stay (1.4 vs 5.1 days) when compared to negative or nontherapeutic laparotomy [2].

Typical conditions in which laparoscopy can be employed include localized peritonitis and acute abdominal pain of uncertain etiology associated with equivocal physical, sonographic, or radiological findings. Acute cholecystitis, acute appendicitis, and acute gynecological pathology are classic examples of clinical disorders that can be diagnosed and managed laparoscopically. Less common or

Table 1. Applications of laparoscopy in source control

Clear indications for laparoscopy	Potential and controversial indications for laparoscopy	Contraindications to laparoscopy
Acute cholecystitis	Perforated peptic ulcer disease	Unstable patient
Acute appendicitis	Perforated colon (diverticulitis, colonoscopic perforation)	Presence of abdominal hypertension
Diagnostic laparoscopy in acute pain of unknown etiology	Intestinal obstruction	Severe established peritonitis
Acute gynecological pathology	Abdominal pain in a pregnant patient	Lack of experience
	Second-look laparoscopy	Elevated ICP (head trauma patient)
	Drainage of intra-abdominal abscess	
	Rule out intra-abdominal source of sepsis in ICU patient	
	Stable trauma patient with no urgent indications for laparotomy	

ICU, intensive care unit; ICP, intracranial pressure.

controversial applications for laparoscopy include inflammatory processes or perforations of the large or small bowel, perforated peptic ulcer, intestinal obstruction, and evaluation of the acute abdomen in the intensive care unit, during pregnancy, and in the stable trauma patient (Table 1).

Absolute contraindications to laparoscopy include hemodynamic instability, severe abdominal distention with signs of intra-abdominal hypertension and established diffuse peritonitis. In these patients, signs of profound systemic inflammatory response (SIRS) or organ dysfunction call for a prompt laparotomy. Abdominal decompression and rapid source control are much more important for favorable outcome than the route of operative access. Increasing the intra-abdominal pressure (with the pneumoperitoneum) and prolonging surgical intervention in this group of sick patients would compromise organ perfusion and impair venous return and cardiac output.

Specific Considerations

Acute Cholecystitis

Acute cholecystitis (AC) is a classic example of a resectable infection. Prompt cholecystectomy for patient suffering from AC is therefore the most rational therapeutic option. Once considered a contraindication to the laparoscopic approach, acute cholecystitis has become one of the most common indications for laparoscopy and studies have confirmed both the safety and feasibility of the laparoscopic approach [3, 4]. The outcome of laparoscopic cholecystectomy is similar to that of elective cholecystectomy [5]. Nonoperative therapy of the acute process, followed by delayed cholecystectomy, offers no advantage [6]. Nevertheless, the rates of conversion to an open procedure and the operating time tend to be increased in patients with acute cholecystitis as compared to elective laparoscopic cholecystectomy [3].

Acute cholecystitis should be treated by laparoscopic cholecystectomy, preferably within the first 72 h. Conversion to an open procedure, when anatomy becomes unclear or dissection difficult is a sign of a good surgical judgment (see Chap. 16).

Acute Appendicitis

The primary advantage of laparoscopic over open appendectomy is its potential to evaluate the entire peritoneal cavity. It is particularly helpful in cases in which the diagnosis is uncertain, for example, in women with right lower quadrant pain [7]. In a study of 100 patients subjected to diagnostic laparoscopy before an open appendectomy, the rate of misdiagnosis was 41% in female patients of reproductive age and 8% in male patients [8]. Findings other than appendicitis permit selection of the optimal incision or a decision for conservative treatment. Ruptured appendicitis with diffuse peritonitis or abscess formation can also be successfully managed by laparoscopy [9,10]. In a meta-analysis of twelve randomized controlled trials of laparoscopic versus open appendectomy [11], fewer wound infections and an earlier return to normal activities were noted in laparoscopic groups. There were no significant differences in mean length of hospital stay, intra-abdominal abscess formation and readmission rates. Mean operating time was significantly longer when the laparoscopic approach was used, and overall conversion to an open procedure was 11%.

Laparoscopic appendectomy is a good alternative to an open appendectomy. The advantages of the laparoscopic approach are particularly evident in female patients and in those in whom the diagnosis is uncertain. Obese patients may also benefit from laparoscopy since the technique facilitates exposure and minimizes wound complications (see Chap. 14).

Perforation of the Colon

Acute diverticulitis and iatrogenic perforation of the colon during colonoscopy are novel examples of successful application of minimally invasive techniques in the management of colonic source. Depending on the nature of the perforation and the severity of peritonitis, simple closure, tangential resection, segmental resection, or creation of a colostomy can all be performed laparoscopically [12]. Laparoscopy-assisted sigmoid resection with anastomosis has been successfully utilized in patients with diverticulitis (Hinchey I patients), with a reduced hospital stay compared to laparotomy [13]. Laparoscopic peritoneal lavage without resection or diversion was described in eight patients with diffuse purulent peritonitis secondary to perforated diverticular disease. All patients made a complete recovery within 5-8 days and no patient required surgical intervention during 12-24 months of follow-up [14]. This innovative approach needs further study to confirm its safety before it can be recommended. Hand-assisted colectomy can combine the advantages of minimally invasive access with preservation of tactile sensation during dissection. This so-called handoscopy technique also offers an intermediate step for surgeons interested in laparoscopic colon surgery. Laparoscopy should not be used in the management of perforated cancer or complex penetrating trauma to the colon.

Perforated Peptic Ulcer Disease. Is Laparoscopy Less Invasive?

Animal studies have shown that minimally invasive techniques result in reduced cytokine production when compared to laparotomy [15]. This, however, may be of secondary importance in peritonitis. In the two randomized studies comparing laparoscopic to an open repair of perforated peptic ulcer [16, 17], there was no difference between the two treatment groups with respect to acute stress response [16]. A study from Hong Kong showed no difference between the laparoscopic and open groups in terms of duration of nasogastric aspiration, duration of intravenous fluids, total hospital stay, time to resumption of a normal diet, morbidity, and reoperation and mortality rates [17]. It suggested that for patients with established peritonitis, the minimal reduction in access-related stress response is largely offset by sepsis, the major contributing factor to the inflammatory response. The requirement for postoperative analgesics was, however, significantly less with the laparoscopic approach to perforated peptic ulcer disease (PUD). One can also expect a reduction in short and long-term wound complications in laparoscopically treated patients (see Chap. 11).

Special Problems Related to Laparoscopy

Increased Intra-abdominal Pressure

Peritoneal insufflation elevates intra-abdominal pressure (IAP) to approximately 15 mmHg and may cause symptoms of intra-abdominal hypertension. This increased pressure, in turn, can adversely affect hemodynamic and respiratory function [18]. Therefore, conditions in which signs of intra-abdominal hypertension exist such as severe peritonitis with visceral edema or the need for massive fluid resuscitation preclude the safe use of laparoscopy. In such patients, the added pressure from the pneumoperitoneum can result in visceral hypoperfusion, decreased cardiac output and venous return and worsening of the overall septic picture [19, 20]. The duration of the laparoscopic procedure and patient comorbidities should also be considered before attempting a laparoscopic approach.

CO$_2$ Pneumoperitoneum and Bacterial Translocation

It has been suggested that CO$_2$ pneumoperitoneum may increase bacterial translocation and aggravate bacteremia and the metabolic and hemodynamic disturbances induced by peritonitis. Animal studies yield divergent results, both positive [21] and negative [22]. It appears, however, that CO$_2$ pneumoperitoneum may play a role in aggravating the severity of peritonitis in cases of advanced peritonitis and prolonged exposure to positive-pressure pneumoperitoneum [20, 21].

Reduced Venous Return and Deep Vein Thrombosis

Reduced venous return during peritoneal insufflation may contribute to the development of deep vein thrombosis (DVT) by producing venous stasis in lower extremities. This theoretical risk can be obviated if adequate prophylaxis in the form of low-dose heparin and sequential compression stockings are utilized [23]. In a prospective study from Australia [24], the incidence of DVT detected on a routine preoperative and postoperative duplex scan was the same among patients undergoing minilaparotomy and laparoscopic cholecystectomy. A collective review of 153,832 patients undergoing laparoscopic cholecystectomy revealed that the rate of fatal pulmonary embolism was 0.02% and total rate of pulmonary embolism was 0.06%. The average rate of reported DVT was 0.03% and seemed to be lower than after conventional cholecystectomy [25].

Laparoscopy in the Pregnant Patient

Approximately 0.2% of pregnant patients require intra-abdominal general surgical intervention during pregnancy. Acute appendicitis and acute cholecystitis are the most common surgical emergencies, occurring in 0.05%-0.1% and 0.05% of pregnancies, respectively. Multiple reports have shown the feasibility and safety of laparoscopic intervention during all trimesters of pregnancy, but the second trimester appears to be the safest [26]. The advantages of laparoscopic intervention are the same as for nonpregnant patients, and no increase in maternal or fetal morbidity or mortality has been identified [27]. There are some concerns, however, that prolonged positive-pressure pneumoperitoneum and hypercapnia may have adverse effects on fetal metabolism. Therefore, close intraoperative maternal and fetal monitoring is advised. Limited working space caused by an enlarging uterus and more difficult access render the laparoscopic technique in a pregnant patient a challenge.

Controversies

Since laparoscopic techniques are continuously expanding, there are an increasing number of controversies regarding their use. Most of the relevant studies represent clinical reviews rather than randomized trials. The problem of data analysis is often biased by selection criteria and surgeon experience. The question also remains whether the benefits of minimally invasive access outweigh its potential shortcomings, including the need for positive-pressure pneumoperitoneum and a duration of laparoscopic intervention. The main controversies can be summarized as follows:

- Is laparoscopy better than laparotomy in treating patients requiring source control intervention?
- Is laparoscopy adequate to determine the source of abdominal infection?
- Who is an appropriate candidate for the laparoscopic approach?
- Does laparoscopy provide adequate source control?
- Is it safe and effective in the pregnant patient?
- Are the adverse effects of CO_2 pneumoperitoneum and elevated intra-abdominal pressure clinically significant?
- Who is qualified to perform the procedure?

Critical Factors and Decision Making

Laparoscopy has become a valid tool in the management of the patient requiring source control intervention. Its primary role is to decrease the morbidity of a negative or nontherapeutic laparotomy and to provide a diagnosis of abdominal pain of unclear etiology. It has an established role in the management of common

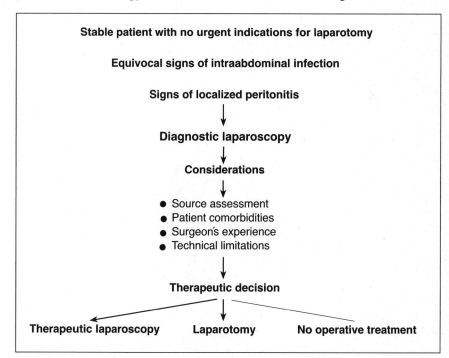

Diagram 1. Algorithm for application of laparoscopy in source control

infections such as acute cholecystitis, appendicitis, and gynecological pathology. Source control in early perforated peptic ulcer or early colonic perforation has demonstrated the benefits of minimally invasive access. Other potential applications for laparoscopy have been reported (Table 1). Laparoscopy should not be used in patients with severe established peritonitis, especially those with pre-existing abdominal hypertension or hemodynamic instability. Surgeons interested in emergency laparoscopy should know their technical limitations, and should have experience in elective laparoscopy.

References

1. Salky BA, Edye MB (1998) The role of laparoscopy in the diagnosis and treatment of abdominal pain syndromes. Surg Endosc 12:911–914
2. Sosa JL, Baker M, Puente I, Sims D, Sleeman D, Ginzburg, Martin L (1995) Negative laparotomy in abdominal gunshot wounds: potential impact of laparoscopy. J Trauma 38:194–197
3. Pessaux P, Tuech JJ, Rouge C, Duplessis R, Cervi C, Arnaud JP (2000) Laparoscopic cholecystectomy in acute cholecystitis. A prospective comparative study in patients with acute vs chronic cholecystitis. Surg Endosc 14:358–361
4. Lo CM, Liu CL, Lai EC, Fan ST, Wong J (1996) Early versus delayed laparoscopic cholecystectomy for treatment of acute cholecystitis. Ann Surg 223:37–42
5. Lujan JA, Parrilla P, Robles R, Marin P, Torralba JA, Garcia-Ayllon J (1998) Laparoscopic cholecystectomy vs open cholecystectomy in the treatment of acute cholecystitis: a prospective study. Arch Surg 133:173–175
6. Lai PB, Kwong KH, Leung KL, Kwok SP, Chan AC, Chung SC, Lau WY (1998) Randomized trial of early versus delayed laparoscopic cholecystectomy for acute cholecystitis. Br J Surg 85:764–767
7. Ou CS, Rowbotham R (2000) Laparoscopic diagnosis and treatment of nontraumatic acute abdominal pain in women. J Laparoendosc Adv Surg Tech A 10:41–45
8. Tytgat SH, Bakker XR, Butzelaar RM (1998) Laparoscopic evaluation of patients with suspected acute appendicitis. Surg Endosc 12:918–920
9. Yao CC, Lin CS, Yang CC (1999) Laparoscopic appendectomy for ruptured appendicitis. Surg Laparosc Endosc Percutan Tech 9:271–273
10. Paya K, Rauhofer U, Rebhandl W, Deluggi S, Horcher E (2000) Perforating appendicitis. An indication for laparoscopy? Surg Endosc 14:182–184
11. Temple LK, Litwin DE, McLeod RS (1999) A meta-analysis of laparoscopic versus open appendectomy in patients suspected of having acute appendicitis. Can J Surg 42:377–383
12. Wullstein C, Koppen M, Gross E (1999) Laparoscopic treatment of colonic perforations related to colonoscopy. Surg Endosc 13:484–487
13. Sher ME, Agachan F, Bortul M, Nogueras JJ, Weiss EG, Wexner SD (1997) Laparoscopic surgery for diverticulitis. Surg Endosc 11:264–267
14. O'Sullivan GC, Murphy D, O'Brien MG, Ireland A (1996) Laparoscopic management of generalized peritonitis due to perforated colonic diverticula. Am J Surg 1171:432–434
15. Iwanaka T, Arkovitz MS, Arya G, Ziegler MM (1997) Evaluation of operative stress and peritoneal macrophage function in minimally invasive operations. J Am Coll Surg 184:357–363
16. Lau WY, Leung KL, Kwong KH, Davey IC, Robertson C, Dawson JJ, Chung SC, Li AK (1996) A randomized study comparing laparoscopic versus open repair of perforated peptic ulcer using suture or sutureless technique. Ann Surg 224:131–138
17. Lau JY, Lo SY, Ng EK, Lee DW, Lam YH, Chung SC (1998) A randomized comparison of acute phase response and endotoxemia in patients with perforated peptic ulcers receiving laparoscopic or open patch repair. Am J Surg 175:325–327
18. Schein M, Wittmann DH, Aprahamian CC, Condon RE (1995) The abdominal compartment syndrome: the physiological and clinical consequences of elevated intra-abdominal pressure. J Am Coll Surg 180:745–753

19. Schein M, Ivatury R (1998) Intra-abdominal hypertension and the abdominal compartment syndrome. Br J Surg 85:1027–1028
20. Schulman CI (2000) Abdominal compartment syndrome mimicking sepsis. Infect Med 17:745–757
21. Bloechle C, Emmermann A, Treu H, Achilles E, Mack D, Zornig C, Broelsch CE (1995) Effect of a pneumoperitoneum on the extent and severity of peritonitis induced by gastric ulcer perforation in the rat. Surg Endosc 9:898–901
22. Gurtner GC, Robertson CS, Chung SC, Ling TK, Ip SM, Li AK (1995) Effect of carbon dioxide pneumoperitoneum on bacteraemia and endotoxaemia in an animal model of peritonitis. Br J Surg 82:844–848
23. Schwenk W, Bohm B, Fugener A, Muller JM (1998) Intermittent pneumatic sequential compression (ISC) of the lower extremities prevents venous stasis during laparoscopic cholecystectomy. A prospective randomized study. Surg Endosc 12:7–11
24. Lord RV, Ling JJ, Hugh TB, Coleman MJ, Doust BD, Nivison-Smith I (1998) Incidence of deep vein thrombosis after laparoscopic vs minilaparotomy cholecystectomy. Arch Surg 133: 967–973
25. Lindberg F, Bergqvist D, Rasmussen I (1997) Incidence of thromboembolic complications after laparoscopic cholecystectomy: review of the literature. Surg Laparosc Endosc 7:324–331
26. Curet MJ (2000) Special problems in laparoscopic surgery. Previous abdominal surgery, obesity, and pregnancy. Surg Clin North Am 80:1093–1110
27. Gurbuz AT, Peetz ME (1997) The acute abdomen in the pregnant patient. Is there a role for laparoscopy? Surg Endosc 11:98–102

Invited Commentary

Zygmunt H. Krukowski

Laparoscopy is a large component of my elective practice but I use it relatively infrequently in emergency circumstances. With few exceptions, in a genuine emergency, as opposed to scheduled operation, the need to achieve all the therapeutic objectives can only be achieved by an adequate laparotomy.

Diagnostic Laparoscopy

The diagnostic potential of laparoscopy is clear but its role remains controversial. A firm diagnosis is only necessary if it impacts on management. Several self-limiting and relatively minor conditions, which may present with abdominal signs insufficient to merit early intervention, are satisfactorily managed by active observation. The comparative risk of a period of observation versus a *controlled episode of penetrating abdominal trauma* (i.e., diagnostic laparoscopy) is no contest in my view. This is not to say that there are no indications for diagnostic laparoscopy in a subgroup of patients in whom continuing symptoms merit intervention when resolution has not followed noninvasive assessment. By itemizing the absolute contraindications to laparoscopy in emergency surgery, Dr. Gorecki has, by my reckoning, defined the precise indications for emergency surgery requiring source control.

Therapeutic Laparoscopy

A laparoscopic approach has an established role in appendicitis and cholecysti-tis. The relative benefits are greatest in the heavily muscled or obese patient in whom open access requires a larger incision or more aggressive retraction with consequent wound trauma and increased risk of wound sepsis. Similarly, a lapa-roscopic approach to insert the few sutures required to seal the majority of per-forated peptic ulcers is superficially attractive but the relative difficulty of a thorough peritoneal toilet in established peritonitis means that it is most effec-tive when the perforation is recent and contamination more limited. Nonrando-mized series confirm the technical feasibility of laparoscopic closure but rando-mized study suggests that there may be a higher incidence of postoperative peritoneal abscess. It may also be hard for the surgical psyche to admit "defeat" and change from a laparoscopic to an open approach to achieve optimal perito-neal toilet.

A flood of supportive documentation has not followed the pilot report of managing generalized peritonitis due to diverticular disease. A conservative approach to sepsis secondary to sigmoid diverticulitis is well documented. Esti-mating the extent of peritoneal reaction without surgery is speculative. If all pa-tients with a clinical and/or radiological diagnosis of acute diverticulitis were subjected to surgery the extent of inflammatory response would often be consi-derable, but we know that the majority resolve without intervention. Resolution after laparoscopic peritoneal lavage may be attributed to this intervention, although a cynic would question this. In the absence of controlled comparative da-ta I would maintain that these patients would have settled without the intervention.

The possibility of laparoscopic management of an instrumental colonic per-foration would depend on the site and size of the perforation. If intervention is required to control contamination and a major resection is not indicated then this seems a reasonable suggestion. The few colonoscopic perforations I have ma-naged have been treated without operation albeit with an anxious few days for the colonoscopist.

Dr. Gorecki does not mention laparoscopy-assisted minimal access approa-ches to pancreatic abscess and necrosectomy. There are encouraging reports of successful management of severe retroperitoneal sepsis by a laparoscopic extra-peritoneal rather than transperitoneal route and our limited experience suggests that this is a very promising development [1, 2].

In summary, source control is most necessary for patients with the most se-vere assault on their peritoneal defense mechanisms and systemic sepsis. These, however, are the patients least likely to do well with a laparoscopic approach.

References

1. Carter CR, McKay CJ, Imrie CW (2000) Percutaneous necrosectomy and sinus tract endoscopy in the management of infected pancreatic necrosis: an initial experience. Ann Surg 232:175–180
2. Alverdy J, Vargish T, Desai T, Frawley B, Rosen B (2000) Laparoscopic intracavitary debride-ment of peripancreatic necrosis: preliminary report and description of the technique. Sur-gery 127:112–114

Editorial Comment

The role of laparoscopy in the diagnosis and treatment of nontraumatic abdominal emergencies is evolving. Hitherto, it has reached wide acceptance in acute cholecystitis and gynecological conditions. There is a strong rationale for laparoscopy when the source of right lower quadrant pain is questionable – especially in a female patient.

We find that insertion of the laparoscope prior to an exploratory laparotomy for clinical diffuse peritonitis allows for a more direct and less traumatic access: a smaller transverse incision directly over the source – identified during the laparoscopy – is easier on the patient than the classic long midline laparotomy with its inherent tendencies to dehisce and herniate. However, a "negative" laparoscopy in a patient with clinical acute peritonitis is an indication to convert to a laparotomy, for sometimes the tactile sense is indispensable (e.g., a diverticular abscess hidden within the leaves of the mesocolon).

In order to be able and confident to tackle other conditions through the laparoscope, one has to be able to laparoscopically explore the various spaces and corners of the peritoneal cavity. One has to be skilled in advanced laparoscopic techniques and intracorporeal suturing techniques to deal laparoscopically with more complicated situations such as the perforated peptic ulcer.

Professor Krukowski emphasizes that by listing the contraindications to laparoscopy one understands the indications. Clearly, the acutely ill patient is not a suitable guinea pig for budding laparoscopic ambitions. The sicker the patient, the more diffuse the peritonitis, the less suitable the patient is for the magic lenses and trocars. One has to be selective and balanced.

37 Pediatric Surgery

GRAEME PITCHER

Key Principles

- The systemic response to sepsis in early life is different.
- The main challenge in abdominal source control is necrotizing enterocolitis.
- Empyema and mediastinitis occur after surgery for esophageal atresia, trauma, and pneumonia.

General Approach

Management of the child with a surgical focus of infection differs considerably from that of the adult. A different spectrum of diseases presents to the pediatric surgeon and children manifest different immunological and metabolic responses to systemic infection. This is particularly true in the neonatal period, and the challenges of source control differ between the neonate and the older child (Table 1). The neonate or infant with serious surgical infection should ideally be managed by a specialized pediatric surgical service.

This chapter concentrates on the spectrum of conditions commonly treated by pediatric surgeons.

Table 1. Surgical abdominal conditions requiring source control in childhood

Neonate	Infant and child
Necrotizing enterocolitis	Appendicitis
Hirschsprung's enterocolitis	Intussusception
Complications of abdominal surgery	Meckel's diverticulitis
Leaking enteric anastomoses	Bowel perforations
Abdominal wall defects	Solid visceral abscesses
Miscellaneous bowel perforations	Complications of abdominal surgery
Urinary tract obstruction with infection	Leaking enteric anastomoses
Meconium peritonitis	Crohn's disease
	Obstructive uropathy with infection
	Urachal remnants
	Infected pancreatic pseudocysts
	Cholecystitis

The Inflammatory Response

The neonate, particularly the premature infant, is immunologically immature. Maternal IgG crosses the placenta and is present from birth. Levels drop during the first 30 days of life so that there is a relative hypogammaglobulinemia during the second and third months of life. In addition, certain subclasses of IgG namely IgG2 and IgG4 cross the placenta relatively poorly. As a result, the neonate is more susceptible to infection with Group B *Streptococci* because of a reduced response to the polysaccharide capsule. IgM and IgA are absent unless their production has been stimulated prenatally by active infection during the pregnancy.

The newborn's lymphocytes have an impaired ability to differentiate into plasma cells and produce immunoglobulin [1]. Helper T cells are also deficient and this deficiency contributes to poor immunoglobulin production. Even during overwhelming infection, neonates do generally not produce type specific antibody [2].

Some aspects of cell-mediated immunity are normal in the newborn, whereas others such as the production of IL-2 may be deficient. Cytokine production differs from that of the adult and is affected by insults such as fetal distress and prolonged labor [3]. Neonates have both quantitative and qualitative neutrophil defects, with decreased bone marrow neutrophil storage reserves, an inability to increase neutrophil production, and defective neutrophil functional activity. They respond to overwhelming sepsis with depletion of the storage pool and the development of peripheral neutropenia [4]. As a result of all of these factors, neonates are at particular risk of serious life threatening infections and experience increased mortality and morbidity from such infections.

The clinical response to life threatening infection differs from that of the adult. The neonate typically exhibits such nonspecific signs as lethargy, poor feeding, abnormalities of temperature control (often hypothermia rather than fever), and apneic spells, followed by acidosis, oliguria, and circulatory collapse. The elevated white cell count seen in the adult is frequently not seen in the neonate. Neutropenia commonly accompanies severe neonatal sepsis and is often associated with thrombocytopenia due to dysregulation of the neonatal hematopoetic response [5]. The overstimulation of the cytokine cascade that characterizes the systemic inflammatory response syndrome (SIRS) – so well recognized in adults – seems to be severely attenuated in the neonatal period. Proinflammatory cytokine production is impaired, a factor that likely contributes to an altered clinical response. In states of overwhelming infection, neonates tend to develop severe acidosis and circulatory collapse of frank septic shock; the insidious progressive organ dysfunction (often in the absence of identifiable infection) that characterizes SIRS in the adult is rare in the neonate.

The Abdomen

The abdomen is the commonest site of infection that requires source control in the neonate. Necrotizing enterocolitis (NEC) continues to pose a significant challenge to neonatologists and pediatric surgeons worldwide.

Aspects of the management of neonatal NEC remain controversial. Early treatment is nonsurgical and based on resuscitation, bowel rest and decompression, and antibiotic therapy. As the majority of cases of NEC resolve on conservative treatment, surgery is reserved for bowel perforation or nonrecoverable segmental necrosis. Some centers advocate an aggressive approach with early surgery [6] prompted by clinical and biochemical markers of severe disease, while others practice conservatism with aggressive systemic support and delayed surgery [7]. NEC is a heterogeneous disease and accurate markers for irreversible bowel ischemia and necrosis have not as yet been clearly established. In addition, practices vary according to the standards of supportive care available. The key principles of the surgical management of NEC are:

- Operation or drainage to control enteric contamination in cases of perforation
- Resection of definitely necrotic bowel
- Preservation of maximal bowel length including the ileocecal valve if possible
- Drainage of localized intraperitoneal infection
- "Defunctioning" of severely involved bowel that has the potential to recover
- Management of late complications such as stricture

The neonatal peritoneal cavity can be effectively drained by the insertion of a soft drain through the abdominal wall, an intervention that can be performed at the bedside in the intensive care unit. This maneuver can relieve abdominal distension that may compromise ventilation in patients with intestinal perforation, and can be an effective adjunct to resuscitation in babies being prepared for laparotomy. Many centers have shown that drainage alone can suffice as definitive treatment (particularly in the ultra low-birth-weight baby < 1,000 g).

Resection of severely affected, nonrecoverable bowel is the most effective modality of treatment, but is limited by the need to preserve maximal bowel length. The length of the small bowel is approximately 115 cm at 27 weeks and increases to 250 cm at term [8]. In order to prevent short bowel syndrome, a length of 30-60 cm including the ileocecal valve should be preserved. In patients with short segment, localized disease segmental resection and primary resection can be applied, usually with good results.

Patients with pan-intestinal disease involving more than 75% of the small bowel length comprise about 20% of cases of NEC. They pose a particularly difficult problem. If the affected bowel is resected the patient is doomed to suffer from short bowel syndrome. Under these circumstances, and when there is patchy, segmental involvement, it is necessary to leave inflamed potentially nonviable bowel in the abdomen. While this approach may appear to breach key principles of surgical dogma, it may offer the only chance of recovery with an adequate length of viable bowel. Many innovative techniques have been described. A proximal diverting stoma [9] may allow distal bowel to recover. Moore described the "patch, drain, and wait" procedure where perforations are patched by suture closure, the abdomen is closed with a Penrose drain in each lower quadrant, and the patient is then treated supportively with parenteral nutrition in the hope that there will be a recovery of affected bowel and preservation of bowel length [10]. A "clip and drop back" technique [11] allows segments of bowel to be "defunctioned" between surgical clips and returned to the abdomen and reassessed at a later operation – when their viability has been confirmed, and continuity restored at that time.

All of these operations leave potentially nonviable bowel in situ, tissue that may act as an ongoing nidus for inflammation and infection. Yet this violation of a general principle of surgical source control is necessary because of the potential for recovery of the affected bowel and the need to conserve bowel length. In many instances, with modern supportive therapy, patients tolerate this treatment. In some cases overwhelming sepsis occurs, but were it not for these innovative approaches, more babies would succumb to the complications of short bowel syndrome, thus justifying this apparently paradoxical approach.

Hirschsprung's Disease

The most common source control problem in the surgical treatment of Hirschsprung's disease (HD) is the management of anastomotic problems after definitive coloanal pullthrough surgery. One-stage pullthrough without covering colostomy has become common practice, but regardless of the type of operation used, an anastomotic leak poses a major threat to the patient, both in immediate morbidity and long term functional results. Reexploration is indicated at the earliest sign of anastomotic leak (lower abdominal pain, tenderness and fever), and diversion performed to avoid the disastrous complications of stricture, frozen pelvis, and poor anorectal function.

The Chest

Conditions requiring thoracic source control are:
- Anastomotic leaks from repair of esophageal atresia
- Mediastinitis or empyema following esophageal injury, instrumentation, or dilatation
- Empyema complicating pneumonia
- Empyema following trauma

Esophageal Atresia

As a result of the use of modern surgical techniques, magnification, and monofilament suture materials, anastomotic leaks complicating operations for esophageal atresia have become rare. The incidence is reported from 0% [12] in a series from Minneapolis, including wide gap so-called pure esophageal atresia without fistula, to 6%-12% in some series. A 0% leak rate may be difficult to sustain in a larger series, but all cases of esophageal atresia and tracheoesophageal fistula should be amenable to uncomplicated primary anastomosis. Our own unpublished experience has been 3 leaks in over 250 cases. Survival of infants with esophageal atresia is now dependent on other factors such as associated cardiac and chromosomal abnormalities.

Extrapleural surgical repair with para-anastomotic drainage limits and effectively contains the sequelae of minor anastomotic leaks. The findings on a water-soluble contrast study guide the management of the leaking anastomosis. Minor extrapleural leaks with esophageal continuity can be treated expectantly. Major leaks with loss of esophageal continuity (complete anastomotic disruption), or associated with pneumothorax and pleural contamination, require reexploration. Partial anastomotic breakdown may be managed by suture or by T-tube drainage to establish a controlled fistula. Complete disruption usually requires a cervical esophagostomy and the "abandonment" of the esophagus.

Empyema

Empyema remains the most common intrathoracic infection presenting to the pediatric surgeon (see Chap. 21). It is usually a sequel of pneumonia, but may follow thoracic trauma or esophageal perforation. Empyema is classified by the American Thoracic Society as exudative, fibrino-purulent, and organizing.

The mainstay of source control intervention has been tube drainage, with open thoracotomy and formal decortication reserved for those cases that do not resolve with tube thoracostomy. The requirement for decortication is reported as 18%, or 7 of 39 cases of fibrino-purulent empyema reported in a large series [13]. In our own experience formal decortication has never been necessary for postpneumonic empyema in young, rapidly growing infants and children, and is rarely required for empyema following esophageal perforation. Most cases resolve with tube thoracostomy drainage and prolonged intravenous antibiotic therapy.

Newer strategies include early thoracoscopy to break down loculations and drain empyema cavities, and the use of a fibrinolytic agent such as urokinase instilled directly into the empyema cavity [14]. These approaches are most beneficial when used early in the treatment of empyema and have been shown to significantly shorten time to resolution and to decrease the requirement for thoracotomy and decortication. However when thoracoscopy is used later for nonresolution, it has proven less beneficial [15].

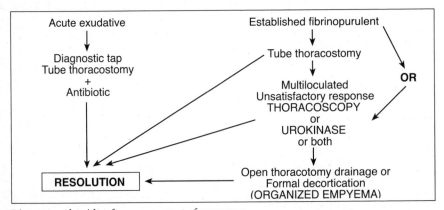

Diagram 1. Algorithm for management of empyema

Current approaches favor early active intervention by thoracoscopy rather than the alternative of prolonged hospitalization or extended outpatient intravenous antibiotic therapy. However, this strategy may result in many unnecessary interventions for the gain of shorter hospitalization times. The algorithm in Diagram 1 is applicable.

References

1. Hayward AR, Lawton AR (1977) Induction of plasma cell differentiation of human fetal lymphocytes: evidence for functional immaturity of T and B cell. J Immunol 115:1213–1217
2. Mills EL (1983) Mononuclear phagocytes in the newborn: their relation to the state of relative immunodeficiency. Am J Pediatr Haematol Oncology 5:189–198
3. Jokic M, Guillois B, Cauquelin B, Giroux JD, Bessis JL, Morello R, Levy G, Ballet JJ (2000) Fetal distress increases interleukin-6 and interleukin-8 and decreases tumour necrosis factor-alpha cord blood levels in noninfected full-term neonates. BJOG 107:420–425
4. Bracho F, Goldman S, Cairo MS (1998) Potential use of granulocyte colon-stimulating factor and granulocyte-macrophage colony-stimulating factor in neonates. Curr Opin Hematol 5:215–220
5. Rosenthal J, Cairo MS (1995) The role of cytokines in modulating neonatal myelopoiesis and host defense. Cytokines Mol Ther 1:165–176
6. Kosloske AM (1994) Indications for operation in necrotizing enterocolitis revisited. J Pediatr Surg 29:663–666
7. Badowicz B, Latawiec-Mazurkiewicz I (2000) Necrotising enterocolitis (NEC) – methods of treatment and outcome: a comparative analysis of Scottish (Glasgow) and Polish (Western Pomerania) cases. Eur J Pediatr Surg 10:177–181
8. Touloukian RJ, Smith GJ (1983) Normal intestinal length in preterm infants. J Pediatr Surg 18:720–723
9. Martin LW, Neblett WW (1981) Early operation with intestinal diversion for necrotizing enterocolitis. J Pediatr Surg 16:252–255
10. Moore TC (1989) Management of necrotizing enterocolitis by "patch drain and wait". Pediatr Surg Int 4:110–114
11. Vaughan WG, Grosfeld JL, West W, et al (1996) Avoidance of stomas and delayed anastomosis for bowel necrosis: the "clip and drop-back technique." J Pediatr Surg 31:542–545
12. Foker JE, Linden BC, Boyle EM, et al (1997) Development of a true primary repair for the full spectrum of esophageal atresia. Ann Surg 226:533–543
13. W. Chan et al (1997) Empyema thoracis in children: a 26 year review of the Montreal Children's Hospital experience. J Pediatr Surg 32: 870–872
14. Komecki A, Sivan Y (1997) Treatment of loculated pleural effusion with intrapleural urokinase in children. J Pediatr Surg 32:1473–1475
15. Kern JA, Rodgers BM (1993) Thoracoscopy in the management of empyema in children. J Pediatr Surg 28:1128-1132

Invited Commentary

Wojciech J. Górecki

The management of a child with a surgical infection does not differ from that of an adult. What makes the philosophy of source control in pediatric surgery considerably different is the approach to the newborn, in particular the premature infant.

Although there is a different spectrum of diseases presenting in childhood, the principles of treatment of conditions itemized in the second column of Table 1 remain the same. It must be emphasized that in infants, *intussusception* is the most common abdominal emergency. Early intussusception, without bowel necrosis, should be reduced conservatively with pneumatic [1] or hydrostatic pressure [2]. The resulting transitory bacteremia [3] represents contamination rather than infection [4] and can be treated with a short course of antibiotics, or no antibiotics at all.

In a child with a nontraumatic acute abdomen, *appendicitis* should be considered the responsible diagnosis until proven otherwise. In children, a nonoperative approach with prolonged antibiotics may be effective in the treatment of postappendectomy, intraperitoneal abscesses [5, 6]. This approach, however, is based on retrospective analyses, and may include sterile collections found on ultrasound or CT that require no therapy [7]. Acute cholecystitis is rare in children [8].

There are a number of soft tissue infections in pediatric patients that are not discussed in this chapter. Some are unique to the newborn (e.g., omphalitis, neonatal mastitis), but again are treated with a nonspecific approach. One of the most common in children – *submental suppurative adenitis* – may by mimicked by inflammation of congenital cysts of the neck; the former requires incision and drainage, whereas the latter can be excised electively, after inflammation subsides.

The immunological immaturity of the newborn is described in detail, without however, clear therapeutic suggestions. Management is controversial. Some authors recommend supplementation of immunoglobulins in neonatal infections [9, 10], and a prospective, placebo-controlled trial demonstrated a reduction in postoperative respiratory and urinary infections with intravenous immunoglobulin administration [11]. On the other hand, on the basis of evidence of the benefit of breast-feeding in preventing NEC, oral administration of an IgA-IgG preparation was shown to prevent the development of NEC in premature newborns [12]. The description of a different pattern of SIRS in neonates is of great importance, but may have other causes than attenuation of the cytokine cascade, as elevated serum interleukin-6 levels are also observed in fetuses with fetal inflammatory response syndrome [13].

NEC represents the main challenge in newborn source control and the basic difference between adult and pediatric surgery. Aspects of surgical management of NEC listed by Dr. Pitcher remain controversial, however, sound surgical common sense favors resection of necrotic bowel with primary anastomosis [14,15]. It does not appear that the outcome is influenced by the presence of the ileocecal valve [14,16]. Ideally resection should be done before intestinal perforation occurs [17]. While it is true that accurate markers for bowel necrosis have not yet been clearly established, the following criteria have been suggested: positive paracentesis, radiological signs of portal venous gas and fixed intestinal loop, erythema of the abdominal wall, palpable abdominal mass [17], and a scoring scale based on laboratory tests [18] or plasma IL-6 levels [19]. There is no doubt that intervention is required in cases of intestinal perforation. It is very easy to put a drain through the abdominal wall at the bedside in the ICU, and it may stabilize a very sick baby before operation. However, I agree with Dr. Pitcher that drainage as the definitive treatment should be reserved for very low-birth-weight newborns [20-22] that, may require further surgery to survive [23].

Babies with potentially nonviable bowel left in situ treated as described by Dr. Pitcher – against all dogmas of surgical source control – require a prolonged ICU stay and are subjected to the iatrogenic ravages of a prolonged central venous line, TPN, ventilators, antibiotics, blood products, and opportunistic infections. Whether this is superior to early resection of gangrenous bowel is controversial.

References

1. Yoon CH, Kim HJ, Goo HW (2001) Intussusception in children: US-guided pneumatic reduction – initial experience. Radiology 218:85–88
2. Duncan ND, Dennis W, Reid V, et al (1998) Hydrostatic reduction of acute intussusception: a prospective study. West Indian Med J 47:31–33
3. Luks FI, Yazbeck S, Brandt ML, et al (1990) Transient fever associated with a reduction of intestinal invagination. Chir Pediatr 31:157–159
4. Somekh E, Serour F, Goncalves D, et al (1996) Air enema for reduction of intussusception in children: risk of bacteremia. Radiology 200:217–218
5. Okoye BO, Rampersad B, Marantos A, et al (1998) Abscess after appendicectomy in children: the role of conservative management. Br J Surg 85:1111–1113
6. Lee MJ, Lee HC, Young W, et al (1998) Conservative treatment of intra-abdominal abscess in children. Zhonghua Min Guo 39:301–305
7. Schein M (2001) Management of intraabdominal abscesses. In: Holzheimer RG, Mannick JA (eds) Surgical treatment – evidence-based and problem-oriented. Zuckschwerdt Verlag, München, pp 695–702
8. Holcomb GW, Sharp KW, Neblett WW, et al (1994) Laparoscopic cholecystectomy in infants and children: modifications and cost analysis. J Pediatr Surg 29:900–904
9. Sidiropoulos D, Boehme U, Von Muralt G, et al (1986) Immunoglobulin supplementation in prevention or treatment of neonatal sepsis. Pediatr Infect Dis 5:S193–S194
10. Hoffmann P, Franz A, Sigge W, et al (1986) Omphalocele and gastroschisis: problems in intensive medical treatment. Zentralbl Chir 111:448–456
11. Scielzo R, Caramazza L, Circone R, et al (1992) Intravenous immunoglobulin in the prevention of infections in high-risk pediatric neurosurgery. Minerva Anesthesiol 58:235–238
12. Eibl MM, Wolf HM, Furnkranz H, et al (1988) Prevention of necrotizing enterocolitis in low-birth-weight infants by IgA-IgG feeding. N Engl J Med 319:1–7
13. Gomez R, Romero R, Ghezzi F, et al (1998) The fetal inflammatory bowel syndrome Am J Obstet Gynecol 179:194–202
14. Fasoli L, Turi LA, Spitz L, et al (1999) Necrotising enterocolitis: Extent of disease and surgical treatment. J Pediatr Surg 34:1096–1099
15. Harberg FJ, McGill CW, Saleem M, et al (1983) Resection with primary anastomosis for necrotising enterocolitis. J Pediatr Surg 18:743–745
16. Bianchi A (1997) Longitudinal intestinal lengthening and tailoring: results in 20 children. J R Soc Med 90:429–432
17. Kosloske AM (1994) Indication for operations in necrotising enterocolitis revisited. J Pediatr Surg 29:663–666
18. Gupta S, Burke G, Herson VC (1994) Necrotising enterocolitis: laboratory indicators of surgical disease J Pediatr Surg 29:1472–1475

19. Morecroft JA, Spitz L, Hamilton PA, et al (1994) Plasma interleukin-6 and tumour necrosis factor levels as predictors of disease severity and outcome in necrotising enterocolitis. J Pediatr Surg 29:798–800

20. Lessin MS, Luks FI, Wesselhoeft CW, et al (1998) Peritoneal drainage as definitive treatment for intestinal perforation in infants with extremely low birth weight (<750 g) J Pediatr Surg 33:370–372

21. Morgan LJ, Shochat SJ, Hartman G (1994) Peritoneal drainage as primary management of perforated NEC in the very low birth weight infant. J Pediatr Surg 29:310–315

22. Takamasu H, Akiyama H, Ibara S, et al (1992) Treatment for necrotising enterocolitis perforation in the extremely premature infant. J Pediatr Surg 27:741–743

23. Ahmed T, Ein S, Moore A (1998) The role of peritoneal drains in treatment of perforated necrotising enterocolitis: recommendations from recent experience. J Pediatr Surg 33:1468-1470

38 The AIDS Patient

Sai Sajja, Vellore Parithivel

Key Principles

- The general principles of source control are applicable to the HIV/AIDS patient; however, a thorough understanding of the natural history and spectrum of HIV disease is essential. The pathology may or may not be related to HIV status.
- Abdominal complaints are extremely common in the HIV population and clinical evaluation is often difficult. Serial clinical evaluation and frequent use of the CT scan are essential to prevent nontherapeutic interventions.
- Early diagnosis and prompt intervention are essential for non-HIV-related surgical disorders such as acute appendicitis and cholecystitis. Surgical intervention is also essential for complications of opportunistic infections such as cytomegalovirus (CMV) perforation. The morbidity and mortality of surgical procedures depends on the stage of the HIV disease and the nature of pathology.
- Surgical interventions should not be denied to this population because of the risk of occupational transmission and the fear of high complication rates. Relief of symptoms and improvement in quality of life are the chief considerations.

General Approach

Human immunodeficiency virus (HIV) infection and its inevitable consequence of acquired immunodeficiency syndrome (AIDS) is a major public health problem worldwide that has affected the way surgery and medicine is practiced. As of the end of 2000, according to the Joint United Nations Program on HIV/AIDS, there were 36.1 million people living with HIV/AIDS, 95% of whom live in the developing world [1]. In the United States, according to the Center for Disease Control (CDC), there are an estimated 800,000-900,000 people living with HIV, with 40,000 new HIV infections occurring each year [1]. With the advances in medical treatment, people infected with HIV are living longer; thus it is likely that most of the surgeons, wherever they practice, will encounter and treat patients with HIV/AIDS. While the general principles of source control described in this book are relevant to the HIV patient, we will emphasize the interventions for infections that are unique to this population. It is important to understand the natural history and the disease spectrum, which ranges from asymptomatic HIV infection to advanced AIDS, with a variety of opportunistic infections that potentially afflict this population.

Natural History and Surveillance Case Definition of AIDS

Acute infection with HIV leads to a self-limited, nonspecific illness consisting of fever, lymphadenopathy, pharyngitis, and arthralgias, after an incubation period of 6 days to 6 weeks. HIV has profound affinity for $CD4^+$ lymphocytes and causes their gradual destruction. Depending on the $CD4^+$ count, HIV disease is categorized as early stage ($CD4^+ > 500/\mu l$), mid stage ($CD4^+$ count 200-499/μl), advanced stage ($CD4^+$ 50-200/μl) and terminal ($CD4^+ < 50/\mu l$). The median time from acute infection to the development of AIDS is 8-10 years [2]. Since the introduction of effective antiretroviral therapy and prophylaxis against opportunistic infections, the morbidity and mortality has decreased. A thorough understanding of the stage of HIV disease is essential, as it has important implications for diagnosis, work-up, treatment, and prognosis. In 1993, the CDC modified the case definition of AIDS. Recurrent pneumonias, pulmonary tuberculosis, and invasive cervical cancer were added to the previous list of AIDS-defining illnesses. In addition, $CD4^+$ cell count was included in the case definition. A $CD4^+$ count of less than 200/μl now is defined as AIDS irrespective of the presence of symptoms or other illnesses [3]. Table 1 shows the AIDS indicator conditions and Table 2 shows the revised classification system for HIV infection based on $CD4^+$ cell count.

Table 1. AIDS indicator conditions in the 1993 AIDS surveillance case definition [3]

Candidiasis of bronchi, trachea and lung
Candidiasis, esophageal
Cervical cancer, invasive
Coccidioidomycosis, disseminated or extrapulmonary
Cryptococcosis, extrapulmonary
Cryptosporidiosis, chronic intestinal
Cytomegalovirus disease other than liver, spleen, and nodes
Cytomegalovirus retinitis
Encephalopathy, HIV-related
Herpes simplex, chronic ulcers, bronchitis, pneumonitis, or esophagitis
Histoplasmosis, disseminated or extrapulmonary
Isosporiasis, chronic intestinal
Kaposi's sarcoma
Lymphoma, Burkitt's or equivalent term
Lymphoma, immunoblastic
Lymphoma, primary, of brain
Mycobacterium avium complex (MAC), disseminated or extrapulmonary
Mycobacterium tuberculosis, any site
Pneumocystis carinii pneumonia
Progressive multifocal leukoencephalopathy
Salmonella septicemia, recurrent
Toxoplasmosis of brain
Wasting syndrome due to AIDS

Table 2. 1993 Revised classification system for HIV infection for adolescents and adults (from [3])

CD4+ T-Cell categories	(A) Asymptomatic acute (primary) HIV or persistent generalized lymphadenopathy	(B) Symptomatic, not (A) or (C)	(C) AIDS indicator conditions (Table 1)
(1) > 500	A1	B1	C1
(2) 200-499	A2	B2	C2
(3) < 200	A3	B3	C3

As of January 1, 1993, categories A3, B3, C1, C2, C3 are reportable as AIDS.

Intra-abdominal Complications

Abdominal Pain

Abdominal pain and nonspecific gastrointestinal complaints are common in patients with HIV/AIDS. Clinical evaluation can be difficult. Many patients suffer from chronic abdominal symptoms and for the physician encountering the patient for the first time, the baseline status for the patient may appear very abnormal. The list of differential diagnoses is larger in this population. The white blood cell count, which is a valuable marker of acute inflammation in an uninfected population, may be unreliable because of preexisting leukopenia. Patients often have coexisting infections of the central nervous system, which makes evaluation of the abdominal pain difficult. Antiviral medications frequently cause chronic abdominal symptoms. A thorough history, including the stage of the HIV disease, the presence of opportunistic infections, and the use of antiretroviral therapy, and a careful physical examination along with an erect chest X-ray and abdominal X-rays and routine laboratory tests, including serum amylase and lipase, form the basis on which further management is planned.

When the initial examination is inconclusive, serial examinations often yield valuable information. In the absence of clinical peritonitis, free intraperitoneal air and exsanguinating hemorrhage, a CT scan of the abdomen and pelvis is an indispensable investigation [4]. It often identifies nonsurgical pathology and avoids a nontherapeutic laparotomy. Table 3 summarizes causes of abdominal pain in HIV/AIDS.

Acute Appendicitis

AIDS does not render a patient immune to acute appendicitis, which in the general population is one of the common abdominal emergencies. The incidence of appendicitis in hospitalized HIV patients appears to be higher than in the general population (0.5% vs 0.1-0.2%) [5]. The diagnosis is challenging: while some patients present with typical symptoms and localizing signs in the right lower quadrant, the presentation is often atypical. Diarrhea and vomiting are

Table 3. HIV-related and HIV-unrelated causes of abdominal pain according to the need for source control

	HIV-related conditions	HIV-unrelated conditions
Source control necessary	CMV perforation	Appendicitis
	CMV-related toxic megacolon	Cholecystitis
	Acalculous cholecystitis	Secondary peritonitis
	KS, lymphoma with perforation	Intra-abdominal abscesses
	Splenic abscess	Intestinal ischemia
		Trauma
Nonsurgical	Uncomplicated CMV infection	Organomegaly
	MAC	Constipation
	MTB	Uncomplicated peptic ulcer disease
	Pancreatitis, infectious (CMV, MAC), drug-induced (pentamidine, dideoxyinosine, Trimethoprim-sulphamethaxazole)	Uncomplicated pelvic inflammatory disease

KS, Kaposi's sarcoma; MAC, *Mycobacterium avium* complex; MTB, *Mycobacterium tuberculosis*.

seen more frequently, while fever and leukocytosis are not very reliable. CT scan is the diagnostic imaging study of choice when the clinical presentation is atypical [6]. Diagnostic laparoscopy may facilitate an early and more accurate diagnosis.

CMV infection and Kaposi's sarcoma of the base of the appendix have been reported to cause appendicitis [6, 7]. CMV infection can cause vasculitis with occlusion of the appendicular artery, leading to ischemia and perforation. The operative and postoperative management is similar to the non-HIV population. The high morbidity and mortality seen in early series by LaRaja et al. [8] and Burack et al. [9] likely reflects the late clinical presentation. In a recent review of 55 patients, Flum et al. [10] reported 100% 30-day survival. Prolonged postoperative fever was the most frequent complication in this study. Thus, a high index of suspicion and early clinical evaluation along with appropriate use of CT scan and diagnostic laparoscopy should lead to early diagnosis and a better postoperative outcome.

Cytomegalovirus

While 80% of adults over the age of 35 years show evidence of infection with CMV, it is of clinical consequence only in the immunosuppressed patient. In the AIDS patient, CMV is found in every organ system in the body, is the most common opportunistic infection of the GI tract, and often involves the colon – causing fever, diarrhea, and abdominal pain [4]. CMV infects endothelial cells, leading to thrombosis of the submucosal blood vessels and resulting in mucosal ischemia, ulceration, hemorrhage, perforation, and toxic megacolon. Diagnosis is established by colonoscopy and biopsy, which shows characteristic intranuclear inclusion bodies. CT scan findings of thickening of the bowel wall and mural ulceration are nonspecific [11]. Once the diagnosis is established, treatment with ganciclovir or foscarnet is started. It is very important to keep these patients under close observation while they are on medical therapy, to identify the development of complications. Despite aggressive medical management, some patients develop perforation, toxic megacolon, and hemorrhage – complications that require urgent surgical intervention. The perforations related to CMV appear punctate when viewed from the serosal surface [4]. Resection of the involved segment of bowel and formation of a colostomy or ileostomy is the treatment of choice. Primary anastomosis is to be avoided. These patients are prone to perforations of other parts of the bowel due to diffuse CMV enteritis, and fecal diversion might decrease the risk of perforation in the defunctioned bowel. When operating for toxic megacolon, a subtotal colectomy and ileostomy is the treatment of choice. The results of surgical therapy were disappointing in early series with mortality rate of 71% [12]. However, in a series of 28 patients undergoing emergency laparotomy for toxic megacolon, small-bowel obstruction, perforated viscus, and appendicitis, Davidson et al. showed a mortality rate of 11% [13].

Acute Cholecystitis

Right upper quadrant abdominal pain associated with fever, nausea, and vomiting is a common complaint in patients with HIV/AIDS. While the cause of this pain may be due to hepatomegaly associated with granulomatous infiltration or colitis, biliary pathology needs to be investigated. Gallstones are present in 27%-70% of patients with HIV/AIDS undergoing cholecystectomy [14]. Patients with HIV/AIDS have a high incidence acalculous cholecystitis in comparison with the general population. CMV and *Cryptosporidium* are the most common opportunistic microorganisms isolated [4]. In HIV/AIDS, overwhelming growth of pathogens seems to be the cause of inflammation and functional obstruction, rather than hypotension, ischemia, and sepsis, the typical causes of acalculous cholecystitis in non-HIV critically ill patients.

Ultrasound is the initial imaging study of choice. The presence of gallstones, the diameter of the common bile duct, gallbladder wall thickness, and the presence of pericholecystic fluid and intramural air can all be demonstrated. CT scans and HIDA scans are useful when the sonogram is inconclusive. As the pathogenesis of acalculous cholecystitis may not involve cystic duct obstruction, a HIDA scan may demonstrate gallbladder filling.

Once the diagnosis is established, depending on the overall condition of the patient, surgical intervention is recommended. Laparoscopic cholecystectomy can be safely performed, as experimental observations have not substantiated concerns regarding aerosolization of HIV in the laparoscopy gas [15]. To prevent blood spray during the retrieval of the gallbladder, pneumoperitoneum must be evacuated first. Routine use of specimen bags is recommended to prevent the accidental spillage of infected contents. A high mortality rate (33%) was observed in early series [8]. More recent results, however, have demonstrated a mortality of 7%-9% [14]. The relatively high mortality rates reflect the fact that acalculous cholecystitis occurs in the more advanced stage of AIDS.

AIDS Cholangiopathy

Opportunistic pathogens cause a spectrum of extrahepatic biliary pathology in patients with AIDS [16], characterized by marked elevation of the alkaline phosphatase with mild elevation of bilirubin and transaminases. *Cryptosporidium*, CMV, *Microsporidia*, and *Mycobacterium avium* complex (MAC) are the most common pathogens identified [17]. Cello described four types of cholangiopathy in HIV patients, based on endoscopic retrograde cholangiopancreatogram (ERCP) findings [16]; these are shown in Table 4.

Table 4. AIDS-related cholangiopathy [16]

Papillary stenosis	CBD> 8 mm Contrast material empties in > 30 min Sphincter of Oddi pressure > 40 mmHg 2-4 mm tapering of the distal CBD
Sclerosing cholangitis	Focal strictures of intra- and extrahepatic bile ducts
Papillary stenosis and sclerosing cholangitis	Features of papillary stenosis and sclerosing cholangitis.
Extrahepatic bile duct strictures	1-2 cm extrahepatic bile duct stricture No prior CBD disease Normal pancreatic duct

Antimicrobial therapy is ineffective in the management of AIDS cholangiopathy. In the presence of papillary stenosis, sphincterotomy offers pain relief but will not alter the progression of the disease. As cholangiopathy occurs during the advanced stage of HIV disease, survival beyond 1 year is unusual.

Splenic Abscess

Splenic abscess is more common in patients with HIV/AIDS [18]. Metastatic spread from other infections, secondary infection of an infarct, and contiguous spread from an adjacent organ are the usual mechanisms of its development. CT scan or ultrasound establishes the diagnosis. In the absence of loculations, percutaneous CT-guided drainage of splenic abscess has a success rate of 65%-75% [18]. Splenectomy is the definitive treatment when radiological features do not favor percutaneous drainage or when radiological intervention has failed.

Perianal Sepsis

Anorectal problems are common in the HIV/AIDS population, especially in those who practice anal-receptive intercourse [12]. Fifty to 85% of all operations performed on HIV-positive patients involve the anorectum [19]. While being susceptible to anorectal problems found in the general population, HIV/AIDS patients are prone to a variety of opportunistic infections such as CMV and herpes, and to benign and malignant neoplasms of the perianal area [20]. Careful inspection of the perianal area, gentle digital rectal examination and a proctoscopic visualization will identify the perianal condition. Examination under anesthesia is an essential part of evaluation before definitive surgical therapy. As in the non-HIV population, perianal sepsis in this population could result from cryptoglandular disease, but it may also be associated with HIV-related anorectal ulcers or result from secondary infection of anal proliferative lesions. The abscesses associated with HIV-related anorectal ulcers tend to be very deep – transgressing the sphincter planes – with variable destruction of the sphincter mechanism [19]. Surgical intervention is usually necessary: abscesses should be liberally drained and specimens should be obtained for acid fast staining and culture. Biopsy is done if underlying malignancy is suspected. The principles of treatment are similar to the management of perianal sepsis in Crohn's disease. Damage to the sphincters is avoided and noncutting setons and drains are used liberally. Delayed wound healing was a major concern in early reports, but recent reports suggest results that are more favorable [12, 20, 21]. Of the factors related to HIV disease, a $CD4^+$ cell count of less than $50/\mu l$ was identified as a predictor of delayed wound healing [21].

Skin and Soft Tissue Infections

Injectable drugs are one of the major risk factors for HIV/AIDS and these patients are prone to soft tissue infections at the injection sites. They are also prone to a variety of dermatological conditions with secondary pyogenic infections. While clinical evaluation may suffice to differentiate simple cellulitis from an underlying abscess, the best diagnostic test is exploration in the operating room. Plain X-rays may detect gas in the soft tissues and occasionally advanced imaging with CT scan or MRI may be of value when a deep intramuscular abscess is suspected. At the time of debridement, all necrotic tissue should be excised. When suppurative thrombophlebitis is suspected and pus expressed from the puncture site, excision of that segment of the vein should be performed.

Thoracic Empyema

Pulmonary complications are a major cause of morbidity in patients with HIV/AIDS. In a review of 1097 HIV patients, pleural effusion was found in 14.7% [22]. Pleural effusions may develop in response to intra-abdominal or pulmonary disease. Thoracentesis helps to identify the nature of the effusion (exudate vs transudate) and to diagnose empyema. CT scan of the chest is particularly useful in identifying loculated collections [23]. As in non-HIV patients, the method of source control depends on the stage of empyema. Thoracentesis is rarely effective in draining all the fluid, even in the early exudative phase, and tube thoracostomy is needed. If a chest tube fails to evacuate the fluid in 3-5 days or when the patient is first seen during the organized phase of empyema, thoracoscopy should be performed early before the development of a thick pleural peel. If adequate decortication cannot be achieved by video-assisted thoracoscopy, conversion to thoracotomy is essential [23]. All fibrinous membranes and necrotic debris must be removed to allow the lung to expand. Rib resection and open drainage may be needed when patients present late or for the management of residual disease following other forms of source control.

The Risk of Occupational Exposure

While surgeons have always been exposed to the risk of such blood-borne infections as hepatitis B and hepatitis C, the inevitably fatal consequences of HIV infection have increased their awareness of this ubiquitous risk. The prevalence of HIV infection in healthcare workers is not higher than in the general population and only 5% of healthcare workers have no identifiable risk factors. Surgical personnel have a low prevalence of occupational infection despite the frequency with which they are exposed to blood and other body fluids. To date, there has been no documented case of occupational HIV transmission to a surgeon in the United States [24]. The risk of seroconversion after a needle-stick injury is estimated at 0.3% and all documented cases have followed hollow needle injuries; none have been documented from solid suture needles [25]. This low risk likely reflects the low dose of the inoculum and the fact that the glove material wipes the needle. Strict adherence to universal precautions and effective operative technique, for example, avoidance of hand-to-hand passing of sharp instruments, would decrease the risk of injury to the operating team.

Controversies

Patients with complications of CMV infection who require emergency intervention have a high morbidity and mortality. If patients can be operated on at a relatively early stage before the development of catastrophic complications, a more favorable outcome may be possible. Soderlund et al. [26] advocate early operation for the localized form of CMV colitis refractory to medical therapy, before the development of complications. They have operated on eight patients with CMV colitis limited to the right side of the colon. Four patients underwent ileocecal resections, while the remaining four had a formal right hemicolectomy. Primary anastomosis was performed in all patients. There were two deaths, both unrelated to surgery. Complete or partial palliation was achieved in the remaining patients for a mean of 14 months. Further studies need to be done to validate the utility of early intervention in these patients.

Table 5. Clinical staging of HIV disease and surgical mortality [28]

Stage of HIV disease	CDC class (1993)	CD4 count (cells/mm^3)	Estimated surgical mortality (30 days)
Early	A	> 500	0%-3%
Middle	B	200-499	3%-5%
Advanced (terminal)	C	< 200 (< 50)	1%-23%

Perioperative risk assessment for HIV/AIDS patients has been a complex and controversial issue. While early studies [9] showed high morbidity and mortality, more recent studies contradict these conclusions [27]. The factors that increase morbidity and mortality in this population include the stage of HIV disease, the presence of opportunistic infection, a serum albumin concentration of less than 2.5 g/dl, and the presence of concurrent organ failure [28]. In addition, the presence of AIDS-related pathology as the cause of emergency abdominal surgery increases morbidity and mortality by three- to fourfold. However, it is important to note that for two-thirds of HIV/AIDS patients undergoing emergency laparotomy, the problem is not AIDS-related [28]. Table 5 shows surgical mortality according to the stage.

Critical Factors and Decision Making

Patients with HIV/AIDS are susceptible to surgical conditions that may or may not be related to their underlying HIV infection. Clinical evaluation is often dif-

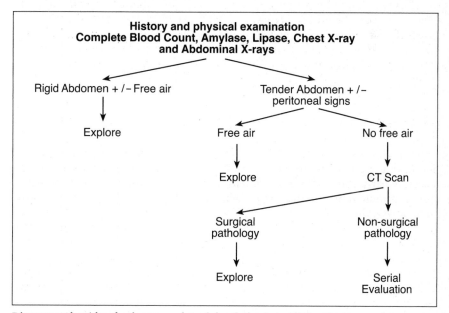

Diagram 1. Algorithm for the approach to abdominal pain in AIDS patients

ficult and imaging studies are used more frequently. When interventions are appropriately performed, complication rates are similar to those reported for other immunosuppressed and malnourished patients. While the risk of occupational transmission is present, strict adherence to universal precautions and appropriate modifications of surgical practice minimizes the risk. As patients with HIV live longer because of advances in medical management, it is likely that many of them will need surgical treatment for unrelated pathology in the years to come. Surgeons must be aware of the natural history and the unique challenges in the management HIV-infected patient.

References

1. Joint United Nations Program on HIV/AIDS, Centers for Disease Control and Prevention, National Center for HIV, STD, and TB prevention. (2001) The global HIV and AIDS epidemic. MMWR Rep 50:434–439
2. Vergis EN, Mellors JW (2000) Natural history of HIV-1 infection. Infect Dis Clin North Am 14:809–825
3. 1993 Revised classification system for HIV infection and expanded surveillance case definition for AIDS among adolescents and adults (1992) MMWR 41:1–19
4. Mueller GP, Williams RA (1995) Surgical infections in AIDS patients. Am J Surg 169:34S–38S
5. Wells SB, Beaton HL (1991) Appendicial disease in HIV-infected homosexual men. AIDS Reader 2:173–175
6. Whitney TM, Macho JR, et al (1992) Appendicitis in acquired immunodeficiency syndrome. Am J Surg 164:467–471
7. Bindreow SR, Shaked AA (1991) Acute appendicitis in patients with AIDS/HIV infection. Am J Surg 162:9–12
8. LaRaja RD, Rothenberg RE, et al (1989) The incidence of intra-abdominal surgery in acquired immunodeficiency syndrome: a statistical review of 904 patients. Surgery 105:175–179
9. Burack JH, Mandel MS, Bizer LS (1989) Emergency abdominal operations in the patient with acquired immunodeficiency syndrome. Arch Surg 124:285–286
10. Flum D, Steinberg S, et al (1997) Appendicitis in patients with acquired immunodeficiency syndrome. J Am Coll Surg 184:481–486
11. Murray JG, Evans SJJ et al (1995) Cytomegalovirus colitis in AIDS: CT features. Am J Rad 165:67–71
12. Wexner SD, Smithy WB, et al (1986) The surgical management of anorectal disease in AIDS and pre-AIDS patients. Dis Colon Rectum 29:719–723
13. Davidson T, Allen-Mersh TG et al (1991) Emergency laparotomy in patients with AIDS. Br J Surg 78:924–926
14. Flum DR, Steinberg SD, Sarkis AY, et al (1997) The role of cholecystectomy in acquired immunodeficiency syndrome. J Am Coll Surg 184:233–239
15. Box JC (1997) Laparoscopy in the evaluation and treatment of patients with AIDS and acute abdominal complaints. Surg Endosc 11:1026–1028
16. Cello JP (1989) Human immunodeficiency syndrome cholangiopathy: spectrum of disease. Am J Med 86:539–546
17. Mehajani RV, Uzer MF (1999) Cholangiopathy in HIV-infected patient. Clin Liver Dis 3: 669–684
18. Ooi LL, Leong SS (1997) Splenic abscess from 1987-1995. Am J Surg 174:87–93
19. Viamonte M, Dailey TH, Gottesman L (1993) Ulcerative disease of the anorectum in the HIV+ patient. Dis Colon Rectum 36:801–805
20. Safavi A, Gottesman L, Dailey TH (1991) Anorectal surgery in the HIV+ patient: Update. Dis Colon Rectum 4:299–304
21. Lord RVN (1997) Anorectal surgery in patients infected with human immunodeficiency virus. Factors associated with delayed wound healing. Ann Surg 226:92–107

22. Afesa B, Green W, et al (1998) Pulmonary complications of HIV infection. Chest 113:1225–1229
23. Borge JH, Michavila IA, et al (1998) Thoracic empyema in HIV-infected patients, microbiology management and outcome. Chest 113:732–738
24. Centers for Disease Control and Prevention (1997) HIV/AIDS surveillance report. MMWR 9:15
25. Centers for Disease Control and Prevention (1995) Case control study of HIV seroconversion in health-care workers after percutaneous exposure to HIV infected blood: France, United Kingdom and United States, January 1988–August 1994. MMWR 44:929–933
26. Soderlund C, Bratt GA, Engstorm L, et al (1994) Surgical treatment of cytomegalovirus enterocolitis in severe immunodeficiency virus infection. Dis Colon Rectum 37:63–72
27. Bizer LS, Pettorino R, Ashikari A (1995) Emergency abdominal operations in the patient with acquired immunodeficiency syndrome. J Am Coll Surg 180:205–209
28. Harris HW, Schecter WP (1997) Surgical risk assessment and management in patients with HIV disease. Gastroenterol Clin 26:377–391

Invited Commentary

MARC WALLACK, JOHN DEGLIUOMINI

The human immunodeficiency virus (HIV) has significantly impacted on the practice of surgery. The morbidity and mortality associated with infection has been reduced, paralleling advances made with the development of new antiretroviral agents. Despite these advances surgeons will still encounter patients with various presentations. Infection with HIV, the development of AIDS and subsequent opportunistic infections, and a variety of tumors (such as lymphoma, and Kaposi's sarcoma, for example) has made evaluating the patient with HIV/AIDS ever more challenging.

Gastrointestinal complaints are a frequent patient complaint. In the absence of clinical peritonitis, differentiating the acute abdomen from chronic symptomatology often causes the surgeon to rely on multiple ancillary studies (such as CT scans and radioactive tagged cell scans) as adjuncts to clinical evaluation.

Although the incidence of appendicitis may be slightly higher in the hospitalized HIV/AIDS patient, clinical management has not significantly changed. CT scanning has been reported to have a 93%-98% accuracy rate for diagnosing or excluding appendicitis [1], and provides a noninvasive alternative to diagnostic laparoscopy in the diagnosis of appendicitis. Late presentations of appendicitis, including perforation, phlegmon, and abscess, are not uncommon. In addition to advanced immunodeficiency and a late presentation, poor nutritional status, weight loss, and low serum albumin contribute significantly to mortality and morbidity in patients with HIV/AIDS undergoing emergency surgery [2].

CMV colitis is a commonly recognized cause of abdominal pain in the patient with HIV/AIDS. Although the presentation can vary depending on the severity of the colitis, once the diagnosis is established, close observation is essential because complications such as bleeding and perforation are common. Limited resection and the prudent use of fecal diversion remain the mainstay of surgical treatment.

The introduction of protease inhibitors has significantly and positively changed the outcome of AIDS-associated CMV colitis [3].

Acute cholecystitis is one of the more common indications for abdominal surgery in patients with AIDS. Ultrasound examination remains the initial study of choice. However, given the incidence of acalculous disease [4] in the patient with AIDS and cholecystitis, HIDA and CT scans can be an invaluable tool in confirming the diagnosis. Once the decision for surgical intervention has been made, the approach (either laparoscopic or open) should be individualized to the patient's condition. Laparoscopic cholecystectomy is generally accepted as safe to perform in the patient with AIDS and acute cholecystitis, provided one uses standard precautions.

Opportunistic infections of the biliary tract in immunocompromised patients were first described in the early 1980s [5]. Initial reported cases involved CMV and *Cryptosporidium* infections. Subsequent reports documented intra- and extrahepatic biliary obstruction with concurrent infection of the biliary tree with microsporidia, *Isospora* and *Mycobacterium avium-intracellulare*. The diagnostic features of this entity include abdominal pain, cholestasis without jaundice, and an abnormal ultrasound exam. Medical treatment has not been shown to be effective and for most patients, cholangitis has been shown to progress despite antimicrobial therapy. ERCP is considered the gold standard for diagnostic and therapeutic interventions. Long-term outcome studies show that following ERCP sphincterotomy, pain scores decreased significantly, but serum alkaline phosphatase levels remain unchanged [6]. Cholangiopathy is a manifestation of late-stage AIDS and is associated with poor long-term survival.

The development of splenic abscess in the patient with HIV/AIDS may manifest as fever and left upper quadrant pain. CT scan of the abdomen is the diagnostic modality of choice. Depending on the physical characteristics, the abscess may be amenable to percutaneous drainage; splenectomy is reserved for failure of radiological drainage.

Anorectal pathology in the anal-receptive patient with HIV/AIDS can vary. Although patients are prone to disorders encountered in an uninfected population, many present with herpetic or papillomatous lesions of the anus. Perianal sepsis can result in destruction of the sphincter mechanism. It is generally agreed that the approach to such patients should involve a careful examination – under anesthesia if necessary – and adherence to the same principles of management of perianal sepsis that are used in Crohn's disease. However, some authors advocate an aggressive approach to anorectal disease in the immunocompromised patient, claiming that high rates of healing and low complication rates can be obtained that are similar to those associated with treatment of the same disease process in the general public [7].

The management of skin and soft tissue infections in the HIV/AIDS patient may be complicated by the presence of deep intramuscular abscesses. The best diagnostic test is operative exploration in the operating room.

Pleural effusions are common in patients with HIV/AIDS, the most common cause being bacterial pneumonia [8]. The approach to thoracic empyema should be that employed in the non-HIV patient, with source control dependent on the stage. Thoracotomy and decortication are best reserved for late-stage presentation.

Although surgeons have always been at risk for exposure to blood-borne pathogens, HIV infection and its sequelae have brought about increased awareness within the profession. The fact that the risk of transmission through solid needles is lower may be a result of a smaller inoculum. Strict adherence to proper technique in handling sharp instruments and adherence to universal precautions cannot be overly stressed.

Like any other patient with medical comorbidities presenting for surgery, the patient with advanced HIV/AIDS presents with other factors that contribute significantly to morbidity and mortality. The stage of HIV disease is an important prognostic factor in patients with surgical pathology. Studies have shown poor hospital outcomes in HIV/AIDS patients with a low CD4$^+$ count [9,10]. Moreover, malnutrition, as evidenced by hypoalbuminemia, has long been recognized as a universal risk factor for increased morbidity in patients undergoing surgery, regardless of HIV status. Organ system dysfunction and the presence of opportunistic infection also place the patient at increased risk.

As medical advances in the treatment of HIV infection progress and patients live longer, surgeons will be faced with an aging population of immunosuppressed patients, some with pathology unique to HIV/AIDS and some with pathology common to the general population. The unique challenges of treating HIV/AIDS patients must be learned by surgeons and the appropriate therapeutic approaches adopted.

References

1. Rao PM, Rhea JT, Novelline RA (1999) Helical CT of appendicitis and diverticulitis. Radiol Clin North Am 37:895–910
2. Wittmann MM, Wittmann A, Wittmann DH (1996) AIDS emergency operations and infection control. Infect Control Hosp Epidemiol 17(8): 532–538
3. Bini EJ, Gorelick SM, Weinshel EH (2000) Outcome of AIDS-associated cytomegalovirus colitis in the era of potent antiretroviral therapy. J Clin Gastroenterol 30:414–419
4. Ricci M, Puente AO, Rothenberg RE, Shapiro K, de Luise C, LaRaja RD (1999) Open and laparoscopic cholecystectomy in acquired immunodeficiency syndrome: indications and results in fifty-three patients. Surgery 125:172–177
5. Mahajani RV, Uzer MF (1999) Cholangiopathy in HIV-infected patients. Clin Liver Dis 3:669–684
6. Cello JP, Chan MF (1995) Long-term follow up of endoscopic retrograde cholangiopancreatography sphincterotomy for patients with acquired immunodeficiency syndrome papillary stenosis. Am J Med 99:600–603
7. Munoz-Villasmil J, Sands L, Hellinger M (2001) Management of perianal sepsis in immunosuppressed patients. Am Surg 67:484–486
8. Afessa B (2000) Pleural effusion and pneumothorax in hospitalized patients with HIV infection: the Pulmonary Complications, ICU support, and Prognostic Factors of Hospitalized Patients with HIV (PIP) Study. Chest 117:1031–1037
9. Rosen MJ, De Palo VA (1993) Outcome of intensive care for patients with AIDS. Crit Care Clin 19:107–114
10. Brown MC, Crede WB (1995) Predictive ability of acute physiology and chronic health evaluation II scoring applied to human immunodeficiency virus-positive patients. Crit Care Med 23:848–853

Part IV: Evaluating the Adequacy of Source Control

39 Clinical and Radiographic Assessment

MITCHELL P. FINK

Key Principles

- The initial treatment of intra-abdominal infection typically consists of an operative intervention plus administration of appropriate antimicrobial chemotherapy. Following these initial therapeutic interventions, it is important to determine the adequacy of source control in order make reasonable decisions about the duration of antimicrobial chemotherapy and/or the need for additional interventional radiographic or surgical procedures. Unfortunately, there is no single test that can provide the clinician with a clear answer to the question: Has adequate source control been achieved?

Physical Examination

Physical examination findings (e.g., abdominal tenderness or muscular rigidity) that are useful in the initial evaluation of patients with suspected intra-abdominal infection are much less useful in the postoperative period after laparotomy. Extra-incisional pain and guarding is hard to distinguish from the pain associated with an abdominal incision. Furthermore, patients (particularly ones who are very sick) are often heavily medicated with analgesics, sedatives, and even anesthetics such as propofol. Accordingly, the clinical assessment of the postoperative patient to determine adequacy of source control depends on a combination of softer clinical findings, nonspecific laboratory tests, and imaging procedures.

Fever

The most obvious clinical finding that suggests that source control has been inadequate is the presence of persistent or recurrent fever. Elevation of core body temperature, of course, is a very nonspecific finding that is caused by the action of certain cytokines (particularly, IL-1, TNF, and IL-6) within the hypothalamus [1-3]. Thus, fever is a sign of inflammation, not infection per se. Although lacking diagnostic specificity, measurements of body temperature remain an invaluable component of clinical monitoring.

The value of fever as a sign of persistent intra-abdominal infection after operation (i.e., inadequate source control) was emphasized in a classic report by Lennard et al. from the University of Washington [4]. These investigators prospectively evaluated 65 patients with intra-abdominal sepsis, who underwent an operative procedure and were treated with a reasonable combination of antibiotics (gentamicin plus clindamycin or gentamicin plus choramphenicol). Of these patients, 51 were afebrile at the end of a 10-14-day course of antibiotics, whereas 14 had persistent fever. Among the afebrile subset, evidence of inadequate source control was diagnosed in seven patients (13.7%) and additional operative intervention was undertaken in six. Among the patients who were still febrile at the end of a defined course of antibiotic therapy, 11 (79%) had postoperative infections; eight of these infections were focused in the abdomen. These data clearly support the view that persistent or recurrent temperature elevation after an operation for intra-abdominal infection should raise suspicion of inadequate source control.

In another classic study, Le Gall et al. prospectively evaluated 100 ICU patients with a temperature greater than 39°C between the third and tenth days after laparotomy [5]. Among these patients, 66 had intra-abdominal sepsis; these patients constituted Group I. The remaining 34 patients constituted Group II. In nine of the patients in Group II, no source of infection within the abdomen could be identified either by surgical exploration or autopsy. The remaining 25 patients recovered completely without reoperation or radiological intervention and were therefore classified as not having intra-abdominal sepsis. Among the patients in Group II, 23 had an extra-abdominal focus of infection, whereas no infectious cause of fever was diagnosed in 11. The most common extra-abdominal sites of infection were surgical wounds, intravenous catheters, and the lungs. Prompted by their data, Le Gall and coworkers recommended that when evaluating ICU patients with a high fever after laparotomy, clinicians should attempt to exclude catheter-related sepsis, wound infection, and pneumonia. Negative findings should suggest a high likelihood of intra-abdominal sepsis, and should prompt further efforts to confirm and localize the source of infection.

Leukocytosis

Leukocytosis is the other "classic" sign of persistent intra-abdominal infection. In the previously cited study by Le Gall et al. of ICU patients with postoperative fever [5], the most significant parameter predicting intra-abdominal sepsis was the absence of bacteremia. The *second most* significant predictor of intra-abdominal sepsis (among patients with fever) was a white blood cell count greater than 12,000 μl^{-1}. Lennard et al. reviewed outcomes for 31 patients who were afebrile after operation and a course of antimicrobial chemotherapy for intra-abdominal infection [6]. These authors reported that recurrent or persistent intra-abdominal infection was diagnosed in 13 (68%) of 19 patients with a white blood cell count greater than 10,000 μl^{-1}. Thus, persistent leukocytosis should prompt efforts to confirm or exclude the presence of ongoing intra-abdominal infection.

Acute-Phase Proteins

Fever is a nonspecific finding indicative of inflammation rather than infection. Leukocytosis, a response to various stress-related and acute-phase hormones and cytokines including cortisol, epinephrine, granulocyte colony stimulating factor, tumor necrosis factor, and interleukin-1, is similarly nonspecific. Accordingly, investigators have long sought a blood test that could be used to distinguish patients with infection from those without infection. Two tests, namely those for circulating levels of C-reactive protein (CRP) and procalcitonin (PCT), have undergone extensive evaluation in this regard.

CRP is an acute-phase protein synthesized by the liver. In a study of 108 patients undergoing clean-contaminated or dirty surgical abdominal surgical procedures, Mustard et al. measured circulating levels of CRP on a daily basis for 14 days to assess whether this test could be used to predict the occurrence of septic complications [7]. These authors determined that CRP testing has modest clinical utility as a way to discriminate patients with ongoing infection from those without infection. Another study, which evaluated only patients requiring care in a surgical ICU, also found that CRP testing (using an appropriate cutoff value) had good sensitivity (85%) for detecting infection, but lacked specificity [8]. Yet another study determined that measurement of CRP (using a cutoff value of 100 ng/ml) lacked sufficient sensitivity (74%) and specificity (74%) to be useful for discriminating infection from the systemic inflammatory response syndrome (SIRS) [9].

Currently, there is a great deal of interest, particularly in Europe, regarding the use of PCT as a diagnostic marker of infection. Like CRP, PCT, a 13-kDa propeptide of calcitonin, is an acute-phase protein. Although contrary findings have been reported [9-11], a number of studies that have evaluated the diagnostic utility of PCT measurements have concluded that serum PCT levels greater than 2 ng/ml are a reliable indicator of infection [12-15]. Some studies have concluded that CRP is a more reliable indicator of infection than PCT [11], and some have come to the opposite conclusion [10, 15]. There are insufficient data in the published literature to warrant making strong statements regarding the usefulness of either CRP or PCT measurements for assessing the adequacy of source control after operation for intra-abdominal infection.

Imaging

A variety of imaging approaches have been employed to confirm the diagnosis of intra-abdominal infection after initial laparotomy. These approaches include scintigraphy using leukocytes labeled with [111]Indium [16], scintigraphy using [67]Gallium citrate [17], and abdominal ultrasound [17]. Nevertheless, the imaging procedure of choice remains computed tomography (CT) – although ultrasonography is useful in selected cases, largely because the imaging equipment can be moved to the patient instead of vice versa. CT imaging is not limited by overlying bowel gas as is ultrasound. Proper enteral and intravenous contrast administration and scanning protocols must be followed to permit differentiating fluid-filled loops of bowel from abnormal fluid collections.

In one recent study of patients with suspected intra-abdominal sepsis after major trauma, the sensitivity and specificity of abdominal CT for diagnosing an intra-abdominal focus of infection was 97.5% and 61.5%, respectively [18]. CT (and to a lesser degree, ultrasonography) is so valuable that reoperation should rarely be undertaken unless guided by findings obtained using one or both of these imaging methods [19, 20]. In general, positive findings obtained by CT are much more likely to modify the therapeutic plan than are negative findings [21]. CT is particularly valuable because the anatomical information provided often permits interventional radiological methods to be used to drain suspicious fluid collections, thereby avoiding the need to subject the patient to reoperation [22].

Scintigraphic imaging approaches should be used rarely, being reserved for those cases when CT is negative yet there remains a very strong clinical suspicion of an intra-abdominal abscess. Although more expensive, imaging using ^{111}Indium-labeled white blood cells is preferable to scintigraphy using ^{67}Gallium citrate, since the latter approach requires a minimum of 24 h before diagnostic information is available.

References

1. Cannon JG, Tompkins RG, Gelfand JA, et al (1990) Circulating interleukin-1 and tumor necrosis factor in septic shock and experimental endotoxin fever. J Inf Dis 161:79–84
2. Horai R, Asano M, Sudo K, et al (1998) Production of mice deficient in genes for interleukin (IL)-1a, IL-1 b, IL-1a/b, and IL-1 receptor antagonist shows that IL-1b is crucial in turpentine-induced fever development and glucocorticoid secretion. J Exp Med 187:1463–1475
3. Saper CB, Breder CD (1994) The neurologic basis of fever. N Engl J Med 330:1880–1886
4. Lennard ES, Dellinger EP, Wertz MJ, et al (1982) Implications of leukocytosis and fever at conclusion of antibiotic therapy for intra-abdominal sepsis. Ann Surg 195:19–24
5. Le Gall JR, Fagniez PL, Meakins J, et al (1982) Diagnostic features of early high post-laparotomy fever: a prospective study of 100 patients. Br J Surg 69:452–455
6. Lennard ES, Minshew BH, Dellinger EP, et al (2001) Leukocytosis at termination of antibiotic therapy. Arch Surg 115:918–921
7. Mustard RA, Bohnen JM, Haseeb S, et al (1987) C-reactive protein levels predict postoperative septic complications. Arch Surg 122:69–73
8. Fassbender K, Pargger H, Muller W et al (1993) Interleukin-6 and acute-phase protein concentrations in surgical intensive care unit patients: diagnostic signs in nosocomial infection. Crit Care Med 21:1175–1180
9. Suprin E, Camus C, Gacouin A, et al (2000) Procalcitonin: a valuable indicator of infection in a medical ICU? Intensive Care Med 26:1232–1238
10. Aouifi A, Piriou V, Bastien O, et al (2000) Usefulness of procalcitonin for diagnosis of infection in cardiac surgical patients. Crit Care Med 28:3171–3176
11. Ugarte H, Silva E, Mercan D, et al (1999) Procalcitonin used as a marker of infection in the intensive care unit. Crit Care Med 27:498–504
12. Hatherill M, Tibby SM, Sykes K, et al (1999) Diagnostic markers of infection: comparison of procalcitonin with C reactive protein and leukocyte count. Arch Dis Child 81:417–421
13. Selberg O, Hecker H, Martin M, et al (2000) Discrimination of sepsis and systemic inflammatory response syndrome by determination of circulating plasma concentration of procalcitonin, protein complement 3a, and interleukin-6. Crit Care Med 28:2793–2798
14. de Werra I, Jaccard C, Corradin SB, et al (2001) Cytokines, nitrite/nitrate, soluble tumor necrosis factor receptors, and procalcitonin concentrations: comparisons in patients with septic shock, cardiogenic shock, and bacterial pneumonia. Crit Care Med 25:607–613
15. Muller B, Becker KL, Schachinger H, et al (2000) Calcitonin precursors are reliable markers of sepsis in a medical intensive care unit. Crit Care Med 28:977–983
16. Bearcroft PW, Miles KW (1996) Leukocyte scintigraphy or computed tomography for the febrile post-operative patient. Eur J Radiol 23:126–129

17. Hindsdale JG, Jaffe BM (1984) Re-operation for intra-abdominal sepsis: indications and results in the modern critical care setting. Ann Surg 199:31–36

18. Velmahos GC, Kamel E, Berne TV, et al (1999) Abdominal computed tomography for the diagnosis of intra-abdominal sepsis in critically injured patients: fishing in murky waters. Arch Surg 134:831–838

19. Sinanan M, Maier RV, Carrico CJ (1984) Laparotomy for intra-abdominal sepsis in patients in an intensive care unit. Arch Surg 119:652–658

20. Butler JA, Huang J, Wilson SE (1987) Repeated laparotomy for post-operative intra-abdominal sepsis: an analysis of outcome predictors. Arch Surg 122:702–706

21. McLean TR, Thornby J, Svensson LG (1993) Predicting the results and outcome of patients who undergo abdominal CT scanning while in the surgical intensive care unit. Am Surg 59:610–614

22. Shuler FW, Newman CN, Angood PB, et al (1996) Nonoperative management for intra-abdominal abscesses. Am Surg 62:218–222

Invited Commentary

ROBERT A. MUSTARD JR.

Dr. Fink has provided a succinct and up to date review of the clinical and radiologic assessment of source control for intra-abdominal infections. There are really two clinical problems being addressed here. First, is the source of the infection (e.g., hole in bowel) controlled (closed, exteriorized, etc.)? Second, is the bacterial infection controlled?

Generally speaking, the first question usually arises when the patient is "not doing well" (a concept Dr. Fink makes explicit in this chapter) in the first 5-10 days after surgery. Failure of source control in this sense is usually straightforward to diagnose with modern radiologic investigations. This first aspect of source control is only a problem when it is overlooked as a cause of "not doing well." A patient I recently cared for in the ICU illustrates this point. An 86-year-old lady had undergone total hysterectomy and bilateral salpingo-oophorectomy for carcinoma of the ovary. In the 5 days following her surgery, she developed acute renal failure and then respiratory failure necessitating admission to the ICU. Numerous consultants had seen the patient on the floor, but no consideration had been given to a diagnosis of intra-abdominal sepsis because the patient was afebrile, had a normal white blood cell count, and did not have peritonitis on physical examination. Her first investigation on admission to the ICU was an abdominal CT scan, which showed gross free fluid in the peritoneal cavity which, when aspirated, was bile-stained. Laparotomy revealed a perforated duodenal ulcer. She subsequently recovered from her organ failure.

The second question is more difficult to answer and is reviewed by Dr. Fink in considerable detail. He considers the clinical approach to the diagnosis of intra-abdominal sepsis based on physical examination, fever, and leukocytosis. He points out the difficulties with interpretation of these findings especially in the ICU patient. He also discusses the search for a serum marker for infection [1]. Unfortunately, differentiation of infection from sterile inflammation is unlikely to be possible using host derived products (except for certain antibodies). Of more interest is the future use of polymerase chain reaction technology to look for minute quantities of bacterial products in blood or other fluids [1].

The best diagnostic tool in intra-abdominal sepsis is the third-generation CT scanner. Not only can the scanner detect "leaks," it can also demonstrate rather subtle amounts of edema resulting from inflammation or infection. Modern CT scanning now claims an accuracy rate of 98% for the diagnosis of acute appendicitis [2].

References

1. Reinhart K, Meisner M, Hartog C (2001) Diagnosis of sepsis: novel and conventional parameters. Adv Sepsis 1:42–51
2. Rao PM, et al (1998) The effects of computer tomography of the appendix on treatment of patients and use of ospital resources. N Engl J Med 338:141–146

Editorial Comment

Persistence or recurrence of fever and/or leukocytosis after an operation to control the source of infection suggests the persistence or recurrence of infection *at the site of the operation*. Such findings are not an indication to continue antibiotics or change them for "more powerful" agents – for there is no evidence whatsoever to support the notion that doing so would do anything good. In fact, we suspect that antibiotics masked the clinical picture in the patient described by Dr. Mustard. Clearly, open wounds, drain tracts, granulation tissue, absorbing hematomas, and necrotic tissues can generate local inflammation and SIRS, and produce signs of inflammation which is usually self-limited. *Moreover, the longer one is from the index operation the higher the probability that the inflammation/ infection is remote from the operative site.*

We agree thus with Drs. Fink and commentator Mustard that one has to "suspect, examine, and image." But even third-generation CT scanners, which "demonstrate rather subtle amounts of edema resulting from inflammation or infection," are nonspecific during the first few days after the operation when fluid and inflammatory changes are usually present.

Dr. Fink's concept of the postoperative patient who is "not doing well" should be deeply entrenched within the surgical psyche of all surgeons. But human nature is such that surgeons tend to be blind to their own mistakes: those who use CT indiscriminately *before* the operation fail to do so *after* the operation, or obtain it too late. Who is not familiar with the following scenario?

An elderly patient undergoes extended colectomy for cancer of the rectum. Elevated temperature and white cell counts on postoperative day 3 are blamed on "atelectasis." Abdominal distension and persistent signs of inflammation 2 days later are explained by "ileus" and "pneumonia." Antibiotics are changed. On postoperative day 7 the patient is still on the ventilator; "Shouldn't we obtain a gastrografin enema?" asks the resident, and "Is his anastomosis OK?"

"Wait!" responds the surgeon, "He was dirty, a big operation, enough reasons for a big time ileus...."

Renal dysfunction develops. On postoperative day 8, the ICU doctor suggests a CT. The surgeon shrugs his shoulders, "Be my guest." And to his resident, "Gee, those ICU docs would scan everybody...."

CT is booked during the afternoon, but the patient does not "tolerate" the oral contrast and the waiting list is long. Eventually it is performed (by CT technicians) at 4 A.M. and reported at 11 A.M. on postoperative day 9: "Large amount of free fluid and gas throughout the entire abdomen, thickening and edema of tissue planes (operative site?), metal clips (surgical staples?). Small bowel distended and edematous (ischemia? ileus?)."

The ICU resident gets hold of the surgeon who operates at another hospital and agrees that a diagnostic paracentesis is indicated. It reveals bile-stained fecal material. Laparotomy performed at 1 A.M. on postoperative day 10 (scheduled as number 5 "emergency") reveals a large anastomotic leak and diffuse fecal peritonitis. The patient dies 25 days later.

The above scenario is only too common in the real world, and underlines the importance of the concept of the patient "who is not doing well."

Realistic and self-critical surgeons often ask themselves at the end of the operation: "Am I happy? Am I happy with the source control? With the anastomosis? With the 'toilet'?" At that stage they may decide on a planned reoperation in 48 h or insert in a mental note that "if the patient is not progressing well I'll reexplore him in 2 or 3 days." Selected empirical reexploration during the first few preoperative days, at a time when the intra-abdominal events are a mystery, may save those few patients that we lose today – despite our ICUs and third-generation scanners (see Chaps. 4, 9, 30, 35, 42).

40 Monitoring the Course of Inflammation

Artur Bauhofer, Wilfried Lorenz

Key Principles

- Complications resulting from inadequate source control result in a systemic inflammatory response; this response can be detected through changes in circulating levels of a variety of inflammatory mediators, including cytokines such as procalcitonin (PCT) and interleukin 6 (IL-6).
- Systemic inflammation is also manifest in changes in cellular expression of surface molecules such as HLA-DR and the receptor for TNF, and in the ability to generate cytokines in response to microbial stimulation.
- Immunologic monitoring of the high risk patient holds the promise of earlier detection of correctable complications, and so may lead to improved clinical outcomes.

Introduction

An infection is associated primarily with local inflammation through which the body tries to eliminate microbes with its cellular and soluble defense mechanisms. When local infection is not controlled adequately by either host defenses or the surgeon, a systemic reaction occurs which leads to the development of sepsis. The ACCP/SCCM consensus conference [1] defined sepsis as the systemic inflammatory response (SIRS) to infection.

The SIRS concept developed by Bone [2] is still controversial [3] and very nonspecific, but there is no better definition of systemic inflammation. The consequences of trauma and infection are conceptualized to clarify the complex interactions leading to SIRS and multiple organ failure (MOF). Stimuli such as trauma, operation, or infection evoke a systemic response involving activation of the neuroendocrine, immune, complement, kinin, and clotting systems. The activation of circulating monocytes, granulocytes, and lymphocytes, and of endothelial and epithelial cells leads to mediator release and functional changes. A variety of parameters are altered in the course of infection (Fig. 1). They include cytokines mainly secreted from monocytes (IL-1, IL-6, IL-8, IL-10, IL-18, and TNF-α) [4-7], functional changes of granulocytes (chemotaxis, phagocytosis, oxygen radical formation) [8], release of histamine from mast cells [9], the expression of NO and adhesion molecules on endothelial cells [10], and the release of clotting factors, complement factors, adhesion molecules, and procalcitonin (PCT) from epithelial cells [10-13]. These changes produce biological effects such as fever, metabolic disturbances, formation of microthrombi, disseminated intravascular clotting, vessel dilation, and capillary leak. The biological effects lead in severe cases to classical clinical effects that are routinely monitored by clinicians in the course of infection, including decreased cardiac output, hypotension, hypovolemia, interstitial edema, and multiple organ dysfunction.

Therapeutic decisions may be supported by monitoring the inflammatory status of the patients. Common laboratory parameters such as leukocyte counts and the C-reactive protein are too nonspecific to discriminate between bacterial and nonbacterial infection, and they manifest late, when clinical signs are already evident [7, 13].

Parameters for Monitoring the Immune Response

Biochemical factors may allow a more precise description of the inflammatory state in the individual patient. Choosing the optimal indicator substance or panel of factors is not easy since there are many candidates (Table 1). Potential markers include cytokines, hormones, soluble and cell-bound receptors, components of the clotting system, and assays of cellular function. The results reported in the literature are not always consistent, but the predictive capacity for the development of sepsis may be the best for serum IL-6 [4, 5, 7, 14, 15] and procalcitonin (PCT) [13, 16]. SIRS generally correlates with an increase in levels of PCT to more than 3 ng/ml, and of IL-6 to more than 98 pg/ml, while sepsis results in a level of more than 16 ng/ml for PCT, and 380 pg/ml for IL-6 [7]. In prolonged sepsis, monocyte secretion of TNF-α and HLA-DR antigen presenting capacity are severely depressed, while the production of anti-inflammatory factors like IL-10 and IL-1ra is unaffected. This immunological state has been defined as immune paralysis [17, 18]. Early detection of immune paralysis may give the clinician the opportunity to stimulate the immune system with factors like INF-γ [18] or G-CSF [19].

Systemic or Local Measurement

The easiest approach to measure cytokines is to use peripheral venous blood. Analyses are performed using commercially available immunological assays such as ELISA, RIA; often the assays are automated (e.g., Immulite, DPC-Biermann).

Whole blood [20] or isolated cells (monocytes, granulocytes) can be also stimulated ex vivo with bacterial toxins (LPS, *Staphylococcus aureus* enterotoxin B, lipoteichoic acid) [21, 22] to measure the capacity to release cytokines. The measurement of cell-associated cytokines, either bound to the cell surface or internalized with the receptor, is another approach to measure cytokines [23]. Furthermore, determination of intracellular cytokines by flow cytometry permits differentiation of the cell types where the cytokines were produced or bound. Cytokines can be determined in other body fluids. Cytokine levels in the peritoneal fluid of peritonitis patients have been analyzed by several groups [24–26]. However, a clear advantage of measuring local, rather than circulating cytokine

Table 1. Normal range of immune parameters

Parameter	Normal range (serum/plasma)	Source and literature
IL-1β	50-500 pg/ml	R&D Systems, US
IL-6	< 14 pg/ml	
	< 12 pg/ml	PC Biermann, Germany, [46]
IL-8	< 62 pg/ml	PC Biermann, Germany, [46]
	< 70 pg/ml	
IL-8 (cell bound)	65-210 pg/ml	[23]
IL-10	< 5 pg/ml	BioSource, US, [21]
IL-18	36-260 pg/ml	MBL, Japan
TNF-α	0.5-2 pg/ml	R&D Systems, US
	< 8 pg/ml	PC Biermann, Germany
TNF-α release	265→1,000 pg/ml	DPC Biermann, Germany, [21]
	839±119 pg/ml	
G-CSF	< 40 pg/ml	R&D Systems, US
PCT	< 0.5 ng/ml	Brahms, Germany, [7]
sCD 14	1.4-4.5 ng/ml	IBL, Germany, [46]
sICAM-1	230-410 ng/ml	R&D Systems, US, [10, 47, 48]
LBP (LPS binding protein)	1.8-17 µg/ml	ELISA with antibody 1E8, 2B5 [49, 50]
aPC (activated protein C)	>80 % normal	Chromogenic assay Diagnostica Stago, France, [51]
HLA-DR	18,000-55,000 receptors/cell	Becton Dickenson
Phagocytosis of PMN	90 %-99 % positive	Orpegen Phagotest, Germany
Phagocytosis of monocytes	65 %-99 % positive	Orpegen Phagotest, Germany

levels has not been demonstrated. Cytokines can also be measured in broncho-alveolar fluid. Some factors may be elevated locally that are not changed in the blood [27].

Clinical Factors That Can Alter the Inflammatory Response

Major operations are associated with an increase in circulating TNF-α and IL-6 1 day after operation, with a decrease to normal levels 1 day later in the absence of infection. In most cases PCT does not increase after operation [12], but seems to be more specific for the detection of infections [28]. Anemia induces decreased proinflammatory cytokine production that is further enhanced by blood trans-fusion [29], resulting in an impaired response to microbes [30]. Malnutrition is also associated with significant immunosuppression characterized by atrophy of lymphoid organs, impaired cellular immunity, and increased risk for viral and opportunistic infections [31]. Hyper- and hypoglycemia are associated with inhibition of IL-1 biosynthesis and release from macrophages [32]. The kidney plays a role in the metabolism and clearance of cytokines, and cytokines such as TNF-α, IL-1, and IL-6 are elevated in uremic patients [33]. During renal replacement therapy, including hemodialysis or hemofiltration, cytokine production may be increased if a bio-incompatible membrane such as cellulose is used; but clearance may also be supported by binding of cytokines to the membrane (biocompatible; e.g., polyacrilonitrile) [30, 34].

Cytokine expression and release is also altered by pharmacological interventions [35]. Catecholamines promote the secretion of anti-inflammatory cytokines and suppress the release of proinflammatory cytokines [36]. Antimicrobials have multiple effects on cytokine production, either as a result of the release of endotoxin from Gram-negative bacteria or through direct activity on cytokine expression. In most cases, levels of proinflammatory mediators are increased by the use of antibiotics [35], whereas glucocorticoids and pentoxifylline reduce the formation and release of proinflammatory cytokines into the blood [37, 38]. In addition, analgesics, narcotics, histamine antagonists, anticoagulants, calcium channel blockers and a variety of other drugs may influence the cytokine levels detectable in the blood. For more details see the review of AlKharfy et al. [35]. Other factors that modulate cytokine expression include well known risk factors for an adverse outcome in surgery like high age and trauma, as well as gender and genetic predisposition [39, 40]. These complex interactions should be kept in mind when cytokine data are interpreted.

Immune Monitoring of Two Patients With and Without Complications After Resection for Colorectal Cancer: An Example from a Prospective, Randomized Trial

In a randomized, clinical trial patients with colorectal cancer and increased perioperative risk (ASA 3 and 4) were treated with G-CSF to improve the outcome after surgery [41, 42]. Part of the new three component outcome model used for this trial is immunologic monitoring. The new outcome model, as developed for laparoscopic surgery [43], includes classical, mechanistic endpoints of survival, recovery index (McPeek index), complications, guidelines, and immune status. However, hermeneutic endpoints of the patient, including quality of life, expectations, negative effect, social stigma, and coping, are assessed by psychometric quantitative tests. Those reported and evaluated by the patient are used to judge clinical relevance by formal qualitative methods.

Two patients from this ongoing randomized trial with and without postoperative complication were selected (Table 2) to demonstrate immunological changes observed during the postoperative course. It is probable that both patients were in the treatment group (G-CSF prophylaxis), since they showed leukocytosis with 15 G/l and increased G-CSF levels with more than 3,000 pg/ml (ELISA, R&D Systems) in the plasma on day 1 after operation. However, the blinding of the trial has not yet been opened. No differences were detectable between the two patients in the 6-month follow-up after clinical discharge with regard to the McPeek recovery index and the global quality of life.

Patient 1, a typical patient without complications (Table 2) had only a transient postoperative increase in IL-6 and PCT due to the operative trauma (Fig. 1). Parameters had normalized at day 3. Except for IL-18, all parameters (TNF-α release after whole blood stimulation with LPS, HLA-DR expression on monocytes and phagocytosis of *E. coli* by PMNs) were in the normal range during the whole observation period of 6 days.

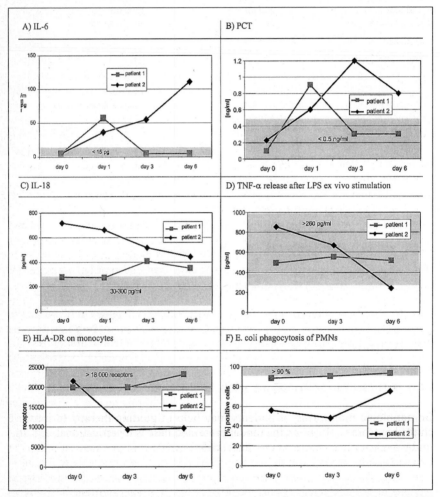

Fig. 1. Immunological parameters of two patients from a randomized clinical trial with G-CSF prophylaxis to improve the postoperative outcome from patients with colorectal cancer and increased perioperative risk (ASA 3 and 4). Patient 1 had no complication and Patient 2 local peritonitis. Normal values are shown in *gray*. At day 0 are baseline values before operation. The other time points are days after operation. Patient characteristics are shown in Table 2

Table 2. Randomized clinical trial with G-CSF prophylaxis

	Patient 1	Patient 2
General data		
Age, sex	90, male	77, Male
Tumor	Rectal cancer	Sigmoid cancer
Grading	pT3, pN1, M0	pT3, pN0, M0
ASA	4	3
Course of the operation		
Operation	Hartmann procedure	Sigmoid resection
Operation time	233 min	160 min
Blood loss	200 ml	1200 ml
Body temperature	36.0°-34.9°C	36.3°-34.8°C
Follow-up		
Survival (6 months)	Yes	Yes
Hospital stay	13 days	20 days
TISS-28	40 points	50 points
Complications	None	Bleeding, local peritonitis at day 7
McPeek index	4 Index points	4 Index points

Patient 2 had a blood loss of 1,200 ml during an operation for colon cancer, but did not receive blood products. The patient developed local peritonitis on day 7, and an anastomotic leak was closed by performing a new anastomosis. The patient was discharged at day 20 in good health.

By immune monitoring, the evolving problem of anastomotic leakage was detectable before clinical signs (fever and hypertension) were evident. At day 3 PCT and IL-6 levels were still elevated (Fig. 1). IL-6 peaked at day 6 with more than 100 pg/ml. The capacity to release TNF-α and the number of HLA-DR receptors on the monocytes declined below normal levels. The PMN phagocytosis rate was suppressed during the whole observation period. The cytokine data of these two patients correlate with the leukocyte counts: in Patient 2 the leukocyte count was normalized at day 4 to 5 G/l while in Patient 1 the leukocyte count was still elevated (day 4 with 14 G/l and day 6 with 12 G/l).

Consequences for Trial Trials and Clinical Practice

Immunologic monitoring of patients may help in guiding therapy to improve clinical outcomes. However, the model presented here is investigational, and still under evaluation in clinical and animal trials. In trials, immune status monitoring helps to explain results and should be included in the outcome concept. This was accomplished in the "three component outcome concept" outlined. Cytokines in this outcome concept will also help to analyze the influence of immune status on the social-psychological status of the patient. There is a close interaction as experienced in several empirical studies in humans [44] and animals [45].

In the future, the immune status may be used to define patient populations who might benefit from immune modulating drugs. This strategy was used with success to define patients with immunosuppression by HLA-DR determination, to include them in a clinical trial with IFN-γ [18]. A similar hypothesis is being tested in the prospective, ongoing trial of G-CSF [41, 42].

Recommendations to measure one specific factor in clinical routine can not be given. In general for immunomonitoring a single factor is not as useful as a combination of factors. Determinations should be performed daily or at relatively frequent intervals of 2 or 3 days. IL-6 and PCT have been the most extensively studied circulating markers in peripheral blood. An increase above normal values (Table 1) indicates the appearance of a problem associated with SIRS and infection. A further increase should notify the clinician that the problem has not yet been solved (for instance adequate source control has not been obtained), and that there is an increased risk of developing an adverse clinical state such as severe sepsis or septic shock. IL-6 and PCT are useful for monitoring the beginning and the progression of the hyperinflammatory state. The late phases of sepsis accompanied with immunosuppression are better detected by the capacity to express and release cytokines like TNF-α after ex vivo stimulation of whole blood, or by the number of HLA-DR found on monocytes. The latter is not as easy to measure since a flow cytometer is needed for the commercially available assay (Orpengen, Germany).

Conclusion

It is still unclear by which factors, at which location, and at which time points the immune status of the patient is best monitored. These factors must be evaluated further, but there are several promising candidates to help define patients who are at risk and may benefit from immediate treatment (surgical and medical). Immune monitoring may be particularly beneficial for postoperative patient management. Immune status has a substantial influence on neuroendocrine function, and so may influence the quality of life of patients.

References

1. Members of the ACCP/SCCM consensus conference committee, Bone RC, et al (1992) American College of Chest Physicians/Society of Critical Care Medicine Consensus Conference: Definitions for sepsis and organ failure and guidelines for the use of innovative therapies in sepsis. Crit Care Med 20:864–874
2. Bone RC (1992) Toward an epidemiology and natural history of SIRS (systemic inflammatory response syndrome). JAMA 268:3452–3455
3. Vincent J-L (1997) Dear SIRS, I'm sorry to say that I don't like you. Crit Care Med 25:372–374
4. Patel RT, Deen KI, Youngs D, Warwick J, Keighley MRB (1994) Interleukin 6 is a prognostic indicator of outcome in severe intra-abdominal sepsis. Br J Surg 81:1306–1308
5. Damas P, Canivet J-C, de Groote D, Vrindts Y, Albert A, Franchimont P, Lamy M (1997) Sepsis and serum cytokine concentrations. Crit Care Med 25:405–412
6. Lin KJ, Lin J, Hanasawa K, Tani T, Kodama M (2000) Interleukin-8 as a predictor of the severity of bacteremia and infectious disease. Shock 14:95–100
7. Selberg O, Hecker H, Martin M, Klos A, Bautsch W, Kohl J (2000) Discrimination of sepsis and systemic inflammatory response syndrome by determination of circulating plasma con-

centrations of procalcitonin, protein complement 3a, and interleukin-6. Crit Care Med 28:2793–2798

8. Rothe G, Kellermann W, Valet G (1990) Flow cytometric parameters of neutrophil function as early indicators of sepsis. J Lab Clin Med 115:52–61

9. Neugebauer E, Lorenz W, Rixen D, Stinner B, Sauer S, Dietz W (1996) Histamine release in sepsis: a prospective, controlled, clinical study. Crit Care Med 24:1670–1677

10. Gearing AJ, Newman W (1993) Circulating adhesion molecules in disease. Immunol Today 14:506–512

11. Fisher CJ Jr, Yan SB (2000) Protein C levels as a prognostic indicator of outcome in sepsis and related diseases. Crit Care Med 28:49–56

12. Reith HB, Mittelkötter U, Wagner R, Thiede A (2000) Procalcitonin (PCT) in patients with abdominal sepsis. Intensive Care Med 26:S166–S169

13. Oberhoffer M, Russwurm S, Bredle D, Chatzinicoulaou K, Reinhart K (2000) Discriminative power of inflammatory markers for prediction of tumor necrosis factor-a and interleukin-6 in ICU patients with systemic inflammatory response syndrome (SIRS) or sepsis at arbitrary time points. Intens Care Med 26:S170–S174

14. Steinmetz HT, Herbertz A, Bertram M, Diehl V (1995) Increase in interleukin-6 serum levels preceding fever in granulocytopenia and correlation with death from sepsis. J Infect Dis 171:225–228

15. Casey LC, Balk RA, Bone RC (1993) Plasma cytokine and endotoxin levels correlate with survival in patients with the sepsis syndrome. Ann Intern Med 119:771–778

16. Herrmann W, Ecker D, Quast S, Klieden M, Rose S, Marzi I (2000) Comparison of procalcitonin, sCD14 and interleukin-6 values in septic patients. Clin Chem Lab Med 38:41–46

17. Döcke WD, Reinke P, Syrbe U, Platzer C, Asadullah K, Krausch D, Zuckermann H, Volk HD (1997) Immunoparalysis in sepsis – from phenomenon to treatment strategies. Transplantationsmedizin 9:55–65

18. Döcke W-D, Randow F, Syrbe U, Krausch D, Asadullah K, Reinke P, Volk H-D, Kox W (1997) Monocyte deactivation in septic patients: restoration by IFN-gamma treatment. Nature Med 3:678–681

19. Hartung T (1999) Immunmodulation by colony stimulating factors. Rev Physiol Biochem Pharmacol 136:1–164

20. de Groote D, Zangerle PF, Gevaert Y, Fassotte MF, Beguin Y, Noizat-Pirenne F, Pirenne J, Gathy R, Lopez M, Dehart I (1992) Direct stimulation of cytokines (IL-1 beta, TNF-alpha, IL-6, IL-2, IFN-gamma and GM-CSF) in whole blood. I. Comparison with isolated PBMC stimulation. Cytokine 4:239–248

21. Astiz M, Saha D, Lustbader D, Lin R, Rackow E (1996) Monocyte response to bacterial toxins, expression of cell surface receptors, and release of anti-inflammatory cytokines during sepsis. J Lab Clin Med 128:594–600

22. Lehner MD, Morath S, Michelsen KS, Schumann RR, Hartung T (2001) Induction of crosstolerance by lipopolysaccharide and highly purified lipoteichoic acid via different toll-like receptors independent of paracrine mediators. J Immunol 166:5161–5167

23. Marie C, Fitting C, Cheval C, Losser MR, Carlet J, Payen D, Foster K, Cavaillon JM (1997) Presence of high levels of leukocyte-associated interleukin-8 upon cell activation and in patients with sepsis syndrome. Infect Immun 65:865–871

24. Scheingraber S, Bauerfeind F, Bohme J, Dralle H (2001) Limits of peritoneal cytokine measurements during abdominal lavage treatment for intraabdominal sepsis. Am J Surg 181:301–308

25. Berge Henegouwen MI, van der PT, Van Deventer SJ, Gouma DJ (1998) Peritoneal cytokine release after elective gastrointestinal surgery and postoperative complications. Am J Surg 175:311–316

26. Schafer K, Schumann RR, Stoteknuel S, Schollmeyer P, Dobos GJ (1998) Lipopolysaccharidebinding protein is present in effluents of patients with Gram-negative and Gram-positive CAPD peritonitis. Nephrol Dial Transplant 13:969–974

27. Mathiak G, Neville LF, Grass G, Boehm SA, Luebke T, Herzmann T, Kabir K, Rosendahl R, Schaefer U, Mueller C, Bohlen H, Wassermann K, Hoelscher AH (2001) Chemokines and interleukin-18 are up-regulated in bronchoalveolar lavage fluid but not in serum of septic surgical ICU patients. Shock 15:176–180

28. Harbarth S, Holeckova K, Froidevaux C, Pittet D, Ricou B, Grau GE, Vadas L, Pugin J (2001) Diagnostic value of procalcitonin, interleukin-6, and interleukin-8 in critically ill patients admitted with suspected sepsis. Am J Respir Crit Care Med 164:396–402

29. Kalechman Y, Gafter U, Sobelman D, Sredni B (1990) The effect of a single whole-blood transfusion on cytokine secretion. J Clin Immunol 10:99–105

30. AlKharfy KM, Kellum JA, Matzke GR (2000) Unintended immuno-modulation: part I. effects of common clinical conditions on cytokine biosynthesis. Shock 13:333–345

31. Deitch EA, Xu DZ, Qi L, Specian RD, Berg RD (1992) Protein malnutrition alone and in combination with endotoxin impairs systemic and gut-associated immunity. JPEN J Parenter Enteral Nutr 16:25–31

32. Hill JR, Kwon G, Marshall CA, McDaniel ML (1998) Hyperglycemic levels of glucose inhibit interleukin 1 release from RAW 264.7 murine macrophages by activation of protein kinase C. J Biol Chem 273:3308–3313

33. Pereira BJ, Shapiro L, King AJ, Falagas ME, Strom JA, Dinarello CA (1994) Plasma levels of IL-1 beta, TNF alpha and their specific inhibitors in undialyzed chronic renal failure, CAPD and hemodialysis patients. Kidney Int 45:890–896

34. Pereira BJ (1995) Cytokine production in patients on dialysis. Blood Purif 13:135–146

35. AlKharfy KM, Kellum JA, Matzke GR (2000) Unintended immune-modulation: part II. effects of pharmacological agents on cytokine activity. Shock 13:346–360

36. van der Pol T, Coyle SM, Barbosa K, Braxton CC, Lowry SF (1996) Epinephrine inhibits tumor necrosis factor-alpha and potentiates interleukin 10 production during human endotoxemia. J Clin Invest 97:713–719

37. Barnes PJ (1996) Molecular mechanisms of steroid action in asthma. J Allergy Clin Immunol 97:159–168

38. Wang P, Ba ZF, Morrison MH, Ayala A, Chaudry IH (1992) Mechanism of the beneficial effects of pentoxifylline on hepatocellular function after trauma hemorrhage and resuscitation. Surgery 112:451–457

39. Grass G, Neugebauer E (2001) Risk and prognosis of sepsis – Current methods on assessment of the immune status. In: Faist E (ed) Immunological screening and immunotherapy in critical ill patients with abdominal infections. pp 1–14

40. Schröder J, Kahlke V, Book M, Stüber F (2000) Gender differences in sepsis: genetically determined? Shock 14:307–310

41. Lorenz W, Stinner B, Bauhofer A, Rothmund M, Celik I, Fingerhut A, Koller M, Lorijn R, Nyström P-O, Sitter H, Schäfer H, Schein M, Solomkin JS, Troidl H, Wyatt J, Wittmann DH, Lucerne Group for Consensus-assisted Development of the Study Protocol on Prevention of Abdominal Sepsis (2001) Example G-CSF, granulocyte-colony stimulating factor in the prevention of postoperative infectious complications and sub-optimum recovery from operation in patients with colorectal cancer and increased preoperative risk (ASA 3 and 4): protocol of a controlled clinical trial developed by consensus of an international study group. Part one: rationale and hypothesis. Inflamm Res 50:115–122

42. Bauhofer A, Lorenz W, Stinner M, Rothmund M, Koller M, Sitter H, Celik I, Farndon JR, Fingerhut A, Hay J-M, Lefering R, Lorijn R, Nyström P-O, Schäfer H, Schein M, Solomkin J, Troidl H, Volk H-D, Wittmann DH, Wyatt J, Lucerne Group for Consensus-assisted Development of the Study Protocol on Prevention of Abdominal Sepsis (2001) Example G-CSF, granulocyte-colony stimulating factor in the prevention of postoperative infectious complications and sub-optimum recovery from operation in patients with colorectal cancer and increased preoperative risk (ASA 3 and 4). Protocol of a controlled clinical trial developed by consensus of an international study group. Part two: design of the study. Inflamm Res 50:187–205

43. Lorenz W, Troidl H, Solomkin JS, Nies C, Sitter H, Koller M, Krack W, Roizen MF (1999) Second step: testing – outcome measurements. World J Surg 23:768–780

44. Kreitler S (1999) Denial in cancer patients. Cancer Invest 17:514–534

45. Dantzer R (1999) Cytokine-induced sickness behavior: where do we stand? Brain Behav Immun 15:7–24

46. Holzheimer RG, Capel P, Cavaillon JM, Cainzos M, Frileux P, Haupt W, Marie C, Muller E, Ohmann C, Schoffel U, Lopez-Boado MA, Sganga G, Stefani A, Kronberger L (2000) Immuno-

logical surrogate parameters in a prognostic model for multi-organ failure and death. Eur J Med Res 5:283–294

47. Kuster H, Weiss M, Willeitner AE, Detlefsen S, Jeremias I, Zbojan J, Geiger R, Lipowsky G, Simbruner G (1998) Interleukin-1 receptor antagonist and interleukin-6 for early diagnosis of neonatal sepsis 2 days before clinical manifestation. Lancet 352:1271–1277

48. Egerer K, Rohr U, Krausch D, Kox W (1997) The circulating adhesion molecules sICAM-1 and sP-selectin in patients with sepsis. Anaesthetist 46:592–598

49. Zweigner J, Gramm HJ, Singer OC, Wegscheider K, Schumann RR (2001) High concentrations of lipopolysaccharide-binding protein in serum of patients with severe sepsis or septic shock inhibit the lipopolysaccharide response in human monocytes. Blood 98:3800–3808

50. Myc A, Buck J, Gonin J, Reynolds B, Hammerling U, Emanuel D (1997) The level of lipopolysaccharide-binding protein is significantly increased in plasma in patients with the systemic inflammatory response syndrome. Clin Diagn Lab Immunol 4:113–116

51. Mesters RM, Helterbrand J, Utterback BG, Yan SB, Chao YB, Fernandez JA, Griffin JH, Hartman DL (2000) Prognostic value of protein C concentrations in neutropenic patients at high risk of severe septic complications. Crit Care Med 28:2209–2216

Invited Commentary

EUGEN FAIST, CHRISTIAN SCHINKEL

A variety of procedures are available to assess the immunological status of critically ill patients. Some parameters such as white cell counts or C reactive protein are well-established components of routine clinical monitoring. Others such as cellular receptor expression, genetic polymorphisms, or a variety of soluble serum factors are recent innovations, and have led to a bewildering profusion of potential diagnostic tools. Moreover, established anatomical and physiological scores often do not provide adequate information to monitor the therapy of the individual patient.

Cells and Cell Function

White blood cell counts and differential cell counts are routine investigations in clinical practice. Both leukocytosis and leukopenia are common in critically ill patients and the parameter is one of the four criteria of the systemic inflammatory response syndrome (SIRS) [1].

A variety of in vitro tests of cell function have been described. Impairment of the ability of lymphocytes to proliferate in response to mitogenic or antigenic stimulation correlates with an increased risk of infectious complications and a poor clinical outcome. The assay is time-consuming and laborious to perform and so has not been evaluated in large patient cohorts, nor adopted into clinical practice. The phagocytic capacity of monocytes or neutrophils can be evaluated by flow cytometry. Phagocytosis is suppressed in sepsis and the degree of suppression correlates with adverse outcome [2].

The ability of the neutrophil to respond to stimulation with respiratory burst activity and production of oxygen intermediates is also impaired in sepsis, although spontaneous respiratory burst activity is enhanced. Neither of these assays of phagocytic cell function is in general clinical use [3, 4].

Immune status in vivo is readily evaluated using delayed hypersensitivity skin testing to common recall antigens. Anergy to recall challenge is associated with an increased susceptibility to infection and with a higher rate of morbidity and mortality after trauma [5].

Diminished expression of MHC class II antigens such as HLA-DR has been documented following surgical or accidental trauma and reduced expression predicts an increased risk of infectious complications. Impaired expression of HLA-DR indicates inadequate monocyte function, likely because of reduced stimulation by interferon gamma. A pilot study showed that interferon gamma treatment of septic patients whose monocytes demonstrated depressed HLA-DR expression resulted in restoration of monocyte function and HLA-DR expression [6].

Finally, changes in lymphocyte subpopulations are evident in critical illness. On the basis of studies in the mouse, T helper lymphocytes are subdivided into Th1 and Th2 populations. Th1 lymphocytes release interleukin-2 and interferon gamma, and support cell-mediated immune responses, whereas Th2 lymphocytes produce interleukin-4 and interleukin-10 and support humoral immune responses. The Th1 response is downregulated following major surgery, and the Th1/Th2 ratio in patients with sepsis is significantly reduced in comparison to healthy controls [7].

Humoral Markers

Protein mediators known as cytokines play critical roles in immune homeostasis, metabolism, wound healing, and organ function. Many of these have been implicated in the pathogenesis of the septic sequel of infection, thus establishing them as potential markers of the host inflammatory response.

Tumor necrosis factor alpha (TNF) levels are increased in the serum of patients following trauma or sepsis and levels correlate with prognosis. The half-life of TNF is relatively short and so serum levels may be unreliable [8]. Interleukin-6 is a very sensitive marker of immune system activation, correlating with the severity of both trauma and sepsis. It appears to be more sensitive than C-reactive protein (CRP); however, it is not specific for an infectious etiology [9].

Acute phase proteins such as CRP are known to remain elevated throughout the course of sepsis. Expression occurs in response to both infection and mechanical trauma; however, levels do not discriminate survivors from nonsurvivors [10].

Neopterin is a product of activated monocytes and macrophages released in response to interferon gamma. Serum or urine levels of neopterin correlate with mortality and the development of organ failure following mechanical or thermal trauma, or in sepsis. It appears to be a reliable marker for risk stratification in surgical patients [11].

Procalcitonin levels are increased in the plasma of patients with bacterial or parasitic infections, sepsis, and organ failure. Several reports have indicated that elevated procalcitonin levels can reliably identify patients with infection and differentiate them from patients with inflammation from noninfectious causes. In patients with septic shock, procalcitonin levels are higher in nonsurvivors than in survivors [12].

Conclusions

There have been a large number of publications relating a wide variety of putative biomarkers to adverse outcome in critical illness. However, none has shown clear utility in guiding therapy in patients with complex infections. The most promising markers appear to be procalcitonin, neopterin, interleukin-6, and monocyte expression of HLA-DR; however, clinical judgment must still take precedence over biochemical monitoring in making management decisions.

References

1. Bone RC, Balk RA, Cerra FB, et al (1992) Definitions for sepsis and organ failure and guidelines for the use of innovative therapies in sepsis. The ACCP/SCCM Consensus Conference Committee. American College of Chest Physicians/Society of Critical Care Medicine. Chest 101:1644–1655
2. Faist E, Ertel W, Salmen B, et al (1988) The immune-enhancing effect of perioperative Thymopentin administration in elderly patients undergoing major surgery. Arch Surg 123:1449–1453
3. Simms HH (1995) Polymorphonuclear leukocytes: their role as central cellular elements in shock pathogenesis. Shock 4:225–231
4. Nast-Colb D, Waydhas C, Gipner-Steppert C, et al (1997) Indicators of the posttraumatic inflammatory response correlate with organ failure in patients with multiple injuries. J Trauma 42:446–454, discussion 454–455
5. Christou NV, Meakins JL, Gordon J, et al (1995) The delayed hypersensitivity response and host resistance in surgical patients 20 years later. Ann Surg 222:534–548
6. Docke WD, Randow F, Syrbe U, et al (1997) Monocyte deactivation in septic patients; restoration by IFN-gamma treatment. Nat Med 3:678–681
7. Zedler S, Bone RC, Baue AE, et al (1999) T-cell reactivity and its predicative role in immunosuppression after burns. Crit Care Med 27:66–72
8. Riche F, Panis Y, Laisne MJ, et al (1996) High tumor necrosis factor serum level is associated with increased survival in patients with abdominal septic shock: a prospective study in 59 patients. Surgery 120:801–807
9. Martin C, Boisson C, Haccoun M, et al (1997) Patterns of cytokine evolution (tumor necrosis factor-alpha and interleukin-6) after septic shock, hemorrhagic shock land severe trauma. Crit Care Med 25:1813–1819
10. Wakefield CH, Barclay GR, Fearon KC, et al (1998) Proinflammatory mediator activity, endogenous antagonists and the systemic inflammatory response in intra-abdominal sepsis. Scottish Sepsis Intervention Group. Br J Surg 86:818–825
11. Strohmaier W, Redl H, Schlag G, et al (1987) D-erythro-neopterin plasma levels in intensive care patients with and without septic complications. Crit Care Med 15:757–760
12. Meisner M, Tschaikowsky K, Hutzler A, et al (1998) Postoperative plasma concentrations of Procalcitonin after different types of surgery. Intensive Care Med 24:680–684

41 Empiric Reexploration – Is There a Role?

PAMELA A. LIPSETT

Key Principles

- Control of surgical infection at the first intervention is optimal.
- The *need* for relaparotomy significantly worsens outcome.
- Planned reexploration of all surgical patients with signs and symptoms of infection will result in a small number of lives saved but at the cost of significant harm to others. Clear indications for planned relaparotomy do not exist.
- Reexploration based on localized radiological or physical findings may be beneficial; directed percutaneous therapy may also be beneficial.
- Undirected relaparotomy for MODS alone without supporting clinical or radiological data results in a 50%-90% rate of negative explorations without clear evidence of benefit. Supportive clinical data include prolonged ileus and pain, wound infection, and positive peritoneal signs. A computed tomographic scan is the most important radiological tool in the decision-making process for relaparotomy.

General Approach

The basic principles in the management of peritonitis – early operation, elimination of the focus, and lavage of the peritoneal cavity – have been practiced for more than a century [1]. Over the last 30 years, more aggressive approaches to the control of abdominal sepsis have been proposed, including continuous postoperative lavage, staged abdominal repair, open abdomen, and scheduled reoperation (*Etappenlavage*). These techniques are discussed elsewhere in this book (Chaps. 5, 7, 9, 10, 12, 30, 35, 39, 42). Conceptually they aim to provide better drainage or cleansing of the peritoneal cavity, earlier detection of possible anastomotic leaks, improved perfusion of the abdominal organs, and improved pulmonary function. However, their merits are still debated and the role of a more conservative approach to the treatment of peritonitis, with reoperation as indicated, has been reexamined (on-demand relaparotomy).

Patients who require relaparotomy have a higher morbidity and mortality than patients who are cured after a single operation. In one large international prospective study, patients who did not require a relaparotomy had a 27% mortality compared to 42% for patients with at least one additional reoperation [2]. Patients undergoing one additional relaparotomy had a mortality of 43%, with a mortality of 40%, 30%, 40%, and 57% for two, three, four and five reoperations, respectively [2].

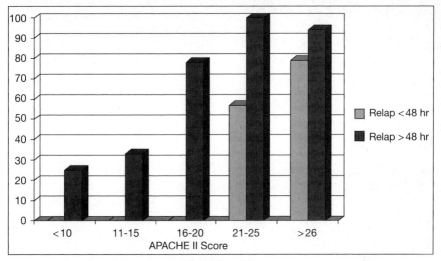

Fig. 1. Mortality after relaparotomy. (Modified from [3])

The prognosis of patients with peritonitis is influenced by the health status of the patient at the time of presentation and by additional concomitant risk factors. Preoperative scoring models such as the APACHE score, the Goris score, and the Mannheim peritonitis index have all been advocated as methods to predict the need for reoperation, quantify disease severity, or aid in comparing outcomes for patients with peritonitis [3, 4]. Koperna and Schulz reported that patients requiring reoperation were sicker as measured by either APACHE II or the Goris score, more likely to be malnourished (albumin < 30 g/l), older than 70 years of age, and more likely to have diffuse peritonitis (49.5% vs 25.6%) when compared with patients who did not require a second operation [3]. The mortality for patients having a second operation was 51% vs 4.3%, when the initial operation successfully controlled the infection. In this study, the lowest mortality for patients requiring relaparotomy was seen in patients who underwent relaparotomy on demand within 48h of the initial operation (see Fig. 1). These patients, however, had a lower APACHE II score (17.6 ± 8) which, more than the treatment decision, may have accounted for the improved clinical outcome. This study also demonstrated the relatively small impact of aggressive, but unsuccessful surgical treatment on outcome. The most important determinant of outcome was a timely index operation with adequate initial source control.

Increased mortality with the on-demand relaparotomy has generally been reported when reoperation is delayed. In the Koperna paper, the mortality of on-demand laparotomy was not different from that of planned relaparotomy (50.6% vs 54.5%) [3].

Clinical Decision Making

There is no standard definition of persistent abdominal sepsis that has been applied across all studies. The concept of persistent abdominal sepsis includes both the macroscopic description of an ongoing inflammatory process and the microbiological detection of organisms. Potential indications for reoperation include clinical deterioration, the development of multiple organ dysfunction syndrome (MODS), failure to improve, radiological evidence of secondary foci, or the suspicion of uncontrolled source in the abdomen. One small retrospective study demonstrated the utility of diagnostic paracentesis, using a positive abdominal fluid aspirate and clinical signs as the indication for operation [5]. The aspirate was considered positive if the fluid was dark, bloody, cloudy, or malodorous. A positive aspirate correlated with intra-abdominal findings, but not necessarily an improved outcome. However, the study was quite small. Certainly paracentesis can add additional information and with the aid of bedside ultrasonography can be easily performed.

Diagram 1 depicts a strategy for relaparotomy on demand within 48 h of the initial surgery, or before MODS has been established and is irreversible. When the initial surgical procedure is considered successful, this decision can be difficult. For patients who do not require ICU care following the initial surgery, use of a scoring system may be helpful. For those who do require intensive care, the only clear-cut indication for relaparotomy is the development or worsening of MODS [6, 7] (see Fig. 2). However, undirected relaparotomy for MODS alone without supporting clinical or radiological data results in a negative exploration rate of 50%-90%. Prolonged ileus and pain, wound infection, and of course, the most important, positive peritoneal signs increase the probability of a positive laparotomy. A computed tomographic (CT) scan is the most important radiological tool in making the decision for relaparotomy. In a recent report of CT scans in critically ill patients with signs and symptoms of sepsis, 7 of 45 examinations demonstrated an intra-abdominal focus of infection, some of which could be managed percutaneously and others of which (perforation and gangrenous colitis) required operation [5].

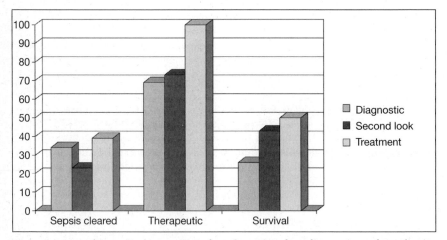

Fig. 2. Outcome of operation by operation class. Operation class: diagnostic, performed to investigate clinical deterioration; second look, planned at previous operation; treatment, to treat a defined surgical condition (drain an identified abscess). (Modified from [7])

Controversies and Changing Practices

Seiler and colleagues [6] have advocated early operation with initial source control and extensive intraoperative lavage (20-60 l) and suggest that initial surgical source control with either resection, repair or decompression of the source is possible in 80 %-90 % of patients. Using this strategy, successful resolution without further operation would be expected in more than 90 % of patients [6]. When initial source control is performed, reoperation has been required in about 10 % of patients, with patients having an abscess, breakdown of an anastomosis, evisceration, or hematoma formation. However, when initial source control is not possible (10 %-15 %) and alternative treatment is employed, these same complications occur with increased frequency (~30 %).

Additional interventions such as continuous postoperative lavage or open packing and scheduled relaparotomy are aimed at the prevention of recurrent infection or secondary foci of infection or necrosis. These aggressive approaches can be associated with considerable treatment-related morbidity and mortality because of secondary complications such as perforation and fistula formation. Hau et al. reported a case-control study of patients who underwent planned laparotomy (PR) vs those who had on-demand relaparotomy (RD) [8]. These authors found no significant difference in mortality (PD 21 % vs RD 13 %). MODS was more frequent in patients with a PR (50 %) when compared with RD (24 %, P = 0.01), as were infectious complications (68 % vs 39 %, P = 0.01). More frequent

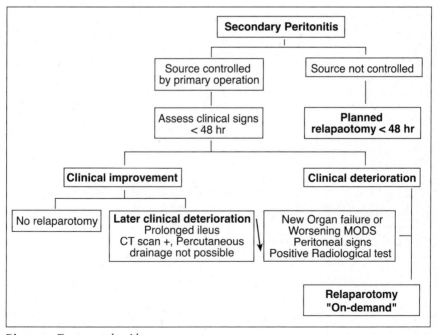

Diagram 1. Treatment algorithm

suture leaks, recurrent intra-abdominal sepsis, and septicemia were all more common in the planned relaparotomy group. These authors suggested that planned relaparotomy for secondary peritonitis should be used with caution until prospective trials have been performed [8)].

It may be unnecessary to reoperate if initial source control is adequate, reserving second operations for clear-cut clinical or radiographic indications; these decisions should be made early, when MODS is developing or worsening. An on-demand approach will reduce the procedure-related morbidity of planned relaparotomy.

References

1. Mikulicz J (1889) Weitre Erfahrungen uber die operative Behanlung der Perforationsperitonitis. Arch Klin Chir (Berl) 39:756–784
   Classic German paper which is among the first to present the principles of managing peritonitis.
2. Christou NV, Barie PS, Dellinger EP, Waymack JP, Stone HH (1993) Surgical Infection Society Intra-abdominal Infection Study. Prospective evaluation of management techniques and outcome. Arch Surg 128:193–199
   Prospective database collected by the SIS of patients with peritonitis.
3. Koperna T, Schultz F (1996) Prognosis and treatment of peritonitis. Do we need new scoring systems? Arch Surg 131:180–186
   Review of the use of the Goris scoring system and the APACHE II score with respect to outcome in patients with peritonitis. The timing of relaparotmy and MODS is discussed.
4. Koperna T, Schulz F (2000) Relaparotomy in peritonitis: prognosis and treatment of patients with persisting intraabdominal infection. World J Surg 24:32–37
   Retrospective case-control study of 523 patients with secondary peritonitis, 105 with relaparotomy. Planned and on-demand relaparotomy compared.
4. Halpern NA, McElhinney AJ, Greenstein RJ (1991) Postoperative sepsis: re-explore or observe? Accurate indication from diagnostic abdominal paracentesis. Crit Care Med 19:882–889
   Small retrospective study of the use of diagnostic paracentesis and subsequent outcome. Patients with a positive paracentesis had an intra-abdominal focus, while those who had a negative paracentesis did not.
5. Barkhausen J, Stoblen F, Dominquez-Fernandez E, Henseke P, Muller RD (1999) Impact of CT in patients with sepsis of unknown origin. Acta Radiolo 40:552–555
   Review of results of CT scan done on critically ill patients with suspected sepsis. Thoracic (5/38) and abdominal CT (7/45) scan identified infectious causes that could be treated either by percutaneous drainage or operation.
6. Seiler CA, Brugger L, Forssmann U, Baer HU, Buchler MW (2000) Conservative surgical treatment of diffuse peritonitis. Surgery 127:178–184
   Prospective study of 258 patients with peritonitis with Mannheim Peritonitis Scoring System. Authors present excellent overall results with aggressive initial operation which includes high-volume lavage in the operating room.
7. Anderson ID, Fearon JCH, Grant IS (1996) Laparotomy for abdominal sepsis in the critically ill. Br J Surg 83:535–539
   60 of 125 ICU patients required relaparotomy for continuing sepsis with only 19 patients surviving to hospital discharge. Outcome of reoperation indication presented.
8. Hau T, Ohmann C, Wolmershauser A, Wacha H, Yang Q (1995) Planned relaparotomy vs relaparotomy on demand in the treatment of intraabdominal infections. The Peritonitis Study Group of the Surgical Infection Society-Europe. Arch Surg 130:1193–1196, discussion 1196–1197
   Short of a randomized controlled study, the best methodology for whether planned relaparotomy vs on-demand relaparotomy should be performed. Convincing data that planned relaparotomy may have a poorer outcome.

Invited Commentary

THOMAS SAUTNER

Although there is broad agreement on the optimal surgical therapy of peritonitis, the concept of intervention to avert imminent failure of this therapy is much less clear. Dr. Lipsett clearly points out that patients successfully managed with a single operation fare better than those who need multiple operations. Fortunately a patient's intra-abdominal infection may be resolved at the first attempt in the majority of cases If, however, the source cannot be controlled early, a scheduled reoperation is indispensable.

The management of patients at risk for failure of initial therapy, and the prevention or early diagnosis of such events is much less well defined. The need for reoperation has been shown to be associated with a number of factors [1]. The risk factors identified in this study (age > 70, diffuse peritonitis, serum albumin levels < 30 g/l, preoperative APACHE II scores > 20, and existing organ failure measured by the Goris score) were, however, not subjected to a multivariate analysis – correcting for the potential interactive effects of factors in one or the other group of patients. Although it seems reasonable that impaired immunocompetence or malnutrition may promote the failure of initial therapy, the data presented in this paper do not provide a sufficiently strong argument to suggest that these factors are causative [1]. Yet these observations may help to identify a subset of patients in need of close attention following the first operation.

Dr. Lipsett pleads for good surgical practice, to examine the patient closely, to consider the need for supportive measures and to employ radiological investigations. This certainly is the approach of choice; however, clinical signs and radiological findings may be difficult to interpret or even misleading, even for surgeons who have considerable experience [2, 3]. Paracentesis may help to identify intra-abdominal infection by interpretation of the aspirate, but *compartmentalized* infection may be missed by this method.

The consequences for the patient depend on the initial source and the extent of peritonitis [4]. Lesions of the upper GI tract and appendicitis seem to result in less morbidity for the patient than large-bowel perforations or postoperative peritonitis. From these observations it is clear that patients at a lower risk of persistent or recurrent infection should be treated with the on-demand approach suggested by Dr. Lipsett. For patients who are at high risk for ongoing infection, who have compromised perfusion of the bowel or intestinal edema, or in whom source control could only be established by intestinal closure with a risk of breakdown, a different approach may be appropriate.

The mortality of patients needing reoperation could be reduced by up to 43 % *if the second operation took place within 48 h* [1]. This was true not only for on-demand relaparotomies but also for planned reexplorations, which made up 41 % of the population [1]. Upon reoperation all patients had persisting peritonitis, a finding that might have been missed without a scheduled reoperation. Considering the risk involved in delaying a necessary reoperation and the increased mortality that has been found to be associated with delay [1], a more aggressive approach of scheduled reexplorations within 48 h might be helpful. This decision should at least be considered whenever the initial surgeon is in doubt as to whether the first operation has definitively resolved the patient's problem [5].

Pathophysiological considerations also influence the decisions for multiple operations in patients with intra-abdominal infections. On the one hand, the increased intra-abdominal pressure following surgery for peritonitis may lead to an abdominal compartment syndrome, and, in turn, to multiple organ failure [6]. Release of the abdominal tension and repeated reoperations with gradual reapproximation of the abdominal wall can avoid the development of intra-abdominal hypertension [7]. On the other hand, an association between repeated operations and an aggravation of the inflammatory response has been established [8]. Clinical studies, however, have not provided convincing evidence of such a "second-hit" effect in peritonitis patients [9]. Finally, it is known that surgery exerts an immunosuppressive effect on the patient [10]. Therefore aggressive surgical management may also be harmful to normal host defenses. These partly contradictory considerations have to be further investigated.

A case-control study by Hau and colleagues on behalf of the Surgical Infection Society Europe [11] provides the only level 3 evidence in comparing on-demand exploration with planned reoperation [12]. The data indicate no advantage for scheduled reoperation, while showing a higher rate of infectious and local complications in the planned relaparotomy group. However, it appears that subgroups of patients who underwent only one scheduled reexploration, or were reoperated in a planned fashion at an experienced center, did as well, if not better, than on-demand patients. It may be that discordant results from less experienced centers contributed to the poor results of planned relaparotomy in this investigation [11].

There is no convincing evidence of the superiority of planned reoperation. Therefore close observation of the patient (until the need for reexploration emerges) is probably the best approach to the treatment of patients with intra-abdominal infection. Whether high-risk patients with certain conditions such as bowel edema, imminent intestinal ischemia, or the risk of anastomotic leaks will benefit from a scheduled second look operation within 48 h deserves to be studied further.

The optimal treatment for patients at high risk of persistent peritonitis may only be identified by a prospective randomized trial. Such a study should compare the best available on-demand approach, supported by a well-defined algorithm defining why and when to reoperate, with a refined type of planned reexploration, for example, staged abdominal repair [7]. Surgical societies devoted to the study of surgical infection should take the lead in promoting such a study.

References

1. Koperna T, Schulz F (2000) Relaparotomy in peritonitis: prognosis and treatment of patients with persisting intraabdominal infection. World J Surg 24:32–37
2. Ferraris VA (1983) Exploratory Laparotomy for potential abdominal sepsis in patients with multiple-organ failure. Arch Surg 118:1130–1133
3. McDowell RK, Dawson SL (1996) Evaluation of the abdomen in sepsis of unknown origin. Inten Care Radiol 34:177–190

4. Bohnen J, Boulanger M, Meakins JL, McLean APH (1983) Prognosis in generalized peritonitis. Arch Surg 118:285–290
5. Götzinger P, Gebhard B, Wamser P, Sautner T, Huemer G, Függer R (1996) Revision bei diffuser Peritonitis: geplant v. on-demand. Langenbecks Arch Chir 381:343–347
6. Schein M, Wittmann DH, Aprahamian CC, Condon RE (1995) The abdominal compartment syndrome: the physiological and clinical consequences of elevated intra-abdominal pressure. J Am Coll Surg 180:745–753
7. Wittmann DH (2000) Staged abdominal repair: development and current practice of an advanced operative technique for diffuse suppurative peritonitis. Acta Chir Austriaca 32:171–178
8. Meldrum DR, Cleveland JC, Moore EE, Patrick DA, Banerjee A, Harken AH (1997) Adaptive and maladaptive mechanisms of cellular priming. Ann Surg 226:587–598
9. Sautner T, Gotzinger P, Redl-Wenzl EM, Dittrich K, Felfernig M, Sporn P, Roth E, Fugger R (1997) Does reoperation for abdominal sepsis enhance the inflammatory host response? Arch Surg. 132:250–255
10. Meakins JL (1989) Host defense mechanisms in surgical patients: effect of surgery and trauma. Acta Chir Scand Suppl 550:43-51, discussion, 51–53
11. Hau T, Ohmann C, Wolmershauser A, Wacha H, Yang Q (1995) Planned relaparotomy vs relaparotomy on demand in the treatment of intraabdominal infections. The Peritonitis Study Group of the Surgical Infection Society-Europe. Arch Surg 130:1193–1196
12. Canadian Task Force on the Periodic Health Examination (1979) The periodic health examination. Can Med Assoc J 121:1193–1254

Editorial Comment

The need for reoperation, be it planned or on demand, identifies a patient at increased risk of morbidity and mortality. When therapeutic (i.e., when correctable pathology is encountered) such a procedure may be life-saving; when negative, however, it may kill the patient. The earlier the therapeutic relaparotomy is carried out, the better. The challenge is how to identify patients who would benefit. Dr. Lipsett advocates on-demand reoperation within 48 h but the question of on-demand for what clinical or radiological findings remains unanswered. Professor Sautner seems to accept cautiously the need for an early planned reoperation in selected patients. He identifies limitations in the study by Hau et al. [1] and hopes for a better prospective randomized study in the future to further enlighten us.

Early reoperation is a double-edged sword; we still have to learn how to use only the edge facing the enemy – the uncontrolled source.

Reference

1. Hau T, Ohmann C, Wolmershauser A Wacha H, Yang Q (1995) Planned relaparotomy vs relaparotomy on demand in the treatment of intraabdominal infections. The Peritonitis Study Group of the Surgical Infection Society-Europe. Arch Surg 130:1193–1196

42 Planned Relaparotomies and Laparostomy

MOSHE SCHEIN, RAMESH PALADUGU

Key Principles

- A planned relaparotomy may be life-saving when the source cannot be adequately controlled during the first or index operation.
- The first week after the index operation – before the infective process has become localized and detectable by CT – offers a window of opportunity for planned relaparotomies.
- When the source is controlled and infection localized, a "directed" or "on-demand" approach is safer.
- Laparostomy is indicated when the abdomen cannot be closed without creating significant intra-abdominal hypertension.
- Excessive or unnecessary relaparotomies may be harmful.

Very little high-level evidence is available concerning the topics discussed in this chapter. The following discussion relies on nonrandomized, usually retrospective, studies, and, in the absence of scientific evidence, we must use a rational individual approach and common sense, both of which will be emphasized.

Definitions and Rationale

Planned Relaparotomy

The policy of planned relaparotomy is decided at the first, or index, operation for peritonitis, when the surgeon decides to reoperate within 1-3 days, irrespective of the patient's immediate postoperative course. The decision to reexplore the abdomen is thus part of the initial management plan. Historically, mesenteric ischemia was the first circumstance for which a planned second look laparotomy was advocated. Penninckx et al. [1] were probably the first to report the use of planned relaparotomies in intra-abdominal infections.

In intra-abdominal infection, the reason for a second look is to better control the source and to repeat the peritoneal toilet, in order to abort or diminish the magnitude of SIRS and multiple organ failure.

Relaparotomy on Demand

The traditional approach to abdominal reexploration following an index operation for peritonitis has been a relaparotomy on demand: the surgeon decides to re-explore the abdomen based on clinical or radiological evidence of persistent or recurrent infection.

Laparostomy

The term "laparostomy," which implies leaving the abdomen open, was coined by P. Fagniez of Paris (personal communication). Pujol was the first to suggest that the severely infected abdomen is best treated openly like an abscess cavity [2]. It has been recognized sporadically throughout the 20th century that peritonitis and its operative treatment often results in increased intra-abdominal pressure (IAP). However, the benefits of the prevention or treatment of intra-abdominal hypertension by with laparostomy have only recently been established [3]. Laparostomy does not eliminate the need for abdominal reexplorations, but these are facilitated by leaving the abdomen open. Thus, in practice, laparostomy has become a corollary to planned relaparotomy: if the abdomen is to be reevaluated 48 h later, why close it at all?

General Approach: Planned Relaparotomy Indications

The indications to embark on planned relaparotomies remain poorly defined and empiric.

- In our experience the best and strongest indication for relaparotomy is failure to obtain adequate source control during the initial operation. A classic example is infected pancreatic necrosis after necrotizing pancreatitis. Another example is an intestinal leak, which cannot be safely repaired or exteriorized, a scenario commonly associated with post-operative peritonitis.
- The necessity to redebride or drain poorly localized, stubborn infective processes, for example, diffuse retroperitoneal fasciitis due to retroperitoneal perforation of the duodenum or colon.
- Diffuse fecal peritonitis is a relative indication [4, 5], with the rationale that massive fecal contamination will require further procedures to achieve an adequate peritoneal toilet.
- Instability of the patient during the initial operation occasionally mandates an abbreviated damage control-type procedure with an obligatory subsequent planned relaparotomy to finish the source control and peritoneal toilet. Obviously, when hemostatic packs must be left in situ, their removal necessitates a relaparotomy [6].

Wittmann, who combines an aggressive policy of planned relaparotomies with laparostomy – calling it staged abdominal repair (STAR) [7], contends that re-operations allow him to assess high-risk anastomoses that previously would have been managed by creation of a stoma.

The Conduct of a Relaparotomy

The surgeon who plans to reenter an abdomen that has recently been operated on must be gentle! The bowel and peritoneal surfaces are edematous, friable, and vascular. Ideally, the surgeon who performed the index procedure should be the one to reoperate. The objective of relaparotomy is to drain all infected collections and control persistent sources of contamination. How thorough the exploration should be depends on the unique circumstances of the individual case. Sometimes several interloop abscesses must be drained and the whole bowel must be carefully unraveled; in other cases, particularly in instances of frozen abdomen, it is sufficient to explore the spaces around the matted bowel (subphrenic spaces, paracolic gutters, pelvis). The decision on the extent of exploration is crucial because the more widespread the exploration, the greater the danger it poses to adjacent structures. Consequently, the extent of exploration depends on whether the operation is directed or nondirected and on its timing.

General Approach: Laparostomy

Indications

Laparostomy may be indicated when the abdomen either cannot be closed or should not be closed.

Abdomen Which Cannot Be Closed

- After major loss of abdominal wall tissue following trauma or debridement for necrotizing fasciitis
- Extreme visceral or retroperitoneal swelling after major trauma, resuscitation, or major surgery (e.g., ruptured AAA)
- Poor condition of fascia after multiple laparotomies

Abdomen Which Should Not Be Closed

- Decision to reexplore within a day or two
- Closure possible only under extreme tension – compromising the fascia and creating intra-abdominal hypertension or abdominal compartment syndrome.

Technical Considerations of Laparostomy

The option of simply covering the exposed viscera with moist gauze packs has been practiced for generations but is not advised. The intestine, if not matted, can eviscerate; moreover, it requires intensive nursing care to keep the patient and his bed clean and dry. Most importantly, it risks creating spontaneous, exposed intestinal fistulas [8]. The exposed bowel, when dilated and friable, tends to tear if repeatedly injured during dressing changes and exposure. Temporary abdominal closing devices to cover the laparostomy wound are therefore highly recommended.

The options for temporary abdominal closure are many and include the Bogota bag fashioned from a large IV fluid bag, a ready-to-use transparent bowel bag, a synthetic mesh (absorbable or nonabsorbable), or a Velcro-type sheath, as advocated by Wittmann [9]. A South American surgeon even uses discarded nylon hose for this purpose. Regardless of the method of closure, a few practical points merit emphasis:

- Try to place the device over the omentum in order to protect the bowel.
- Suture the device to the fascial edges. Large abdominal-wall defects can result because the midline-wound fascial edges tend to retract laterally (note that this is the reason why the abdominal defect resulting from a transverse laparostomy is smaller). The larger the defect, the more problematic its eventual reconstruction.
- Using a permeable material (e.g., mesh) as opposed to a nonpermeable (e.g., Bogota bag) has the advantage of allowing the egress of infected intra-peritoneal fluids.
- Try to adjust the tension of the closure to the intra-abdominal pressure.
- If you plan a relaparotomy within 24-48 h, the type of device used is of little importance and can be replaced at the end of the next laparotomy. The selection of material at the last relaparotomy is crucial; we recommend an absorbable synthetic mesh as discussed below.
- Abdominal reentry is simple: divide the closure material at its center; then, with your finger gently separate the omentum and viscera away from the overlying device. At the end of the procedure resuture the devise with a running suture. Commercial zippers are available but of no additional benefit.

Our choice is the so-called sandwich technique [10] in which absorbable permeable synthetic mesh is sutured to the fascial edges. Two sump drains are placed at the edges of the abdominal defect and over the mesh, brought out through the skin, and connected to suction to collect the abdominal effluent. Sheaths of stoma-adhesive are placed on the healthy skin surrounding the defect; a large adhesive transparent sheath (Steridrape or Opsite) is placed on top to cover the entire abdomen. Hence, the viscera are protected, the laparostomy output is measurable, the patient is clean and dry, and demands on nursing are minimized (Fig. 1).

Terminating the Laparostomy

How should the ensuing abdominal wall defect be managed when the need for laparostomy no longer exists?

- If nonabsorbable material has been used, it must be removed. Retained Marlex mesh results in infected sinuses and even intestinal fistulae.
- Occasionally, a small defect may be closed completely. In most patients recovering from multiple relaparotomies and laparostomy, the defect is too large, however, to allow primary closure of the fascia. Hence, the safest option is to let

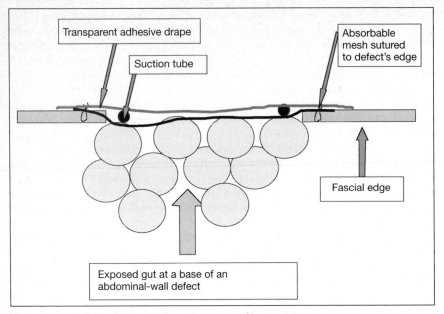

Fig. 1. The sandwich technique in the management of laparostomy

the defect granulate under and over the absorbable mesh. A few weeks after the last laparotomy, when a healthy layer of granulation tissue has covered the now contracting defect and the patient's recovery is well under way, try to mobilize the skin around the defect and to close it at the midline. Relaxing lateral skin incisions may help. If the defect is too large apply split thickness skin grafts on-to the granulation tissue in the bed of the defect. The resulting ventral hernia is usually wide-necked and well tolerated except for its cosmetic appearance. It can be repaired at a later stage.

• Whatever you do with the abdominal-wall defect, remember that your patient has just recovered from the immense stress of peritonitis and multiple opera-tions. Definitive management can be postponed until convalescence has pro-gressed further.

Results and Complications

Since planned relaparotomies are usually combined with laparostomy, it is im-practical, if not impossible, to discuss the results of these modalities separately. Because of the complex nature of the patients, as well as these therapies, rando-mized controlled trials comparing relaparotomy with conventional surgical approaches are probably impossible to perform [11]. The reported mortality for planned relaparotomies or open abdomen approaches has ranged from 30% (Table 1) up to 52% [12].

Hau et al. [13] matched 38 patients undergoing planned relaparotomies by APACHE II score, age, site and cause of infection, and the ability to obtain source control with 38 patients undergoing on-demand relaparotomies. The mortality in the two groups was 21% and 13%, respectively (nonsignificant). Postoperative multiple organ failure was more frequent in the group of patients undergoing planned relaparotomies, compared with the group undergoing on-demand procedures, as were infectious complications (68% vs 39%, respectively). Infectious complications resulted from suture leaks, recurrent intra-abdominal sepsis, and septicemia in the planned group. However, local differences in patient selection and/or local expertise make it difficult to reach definitive conclusions. Another prospective, consecutive, nonrandomized trial by the Surgical Infection Society (SIS) [14] showed no significant difference in mortality when patients treated with a closed-abdomen technique (31% mortality) were compared with those treated with variations of the open-abdomen technique (44% mortality). The authors suggested, as others have done [15], that the outcome in peritonitis depends more on the severity of acute disease and degree of host response than on management strategies or recurrent peritoneal infection.

The largest published clinical experience with planned relaparotomies is by Billing et al. from Munich [16], who treated 377 patients suffering from diffuse peritonitis. The mortality rate for their 152 patients treated with planned relaparotomies was 37.5% as compared to 21% for patients treated conventionally. The mortality for the two treatment modalities in patients in whom source control was achieved during the first operation was 19% and 10%, respectively. However, when source control was not obtained during the initial operation, the mortality rate for patients undergoing planned relaparotomies was 59% as compared to 86% in those treated conventionally. Overall, when source control was successful during the first operation, the mortality rate was 14%, when unsuccessful, it was 64%. This experience points to the crucial importance of source control and suggests that planned relaparotomies may be beneficial when the source is not well controlled during the first operation.

Not surprisingly, the more reoperations one does, the greater the surgical morbidity – usually manifested by intestinal and hemorrhagic complications [4-6, 8,13,14,17]. Reoperation may exacerbate the cytokine-generated local and systemic inflammation [18,19], acting possibly as a "second hit."

Do planned relaparotomies reverse, prevent, or aggravate SIRS and multiorgan dysfunction? Is the benefit/risk ratio favorable? There is no consensus.

Controversies

Are Planned Relaparotomies Beneficial?

Ideally, any surgical maneuver that successfully eliminates the source of infection and/or evacuates contaminants and pus will be beneficial. Planned relaparotomies represent a double-edged sword – achieving the above-mentioned goal, but at a cost to the host. In view of the high morbidity of multiple relaparotomies, we believe that we serve the patient better with an aggressive policy of postoperative, on-demand, percutaneous CT-guided drainage procedures and/or CT-directed, on-demand laparotomies. This more limited strategy spares the rest of the abdomen, and the patient, the trauma of blind exploration.

The first postoperative week, however – before the infective process has become localized – offers a window of opportunity for planned relaparotomies. It is then, when one or two planned relaparotomies may help to better control the source and eliminate heavy contamination. It is our opinion that, at a later phase, intervention should be dictated by the patient's condition, findings on clinical examination (when the abdomen is left open, one can easily place a hand in one of the gutters and gently feel around) and imaging.

Is Laparostomy Beneficial?

The physiological benefits of a decompressing laparostomy for significant intra-abdominal hypertension causing abdominal compartment syndrome are well proven in trauma and general surgical patients [3]. A large body of experimental studies suggests that elevated intra-abdominal pressure promotes systemic absorption of peritoneal endotoxin and bacteria, thus increasing the mortality rate of peritonitis in small and large animals [20]. Although the issue of raised intra-abdominal pressure and its treatment with laparostomy has not been studied specifically in patients with peritonitis, it is clear that reducing elevated intra-abdominal pressure is beneficial. Laparostomy, however, is not free from complications; therefore, though mild elevation of intra-abdominal pressure contributes to the overall morbidity, the risk–benefit ratio of prophylactic laparostomy is not clear. In our practice, we reserve laparostomies for patients with symptomatic abdominal compartment syndrome, those who cannot be closed or those whom we plan to reexplore.

When to Stop?

Planned relaparotomies are classically continued until the abdomen is macroscopically clean. When the source is controlled, however, two or three relaparotomies are sufficient to sterilize the peritoneal cavity [6]. Persistence of SIRS signifies tertiary peritonitis due to opportunistic organisms such as *Candida*. Van Goor et al. [4] suggest that the presence of fewer than 10^5 cfu/ml of micro-organisms in the peritoneal cavity – achieved after an average of three laparotomies – is a useful criterion to stop reoperating. Clearly, the continuation of relaparotomies in a clean abdomen or in the face of tertiary peritonitis is counter-productive.

Antibiotic Therapy

Whether antibiotics should be administered as long as the abdomen remains open is controversial. Obviously, as long as the source is not controlled and the peritoneal cavity grows micro-organisms, antibiotics should be administered.

Microbiological studies in patients undergoing relaparotomies demonstrated that the peritoneal cavity becomes sterile in a few days [4, 20]. Although it has been suggested that fever and leukocytosis at discontinuation of antibiotics predict the recurrence of infection [21], it is far from clear whether continuation of antibiotics could abort such recurrences. In our practice, we stop antibiotics when the source has been controlled and the abdomen is macroscopically clean and culture-negative. An open abdomen, fever, and leukocytosis are not indications to continue administration in the absence of other evidence of ongoing infection. There is some evidence, however, that fluconazole prophylaxis prevents colonization and invasive intra-abdominal *Candida* infections in reoperated patients [21]. Peritoneal *Candida* infections are an independent marker of increased mortality and morbidity [22].

Critical Factors and Decision Making

Relaparotomies and laparostomy are therapeutic measures that are indicated in a minority of patients. Planned relaparotomies are indicated – and probably beneficial – during the early postoperative phase, when the source has not been adequately controlled at the index operation, or when contamination/infection has been extensive or associated with necrotic tissues. Laparostomy is indicated and beneficial when the abdomen cannot be closed or cannot be closed without creating significant intra-abdominal hypertension. Our approach in such selected patients would be to start with one or two planned relaparotomies. Thereafter, once CT imaging becomes accurate, we continue aggressively but selectively – based on clinical judgment and imaging – with *directed* on-demand relaparotomies and/or percutaneous drainage procedures. Directed reoperation guided by CT imaging allows the surgeon to approach the problem through a fresh incision away from the central mass of matted bowel and avoid the potentially damaging effects of one's hands and instruments.

Planed relaparotomies combined with laparostomy represent, for the time being, the heaviest weaponry in the surgeon's mechanical armamentarium for the treatment of severe intra-abdominal infection and other postlaparotomy abdominal catastrophes. Even without level I or II evidence, we are convinced that these therapeutic modalities can be life-saving in a few selected groups of patients. The challenge is to know when to stop and how not to harm (Table 1).

"A negative relaparotomy is better than a positive autopsy but is not, nevertheless, a benign procedure" [23].

Table 1. Laparostomy and planned relaporatomies for intra-abdominal sepsis

	Author	Year	Laparostomy ± planned relaparotomy	APACHE II (mean)	Mortality (%)
1.	Steinberg D et al. [24]	1979	14		7
2.	Casali RE et al. [25]	1980	12		8
3.	Stone HH et al. [26]	1980	124		23
4.	Goris RJA et al. [55]	1980	26		46
5.	Voyles CR et al. [27]	1981	25		24
6.	Duff JH et al. [28]	1981	18		33
7.	Maetani S et al. [29]	1981	13		8
8.	Kendrick JH et al. [30]	1982	21		19
9.	Wouters DB et al. [31]	1983	20		15
10.	Anderson ED et al. [32]	1983	20		55
11.	Broome A et al. [33]	1983	30		0
12.	Penninckx FM et al. [1]	1983	31		29
13.	Hedderich GS et al. [34]	1986	10		20
14.	Teichmann W et al. [35]	1986	61		22.9
15.	Andrus C et al. [36]	1986	34		61.7
16.	Chan STF et al. [37]	1986	14		21.4
17.	Walsh GL et al. [38]	1988	25		32
18.	Ivatury RR et al. [39]	1989	25	16.6	47.7
19.	Bose SM et al. [40]	1991	5		60
20.	Hakkiluoto A et al. [41]	1992	21	22.1	52
21.	Billing A et al. [16]	1992	152	14.5	33.5
22.	Christou NV et al. [14]	1993	18		44
23.	Demmel N et al. [42]	1993	101		32.7
24.	Schein M et al. [43]	1994	43		41.8
25.	Hau T et al. [13]	1995	38	13.1	21
26.	Roeyen G et al. [44]	1996	7	17.7	0
27.	Grunau G et al. [45]	1996	13	17.6	77
28.	Gotzinger P et al. [46]	1996	15	9.8	43
29.	Van Goor H et al. [4]	1997	24	18.7	29
30.	Jiffry BA et al. [47]	1998	52		15.6
31.	Kriwanek S et al. [48]	1998	72	16.3	51.3
32.	Nathens AB et al. [49]	1998	11	21.5	45
33.	Visser MR et al. [50]	1998	41		29.2
34.	Wacha H et al. [51]	1999	55		19.8
35.	Bailey CMH et al. [52]	2000	7	22.7	28.6
36.	Bosscha K et al. [12]	2000	67	13	42
37.	Kriwanek S et al. [53]	2000	145	17	37
38.	Koperna T et al. [54]	2000	22	20.7	54.5

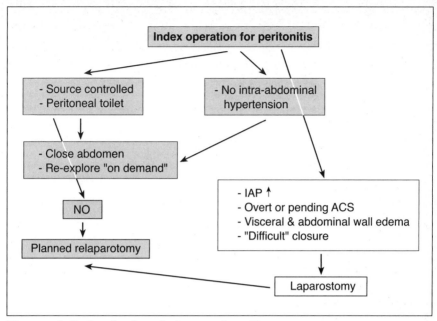

Diagram 1. Indications for planned relaparotomies and laparostomy
IAP, increased intra-abdominal pressure; *ACS*, abdominal compartment syndrome

References

1. Penninckx FM, Kerremans RP, Lauwers P (1983) Planned relaparotomies in the surgical treatment of severe generalized peritonitis from intestinal origin. World J Surg 7:762–766
2. Pujol JP (1975) Thèse pour le Doctorat en Medecine, U.E.R. X Bichat, Paris,
3. Schein M, Wittmann DH, Aprahamian CC, Condon RE (1995) The abdominal compartment syndrome: the physiological and clinical consequences of elevated intra-abdominal pressure. J Am Coll Surg 180:745–753
4. Van Goor H, Hulsebos RG, Bleichrodt RP (1997) Complications of planned relaparotomy in patients with severe general peritonitis. Eur J Surg 163:61–66
5. Schein M (1991) Planned reoperations and open management in critical intra-abdominal infections: prospective experience in 52 cases. World J Surg 15:637–645
6. Wittmann DH, Schein M, Condon RE (1996) Management of secondary peritonitis. Ann Surg 224:10–18
7. Wittmann DH (2000) Staged abdominal repair: development and current practice of an advanced operative technique for diffuse suppurative peritonitis. Acta Chir Austriaca 32:171–178
8. Mastboom WJ, Kuypers HH, Schoots FJ, Wobbes T (1989) Small-bowel perforation complicating the open treatment of generalized peritonitis. Arch Surg 124:689–692
9. Wittmann DH, Aprahamian C, Bergstein JM (1990) Etappenlavage: advanced diffuse peritonitis managed by planned multiple laparotomies utilizing zippers, slide fastener, and Velcro analogue for temporary abdominal closure. World J Surg 14:218–226
10. Schein M, Saadia R, Jamieson JR, Decker GA (1986) The 'sandwich technique' in the management of the open abdomen. Br J Surg 73:369–370
11. Schein M, Assalia A (1994) The role of planned reoperations and laparostomy in severe intro-abdominal infection: is a prospective randomized trial possible? Theo Surg 9:38–42

12. Bosscha K, Hulstaert PF, Visser MR, van Vroonhoven TJ, van der Werken C (2000) Open management of the abdomen and planned reoperations in severe bacterial peritonitis. EurJ Surg 166:44–49
13. Hau T, Ohmann C, Wolmershauser A, Wacha H, Yang Q (1995) Planned relaparotomy vs relaparotomy on demand in the treatment of intra-abdominal infections. The Peritonitis Study Group of the Surgical Infection Society – Europe. Arch Surg 130:1193–1196
14. Christou NV, Barie PS, Dellinger EP, Waymack JP, Stone HH (1993) Surgical Infection Society intra-abdominal infection study. Prospective evaluation of management techniques and outcome. Arch Surg 128:193–198
15. Wickel DJ, Cheadle WG, Mercer-Jones MA, Garrison RN (1997) Poor outcome from peritonitis is caused by disease acuity and organ failure, not recurrent peritoneal infection. Ann Surg 225:744–753
16. Billing A, Frohlich D, Mialkowskyj O, Stokstad P, Schidberg FW (1992) Peritonitisbehandlung mit der Etappenlavage (EL): Prognosekriterien and Behandlungsverlauf. Langenbecks Arch Chir 377:305–313
17. Schein M, Decker GA (1990) Gastrointestinal fistulas associated with large abdominal wall defects: experience with 43 patients Br J Surg 77:97–100
18. Sautner T, Gotzinger P, Redl–Wenzl EM, Dittrich K, Felfernig M, Sporn P, Roth E, Fugger R (1997) Does reoperation for abdominal sepsis enhance the inflammatory host response? Arch Surg 132:250–255
19. Schein M, Wittmann DH, Holzheimer R, Condon RE (1996) Hypothesis: compartmentalization of cytokines in intraabdominal infection. Surgery 119:694–700
20. Schein M, Paladugu R (2000) What's new in pathophysiology of peritonitis? Acta Chir Austriaca 32:162–166
20. Aprahamian C, Schein M, Wittmann DH (1995) Cefotaxime and metronidazole in severe intra-abdominal infection. Diag Microbiol Infect Dis 22:183–188
21. Eggimann P, Francioli P, Bille J, Schneider R, Wu MM, Chapuis G, Chiolero R, Pannatier A, Schilling J, Geroulanos S, Glauser MP, Calandra T (1999) Fluconazole prophylaxis prevents intra-abdominal candidiasis in high-risk surgical patients. Crit Care Med 27:1066–1072
22. Calandra T, Bille J, Schneider R, Mosimann F, Francioli P (1989) Clinical significance of Candida isolated from peritoneum in surgical patients. Lancet 16:1437–1440
23. Saadia R, Schein M (2000) Re-laparotomies and laparostomy for infection. In: Schein, M (ed) Schein's common sense emergency abdominal surgery. Springer Verlag, Heidelberg, NY, pp 321–332
24. Steinberg D (1979) On leaving the peritoneal cavity open in acute generalized suppurative peritonitis. Am J Surg 137:216–220
25. Casali RE, Tucker WE, Petrino RA, Westbrook KC, Read RC (1980) Postoperative necrotizing fasciitis of the abdominal wall. Am J Surg. 140:787–790
26. Stone HH, Fabian TC (1980) Clinical comparison of antibiotic combinations in the treatment of peritonitis and related mixed aerobic-anaerobic surgical sepsis. World J Surg 4:415–421
27. Voyles CR, Richardson JD, Bland KI, Tobin GR, Flint LM, Polk HC Jr (1981) Emergency abdominal wall reconstruction with polypropylene mesh: short-term benefits versus long-term complications. Ann Surg 194:219–223
28. Duff JH, Moffat J (1981) Abdominal sepsis managed by leaving abdomen open. Surgery 90:774–778
29. Maetani S, Tobe T (1981) Open peritoneal drainage as effective treatment of advanced peritonitis. Surgery 90:804–809
30. Kendrick JH, Casali RE, Lang NP, Read RC (1982) The complicated septic abdominal wound. Arch Surg 117:464–468
31. Wouters DB, Krom RA, Slooff MJ, Kootstra G, Kuijjer PJ (1983) The use of Marlex mesh in patients with generalized peritonitis and multiple organ system failure. Surg Gynecol Obstet 156:609–614
32. Anderson ED, Mandelbaum DM, Ellison EC, Carey LC, Cooperman M (1983) Open packing of the peritoneal cavity in generalized bacterial peritonitis. Am J Surg 145:131–135

33. Broome A, Hansson L, Lundgren F, Smedberg S (1983) Open treatment of abdominal septic catastrophes. World J Surg 7:792–796
34. Hedderich GS, Wexler MJ, McLean AP, Meakins JL (1986) The septic abdomen: open management with Marlex mesh with a zipper. Surgery 99:399–408
35. Teichmann W, Wittmann DH, Andreone PA (1986) Scheduled reoperations (etappenlavage) for diffuse peritonitis. Arch Surg 121:147–152
36. Andrus C, Doering M, Herrmann VM, Kaminski DL (1986) Planned reoperation for generalized intraabdominal infection. Am J Surg 152:682–686
37. Chan ST, Esufali ST (1986) Extended indications for polypropylene mesh closure of the abdominal wall. Br J Surg 73:3–6
38. Walsh GL, Chiasson P, Hedderich G, Wexler MJ, Meakins JL (1988) The open abdomen. The Marlex mesh and zipper technique: a method of managing intraperitoneal infection. Surg Clin North Am 68:25–40
39. Ivatury RR, Nallathambi M, Rao PM, Rohman M, Stahl WM (1989) Open management of the septic abdomen: therapeutic and prognostic considerations based on APACHE II. Crit Care Med 17:511–517
40. Bose SM, Kalra M, Sandhu NP (1991) Open management of septic abdomen by Marlex mesh zipper. Aust N Z J Surg 61:385–388
41. Hakkiluoto A, Hannukainen J (1992) Open management with mesh and zipper of patients with intra-abdominal abscesses or diffuse peritonitis. Eur J Surg 158:403–405
42. Demmel N, Osterholzer G, Gunther B (1993) [Differentiated treatment strategy for peritonitis: single stage closure with drainage or open with programmed reintervention/lavage]? Zentralbl Chir 118:395–400
43. Schein M (1991) Planned reoperations and open management in critical intra-abdominal infections: prospective experience in 52 cases. World J Surg 15:537–545
44. Roeyen G, Hubens G, Vaneerdeweg W, Mahieu L, Eyskens E (1996) Scheduled relaparotomies using a zipper system for the treatment of diffuse generalized peritonitis in children. Acta Chir Belg 96:201–205
45. Grunau G, Heemken R, Hau T (1996) Predictors of outcome in patients with postoperative intra-abdominal infection. Eur J Surg 162:619–625
46. Gotzinger P, Gebhard B, Wamser P, Sautner T, Huemer G, Fugger R (1996) [Revision of diffuse peritonitis: planned versus on demand]. Langenbecks Arch Chir 381:343–347
47. Jiffry BA, Sebastian MW, Amin T, Isbister WH (1998) Multiple laparotomies for severe intra-abdominal infection. Aust N Z J Surg 68:139–142
48. Kriwanek S, Gschwantler M, Beckerhinn P, Armbruster C, Roka R (2000) Reconstructive intestinal surgery after open management of severe intraabdominal infection. World J Sur 24:999–1003
49. Nathens AB, Rotstein OD, Marshall JC (1998) Tertiary peritonitis: clinical features of a complex nosocomial infection. World J Surg 22:158–163
50. Visser MR, Bosscha K, Olsman J, Vos A, Hulstaert PF, van Vroonhoven TJ, van der Werken C (1998) Predictors of recurrence of fulminant bacterial peritonitis after discontinuation of antibiotics in open management of the abdomen. Eur J Surg 164:825–829
51. Wacha H, Hau T, Dittmer R, Ohmann C (1999) Risk factors associated with intraabdominal infections: a prospective multicenter study. Peritonitis Study Group. Langenbecks Arch Surg 384:24–32
52. Bailey CM, Thompson-Fawcett MW, Kettlewell MG, Garrard C, Mortensen NJ (2000) Laparostomy for severe intra-abdominal infection complicating colorectal disease. Dis Colon Rectum 43:25–30
53. Kriwanek S, Gschwantler M, Beckerhinn P, Armbruster C, Roka R (2000) Reconstructive intestinal surgery after open management of severe intraabdominal infection. World J Surg 24:999–1003
54. Koperna T, Schulz F (2000) Relaparotomy in peritonitis: prognosis and treatment of patients with persisting intraabdominal infection. World J Surg 24:32–37
55. Goris RJA et al (1980) Ogilvie's method applied to infected wound disruption. Arch Surg 115:1103–1106

Invited Commentary

Harry Van Goor

Surgery to control the source of infection is the cornerstone of initial treatment for secondary peritonitis. The therapeutic dilemma is whether after initial operation, the outcome may be improved by subsequent planned relaparotomy and/or laparostomy and whether the strategy of relaparotomy on demand should be practiced in selected patients.

The surgical strategy of planned relaparotomies in patients with secondary peritonitis is not evidence-based. The majority of studies are retrospective, consist of small numbers of heterogeneous patients, and lack detailed information on definitions, criteria, and interventions used. Criteria for inclusion into the study and choice of therapy, in particular, are not transparent. It is striking to note that in some papers, for example, patients with perforated appendicitis and those with infected pancreatic necrosis are included and that combined results of planned relaparotomies are reported, suggesting that these disease entities, their surgical approaches, complications, and outcomes can be compared. Furthermore, patients initially treated for secondary peritonitis and those referred from other hospitals with established multiple organ dysfunction are combined in one study group.

Necrotizing pancreatitis should be deleted from the discussion of whether or not to perform planned relaparotomies for peritonitis because it is a different disease entity than secondary peritonitis, because of the absence of peritonitis, the inability – per definition – to control the disease in one operation, the initially sterile inflammatory process, and the various secondary operative approaches (continuous postoperative lavage, planned lesser sac explorations, retroperitoneal exploration). Therefore this topic will not be addressed in this invited comment.

Indications for Planned Relaparotomies

Despite the lack of level I and II evidence it, is obvious that a planned relaparotomy is mandatory when the source of infection is not controlled in the first laparotomy. Inability to control the source of infection, however, is rare and occurs only in patients in whom a bowel leak can not be closed, resected, exteriorized, or excluded.

The important question remains whether there are indications for planned relaparotomy in patients in whom the source of infection is adequately controlled. Residual necrosis and debris are reported to be the main indications and these should be removed as thoroughly and rapidly as possible in order to promote the healing process. This debridement is severely hampered by intra-abdominal fibrin. Firstly, fibrin forms adhesions that render abdominal reentry complicated. Adhesiolysis and fibrin peeling causes serosal bleeding, bowel perforation, and fistula formation. Secondly, fibrin localizes infection and is a nidus for abscesses. Thirdly, fibrin impairs host defense mechanisms, which are necessary to clear the abdomen from necrosis, bacteria, and debris. Targeted or nontargeted reduction of fibrinous adhesions would probably render planned relaparotomy used to repeatedly debride the abdomen, superfluous, or at the least would diminish complications associated with planned relaparotomy.

Temporary or Definitive Closure of the Abdomen

Apart from the discussion on indications for planned relaparotomies, there is debate on how to temporarily close the abdomen, when to stop planned relaparotomiesn and how to close the abdomen definitively.

The issue to leave the abdomen open as a laparostomy, viewing the infected abdomen as a huge abscess cavity which should be incised and drained, is settled: *do not do it.* It does not work because proper drainage is impossible as a result of rapid adhesion formation and a laparostomy introduces complications including bleeding, serosal damage, and intestinal fistula.

Temporary closure can be achieved using materials varying from simple sterilized nylon and plastic bags to specially designed Velcro-type sheaths and zippers. Much emphasis is put on closure without tension to avoid abdominal compartment syndrome. It is questionable if temporary closure not approximating fascial edges is necessary and advantageous in most patients with peritonitis – it certainly is harmful. Patients with large granulating defects over an absorbable mesh, receiving split skin grafts, ending up having large ventral hernias with physical and cosmetic complaints are the (silent) witnesses of an unproven method of treatment.

I much agree with doing no more than two or three planned relaparotomies only in the first week after initial operation. In most patients, the source is controlled, necrosis is removed, pus is evacuated, and the initial bacterial load is drastically reduced. Resolution of the inflammatory process takes more time – reflected by "clear" ascites, which often mistakenly is held for infected ascites. This finding is not an indication to continue planned relaparotomy.

In some patients, intra-abdominal inflammation is ongoing and superimposed infections occur – a condition described by the term "tertiary peritonitis" – which never will be cured, but may be aggravated, by repeated surgical interventions and prolonged antibiotic use.

The most frequent scenario – that two or three planned relaparotomies in the first week are adequate to clear the infection – enables closure of the fascia after each laparotomy and avoids complications and the necessity of troublesome secondary closure. Complications associated with raised abdominal tension are the price to pay in a few patients. When primary closure cannot be accomplished, the component separate method as described by Ramirez and currently practiced in our hospital may be used for delayed closure of large defects without the need of foreign material [1].

The Future of Treatment of Frank Peritonitis

There are two important questions with regard to planned relaparotomy. Firstly, how do we identify those patients who will benefit and those in whom one operation is sufficient? Secondly, are there nonsurgical means available as an adjunct to initial surgery that obviate planned relaparotomy?

The answer to the first question is unknown. Well-defined, prospectively gathered, epidemiological data and clinical observations of patients with peritonitis may be of help as shown by the group of Lorenz [2]. Recent findings of genetically determined differences in magnitude of the local and systemic responses to intra-abdominal infection hold promise that gene mapping may help to identify patients who may cope with sequelae of intra-abdominal infection after one laparotomy [3].

The second question is easier to answer. Based on the clinical finding that fibrinous adhesions in particular render planned relaparotomy difficult and introduce complications, fibrinolytic and other adhesion-reducing agents seem logical as an adjunct to initial surgery. After successful animal experiments, the time has come for clinical trials of tissue plasminogen activator (a potent fibrinolytic agent) or hyaluronate derivatives [4].

Recommendations

- Future clinical studies should be prospective, including only patients with colonic perforation and postoperative peritonitis and only patients initially treated in a dedicated center.
- The period of planned relaparotomies should in principle not exceed 7 days.
- The fascia should preferably be closed in a primary fashion. If abdominal compartment syndrome occurs temporary closure is recommended, followed by delayed closure as early as possible using component separation techniques.
- Much effort should be put into targeted medical prevention of intra-abdominal fibrinous adhesions, an important source of residual infection and inflammation.

References

1. De Vries-Reilingh TS, van Engeland MIA, van Goor H, et al (2001) 'Components separation technique' for the repair of large hernias. Br J Surg (in press)
2. Stinner B, Bauhofer A, Lorenz W, et al (2001) Granulocyte-colony stimulating factor in the prevention of postoperative infectious complications and suboptimal recovery from operation in patients with colorectal cancer and increased preoperative risk (ASA 3 and 4). Part three: individual patient, complication algorithm and quality management. Inflamm Res 250:233–248
3. Van Goor H, Goris RJA (2000) Monitoring intra-abdominal infection. In: Tellado JM, Christou NV (eds) Intra-abdominal infections. Harcourt International, Madrid 45–64
4. Reynen MMPJ, Meis JFGM, Postma VA, van Goor H (1999) Prevention of intra-abdominal abscesses and adhesions using a hyaluronic acid solution in a rat peritonitis model. Arch Surg 134:997–1001

43 Antibiotics as an Adjunct to Source Control: Revised Surgical Infection Society Guidelines for Antimicrobial Therapy of Intra-abdominal Infections

John E. Mazuski, Robert Sawyer, Avery Nathens, Joseph DiPiro, Moshe Schein, Kenneth A. Kudsk, Charles Yowler

Key Principles

- Antimicrobial therapy is an adjunct to primary source control procedures in treating patients with intra-abdominal infections.
- Therapeutic antimicrobials (those given for longer than 24 h) are required only for patients with established intra-abdominal infections. Patients with limited exposure to contamination from a perforated viscus and those who have a removable focus of inflammation should be treated with prophylactic antimicrobials only (those given for less than 24 h).
- Therapeutic antimicrobials for intra-abdominal infections should generally be limited to no more than 5-7 days. Ongoing clinical evidence of infection should prompt a search for a new or recurrent infection rather than arbitrary prolongation of antimicrobial therapy with new or different agents.
- Antimicrobial regimens for intra-abdominal infections should cover common aerobic and anaerobic enteric flora. A number of different regimens are available, but the choice of antimicrobials for most patients with community-acquired infections should be dictated primarily by considerations of cost, convenience, and potential toxicity.
- Patients at high risk for therapeutic failure include those with preexisting physiological compromise and those with difficult-to-treat organisms, which many times have been acquired in the hospital. Antimicrobial therapy may need to be intensified in some of these patients to cover resistant Gram-negative aerobic organisms, enterococci, and yeast.

Antimicrobial therapy is an important component in the treatment of patients with intra-abdominal infections. However, the use of antimicrobials should be considered an adjunct to a properly performed surgical or radiologically guided procedure designed to gain control of the infected focus. Even the best antimicrobial therapy has little efficacy if used without an effort to gain adequate source control.

The primary goal of antimicrobial therapy is to prevent the persistence or recurrence of an intra-abdominal infection by eradicating microorganisms remaining after initial efforts at primary source control. A secondary goal of anti-microbial therapy is to prevent dissemination of the infection to other sites, which may occur during or after source control procedures. By assisting in the eradication and control of infecting microorganisms, antimicrobial therapy should limit the patient's systemic response to infection and thereby improve the likelihood of survival and recovery.

The fundamental principles of antimicrobial therapy for intra-abdominal infections were outlined over 25 years ago and have not changed substantially in the interim. These principles were based on experimental models of intra-abdominal infections and clinical studies, which demonstrated the need for coverage of aerobic/facultative anaerobic Enterobacteriaceae and anaerobic organisms, particularly *Bacteroides fragilis* [1, 2]. The initial regimen shown to be efficacious in this regard was an aminoglycoside such as gentamicin, combined with an anti-anaerobic agent such as clindamycin or chloramphenicol. Over the past 2 decades, the repertoire of antimicrobial agents has expanded greatly, and there is a wide variety of single agents or combination regimens currently available for the treatment of intra-abdominal infections.

In 1992 the Antimicrobial Agents Committee of the Surgical Infection Society provided a set of guidelines regarding the use of antimicrobials for intra-abdominal infections [3]. These guidelines have been supplemented by an update undertaken by the Therapeutic Agents Committee, the successor to the Antimicrobial Agents Committee [41]. A summary of these guidelines is included in the appendix of this chapter. However, this recent revision does not supplant the previously published guidelines and the reader is referred both to the original guidelines and the recent update for a full description of the evidence behind the recommendations.

In addition to updating the original guidelines, another goal of the revised document was to describe the evidence behind different recommendations according to evolving terminology of evidence-based medicine. The final recommendations were graded with regard to the quality of evidence that supports them (Table 1). In general, level 1 recommendations were based on two or more well-done, prospective, randomized, controlled studies; level 2 recommendations were based on less well-controlled prospective or retrospective studies; and level 3 recommendations were based on uncontrolled studies and expert opinion. These descriptions were based on those used by the Eastern Association for the Surgery of Trauma [4] and the American Society for Parenteral and Enteral Nutrition [5].

Table 1. Rating scale for recommendations

Level 1.	Recommendation based on consistent, strong research-based evidence. Supported primarily by multiple, relatively homogeneous, prospective, randomized controlled trials.
Level 2.	Recommendation based on fair research-based evidence. Supported by limited data from prospective, randomized controlled trials, or by other prospective or retrospective analyses with good study design.
Level 3.	Recommendation based primarily on limited or uncontrolled data and supported by expert opinion.

While this grading system is somewhat less complex than others, it still allows a straightforward characterization of the strength of the recommendation.

Selection of Patients for Therapeutic Antimicrobial Therapy

Intra-abdominal infections covered by the previous and updated guidelines include those generally described as secondary or tertiary peritonitis and intra-abdominal abscess. The polymicrobial nature of nearly all intra-abdominal infections reflects their origin from an enteric source. Intra-abdominal infections due to primary peritonitis and those associated with indwelling intra-abdominal catheters have a different microbial flora and are not considered further during these discussions. Similarly, specific issues related to pathogens found with primary gynecological disorders preclude further description of antimicrobial treatment of these infections, even though these may involve Gram-negative enteric pathogens and anaerobes.

It is important to identify patients who require therapeutic administration of antimicrobial agents. Although many patients undergoing abdominal procedures receive antimicrobials in the perioperative period, much of this use is intended as prophylaxis to prevent primary superficial surgical site and other infections. Use of prophylactic antimicrobials should not exceed 24 h. Therapeutic antimicrobials, in contrast, are intended to treat established intra-abdominal infections, which are often a result of a pathological process several days in duration. Therapeutic antimicrobials are generally given for several days, as will be discussed below.

Although the distinction between prophylactic and therapeutic antibiotics is clear for most patients, some patients fall into a gray zone. Such patients include those who have significant intra-abdominal contamination sustained shortly before or during an operative procedure and those who have an infected focus within the abdominal cavity that is confined to a specific organ. The current guidelines have attempted to delineate which of these patients should receive therapeutic antimicrobials (Table 2). Several prospective studies have shown that 24 h of antimicrobial therapy is effective for the treatment of patients with bowel injuries as a result of penetrating abdominal trauma, when surgical therapy is undertaken without delay [6-10]. A similar principle should apply to iatrogenic bowel perforations operated on immediately such as endoscopic perforations of the colon or

Table 2. Conditions for which therapeutic antimicrobials (>24 h) are not recommended

Traumatic and iatrogenic enteric perforations operated on within 12 h

Gastroduodenal perforations operated on within 24 h

Acute or gangrenous appendicitis without perforation

Acute or gangrenous cholecystitis without perforation

Transmural bowel necrosis from embolic, thrombotic, or obstructive vascular occlusion without perforation or established peritonitis or abscess enterotomies occurring during surgical interventions. Because of the low bacterial inoculum, most gastroduodenal perforations less than 24 h old do not require therapeutic antimicrobials, although a definitive study of this has never been performed. Small-bowel and colonic perforations greater than 12 h old, and gastro-duodenal perforations greater than 24 h old, are considered to have had sufficient duration to permit an intra-abdominal infection to be established. Thus, therapeutic antimicrobials should be administered for these conditions.

Another group of patients for whom short-term prophylactic antimicrobial therapy is reasonable are those who have an infected focus that can be fully eradicated at the time of surgical intervention. Thus, patients with acute or gangrenous appendicitis or cholecystitis, and those with bowel necrosis due to a vascular accident or strangulation, in whom there is no evidence of perforation or infected peritoneal fluid, can be reasonably treated with 24 h or less of antimicrobials [11, 12]. However, this principle does not apply to those patients whose infection has extended beyond the initial anatomical focus and who clearly have purulent, infected, peritoneal fluid. Since these patients have established peritonitis, therapeutic antimicrobial therapy is warranted.

Duration Of Antimicrobial Therapy

Recommendations vary widely with regard to the duration of antimicrobial therapy for intra-abdominal infections. Nearly all prospective trials have left the duration of antimicrobial therapy to the discretion of the investigator, allowing anywhere from 3 to 14 days of therapy. There have been no large prospective, randomized controlled trials specifically evaluating duration of therapy as a factor in the success or failure of antimicrobial use for intra-abdominal infections.

There is a growing consensus that prolonged antimicrobial therapy is not warranted for most patients with intra-abdominal infections. Bohnen et al. [3] recommended 5-7 days of antimicrobial therapy. Wittman and Schein [11] have proposed even shorter durations of therapy. Using historical data, success rates for protocols that limit the duration of therapy to 3-5 days have been equivalent to those using a longer duration of therapy [12-14].

The risk of treatment failure is quite low in patients who have no clinical evidence of infection at the time of cessation of antimicrobial therapy. This usually implies that the patient is afebrile, has a normal white blood cell count, and is tolerating an oral diet. One prospective randomized study of patients with complicated appendicitis demonstrated that discontinuation of antimicrobials at the time of resolution of clinical signs was as successful as a fixed duration of antimicrobial therapy and resulted in a shorter duration of antibiotic use [15].

The risk of treatment failure, however, is much higher in patients who have persistent signs of infection such as an elevated temperature or white blood cell count at the time that antimicrobials are discontinued [16, 17]. This situation presents a quandary to the clinician and the tendency is to prolong the course of antimicrobials or substitute a different regimen for the one previously employed. However, there have been no prospective studies demonstrating that such an approach actually improves patient outcome. In fact, unresolving clinical signs generally indicate either a persistent or recurrent intra-abdominal infection or the development of a new infection such as a nosocomial pneumonia. Thus, the observation of new or ongoing clinical signs or symptoms of infection should prompt further investigation to identify the source of the problem, rather than simple prolongation of the antimicrobial course with the same or different agents.

There are a few occasions in which a more prolonged course of antimicrobials may be warranted. In a retrospective analysis of patients treated with open abdominal techniques for persistent bacterial peritonitis, Visser et al. [18] identified decreased duration of antimicrobial exposure as a risk factor for failure in these patients. It is generally accepted that when it is not possible to attain optimal primary source control, it may be necessary to rely on prolonged antimicrobial therapy to fully eradicate the intra-abdominal infection. However, such considerations really apply only to the small number of patients in whom primary source control is not feasible or who have tertiary peritonitis after previous treatment failures.

Overall, then, the recommendation is to limit antimicrobial therapy to no more than 5-7 days for most patients with intra-abdominal infections. The duration of therapy should be based on the extent of the infection at the time of the initial source control procedure. At the end of this period of time, or perhaps earlier in patients who have had resolution of all clinical signs of infection, antimicrobials should be discontinued. In patients having persistent clinical signs of infection, an attempt should be made to determine the cause. Patients with persistent or recurrent intra-abdominal infections will likely require additional efforts to attain source control and patients who have infections at other sites will need appropriate antimicrobials for that particular cause. In patients who have persistent clinical evidence of infection, but a negative diagnostic workup, discontinuation of all antimicrobial therapy may be warranted, since the persistent clinical symptoms and signs may be the result of ongoing tissue inflammation (the systemic inflammatory response syndrome) and not a specific infectious disorder. Avoiding indiscriminate use of antimicrobials in this setting should not only decrease the exposure of patients to costly and potentially toxic agents, but also diminish the widespread colonization of patients and the hospital environment with highly resistant organisms.

Antimicrobial Regimens for Intra-abdominal Infections

A number of regimens, both single agents and combinations of antimicrobials, are available for the treatment of patients with intra-abdominal infections. The current recommendations of the Surgical Infections Society are listed in Table 3. All recommended regimens cover both the aerobic/facultative anaerobic Gram-negative bacteria and the anaerobic bacteria commonly associated with intra-abdominal infections. Single agents recommended include second-generation cephalosporins with anaerobic coverage, beta-lactam/beta-lactamase inhibitor agents, and carbapenems. Recommended combination regimens include an aminoglycoside plus an antianaerobic agent (either clindamycin or metronidazole),

Table 3. Recommended antimicrobial regimens for intra-abdominal infection

Single agents:
- Cefoxitin
- Cefotetan
- Ampicillin-sulbactam
- Ticarcillin-clavulanic acid
- Piperacillin-tazobactam
- Imipenem-cilastatin
- Meropenem
- Ertapenem

Combination regimens:
- Aminoglycoside (gentamicin, tobramycin, netilmicin, amikacin)
  plus antianaerobe (clindamycin or metronidazole)
- Cefuroxime plus metronidazole
- Third-/fourth-generation cephalosporin
  (cefotaxime, ceftriaxone, ceftizoxime, ceftazidime, cefepime)
  plus antianaerobe
- Aztreonam plus clindamycin
- Ciprofloxacin plus metronidazole

cefuroxime, or a third or fourth generation cephalosporin plus an antianaerobic agent, aztreonam plus clindamycin, and ciprofloxacin plus metronidazole. It is likely that other agents will be added to this list in the near future, as prospective trials of newer carbapenems and fluoroquinolones become available.

The efficacy of all of the recommended regimens has been confirmed in prospective, randomized, controlled trials. However, it is not possible to identify any specific regimen as superior to another, since these prospective trials have almost always been designed as equivalency trials and have been insufficiently powered to demonstrate superiority. In general, most regimens have shown efficacy rates of 80%-90%, but the actual rates are highly dependent on the selection criteria used to enter patients into the trials. Typically, efficacy rates are higher when many or all of the study patients have perforated appendicitis.

Since all regimens appear to be approximately equivalent, antimicrobial selection should be based on other criteria. With mild to moderate community-acquired infections such as perforated appendicitis, cure is likely with any regimen and antimicrobial agents having a narrower spectrum of activity that are less toxic and less costly are preferable [41]. Such agents might include second-generation cephalosporins with anaerobic coverage, ampicillin/sulbactam, and ticarcillin/clavulanic acid.

The use of oral antibiotics to complete an antimicrobial course also appears reasonable for many patients with intra-abdominal infections. This was specifically demonstrated in a prospective trial of oral ciprofloxacin and metronidazole used as continuation therapy for patients started on intravenous forms of these antibiotics [19]. Oral amoxicillin/clavulanic acid has also been used in several studies, although its efficacy as continuation therapy has not been as well documented. When oral antibiotics have been used, they have not been started prior to 3 days after initiation of therapy and have been used only for patients who are able to tolerate an oral diet.

The use of aminoglycoside-containing regimens has declined substantially in recent years with the availability of other, less toxic agents. A common problem with aminoglycosides is underdosing, and the resultant failure to achieve therapeutic concentrations of these agents. In one study, Solomkin et al. [20] identified subtherapeutic concentrations of aminoglycosides as a likely cause of an increased rate of treatment failures related to the use of these agents. Thus, if these agents are used, it is important to dose them adequately.

Once daily administration of aminoglycosides is an alternative that simplifies their use and may avoid problems of underdosing. Compared to multiple daily dose regimens, once daily administration appears to be associated with equivalent efficacy and possibly decreased side effects [21]. Although daily administration of aminoglycosides has not been studied extensively in patients with intra-abdominal infections, there are sufficient data available to recommend this method for patients with intra-abdominal infections.

Of the recommended regimens, only beta-lactam/beta-lactamase agents and carbapenems routinely cover *Enterococcus*. However, the need for coverage of this organism remains controversial. Prospective trials, which have mainly involved patients with mild to moderate community-acquired infections, have not demonstrated any added clinical benefit for regimens that provide enterococcal coverage when compared to those that do not. For most patients, it does not seem justifiable to use only agents that cover this organism or to routinely add ampicillin or another agent to regimens that do not provide this coverage.

A question as to the adequacy of antimicrobial therapy may arise if final culture results reveal organisms resistant to the initial empiric antibiotic regimen. The need for routine cultures in patients with intra-abdominal infections is controversial, particularly for those with mild to moderate community-acquired infections [22, 23]. However, there seems little justification for altering an initial empiric antibiotic regimen on the basis of culture results if the patient has clinical evidence of an adequate response. Although this might be considered in the patient who is not showing signs of clinical improvement, such a patient is much more likely be benefited by a careful search for another source of an infection, rather than by simple alteration of the antibiotic regimen.

Antimicrobial Therapy for the High-Risk Patient

The identification and optimal treatment of the high-risk patient remains a challenge. First of all, the definition of a high-risk patient is imprecise. Is the high-risk patient one who is simply at increased risk of death, even if that death is due to a perioperative myocardial infarction rather than the intra-abdominal infection itself, or is the high-risk patient one likely to have any infectious complication, even if it is relatively minor such as superficial surgical site infections? Unfortunately, most analyses of risk factors have not clearly separated out the risk of morality from the risk of significant treatment failure, although the latter would be much more likely to be affected by alterations in antimicrobial therapy than the former.

Treatment failure is related both to the extent of the initial infection and to the host's capacity to respond to that infection. Traditionally, the source of the intra-abdominal infection has been thought to influence the risk of treatment failure and death. Mosdell et al. [24] identified patients with perforated appendicitis as having substantially lower mortality than other patients suffering from intra-abdominal infections, whereas patients with colonic perforations not due to diverticular disease were identified as being at particularly high risk for treatment failure and mortality. These latter patients may have had more diffuse peritonitis, in contrast to the localized infections characteristic of diverticular perforations.

However, much of this apparent association between treatment failure and the source of infection more likely reflects preexisting host factors than differences in the virulence of the specific infections. Thus, treatment of perforated appendicitis is generally successful because it is a disease of young, previously healthy patients. It is well recognized that perforated appendicitis is a much more lethal and morbid disorder when it occurs in elderly patients with multiple medical problems.

Several studies have examined risk factors for treatment failure and death using multivariate techniques. Advanced age, poor nutritional status, a low serum albumin concentration, preexisting medical disorders, particularly significant cardiovascular disease, and the use of immunosuppressive medications have all been identified as independent risk factors of mortality [25-30]. Perhaps the most accurate tool for identifying patients at increased risk for adverse outcome is the APACHE II score. This measurement, which is based on both acute and chronic alterations in physiology, correlates well with both the risk of treatment failure and the risk of mortality following treatment of intra-abdominal infections. Unfortunately, this score is somewhat cumbersome to obtain and may not be readily available when initial treatment decisions need to be made.

A few risk factors have been identified that might be pertinent to the selection of antimicrobial therapy for patients at higher risk. Patients who have organisms that are resistant to the initial empiric regimen are more likely to fail therapy than are those with sensitive organisms [31-33]. In many cases, these resistant pathogens are nosocomial in origin and have been acquired during hospitalization prior to a definitive source control procedure. When such resistant organisms are likely, the selection of antimicrobial therapy may need to be modified based on local patterns of pathogens and resistance and the patient's history of prior antimicrobial exposure.

Finally, as has been emphasized earlier, the inability to obtain adequate source control, whether due to a technical problem or the extensiveness of the infection, is a factor that leads to failure of the primary therapy [30]. No antimicrobial regimen will be successful in the face of ongoing contamination or an uncontrolled infectious source within the abdomen.

It is difficult to provide definitive recommendations regarding antimicrobial therapy of high-risk patients with intra-abdominal infections, since comparative trials of antimicrobial agents in this patient population are lacking. Applying the data obtained from most prospective studies of different antimicrobials to high-risk patients is problematic. These trials have primarily involved patients with relatively easy-to-treat community-acquired infections and have specifically excluded patients likely to be at higher risk for failure. Patients with perforated appendicitis are often the predominant population studied. As a result, mortality and failure rates in these trials are generally below those observed in epidemiological studies of patients with intra-abdominal infections. Thus, most recommendations regarding antimicrobial therapy for high-risk patients are based more on expert opinion than objective data.

The current guidelines recommend that patients considered at high risk of failure be treated with antimicrobial regimens having a broader spectrum of activity against most Gram-negative aerobic/facultative anaerobic organisms. Such regimens include extended range beta-lactam/beta-lactamase agents such as piperacillin-tazobactam, carbapenems such as imipenem/cilastatin or meropenem, third- or fourth-generation cephalosporins plus an antianaerobic agent, aztreonam plus clindamycin, and ciprofloxacin plus metronidazole. The use of an aminoglycoside plus an antianaerobe is also reasonable, although adequate doses must be used. High-risk patients may be at increased risk for toxicity from these agents.

The use of aminoglycosides in combination with other agents effective against Gram-negative aerobic/facultative anaerobic organisms has been explored in a few prospective randomized trials. In one study, Dupont et al. [34] found no benefit to the use of the combination of amikacin with piperacillin/tazobactam compared to use of piperacillin/tazobactam alone for patients with both extensive community-acquired and nosocomial intra-abdominal infections. Other studies, which have not been limited exclusively to high-risk patients, have provided some confirmation of this finding [35, 36]. Thus, routine addition of an aminoglycoside to another agent effective against Gram-negative aerobes is not necessary for high-risk patients with intra-abdominal infections.

A further question relates to the use of regimens that have enterococcal coverage. Although, as indicated previously, routine enterococcal coverage is not necessary in most patients, failure due to *Enterococcus* appears to be more prevalent in higher-risk patients [32, 37]. Since regimens such as carbapenems and extended-range beta-lactam/beta-lactamase combinations have enterococcal coverage, it may be reasonable to use such agents in the high-risk patient, although this recommendation can certainly not be considered definitive.

Development of fungal superinfections is also a common problem in the high-risk patient. Eggiman et al. [38] examined the prophylactic use of fluconazole in postoperative patients at high risk for intra-abdominal candidal infections and found a decrease in the incidence of this complication. Although prophylactic therapy with fluconazole may be reasonable in these patients, there is some controversy regarding the adequacy of fluconazole for the treatment of established candidal infections in the peritoneal cavity. Some authorities recommend amphotericin B as the preferred agent instead of fluconazole for these difficult-to-treat infections [39]. Ultimately, the choice of antifungal therapy will be heavily influenced by the risks of toxicity in a given patient.

Few generalizations can be made with regard to antimicrobial therapy for patients with tertiary peritonitis, i.e., those patients who have failed previous attempts at control of intra-abdominal infections. These patients commonly harbor resistant organisms within the infected peritoneal fluid, including coagulase negative *Staphylococcus*, enterococci including those resistant to vancomycin, multiply resistant Gram-negative bacilli, and fungal organisms, including many which are resistant to fluconazole. With tertiary peritonitis, empiric antimicrobial therapy should probably be directed at the nosocomial organisms commonly identified at a particular institution. Empiric therapy should be adjusted according to definitive culture results. Nonetheless, treatment failure is the rule rather than the exception and it is likely that these patients suffer from an overwhelming failure of host defense mechanisms. Ultimately, many of these patients will succumb to or with their infections, regardless of the adequacy of antimicrobial therapy [40].

Conclusions

Antimicrobial therapy for intra-abdominal infections is an adjunct to a properly performed operation or procedure designed to obtain adequate source control. There are a number of antimicrobial regimens suitable for treating patients with intra-abdominal infections and all appear to be of approximately equivalent efficacy. For most patients with mild to moderate community-acquired infections, antimicrobial selection can be based on criteria such as potential toxicity, convenience, and cost. Duration of therapy should generally not exceed 5-7 days. Future improvements in the therapy of these patients will most likely relate to finding more cost-effective means of providing antimicrobial therapy without compromising safety. Thus, future research might focus on the use of narrower spectrum, relatively inexpensive agents, on the adequacy of short duration courses of antimicrobial therapy, and on the use of oral antimicrobial regimens easily administered outside of the hospital setting.

In contrast, for the higher-risk patients and those with more severe infections, there is a dearth of available data with which to make firm recommendations regarding antimicrobial therapy. Generally, these patients require therapy with broader-spectrum antimicrobials, which may have to be tailored to the specific pathogens encountered. In some patients, prolonged therapy may be needed if primary source control cannot be achieved. Improved outcome in these patients is likely to come from further investigation into defining who is at high risk for failure, delineating what antimicrobial regimens should be used, and determining how long therapy should be continued. Newer antimicrobial agents are likely to be needed in these patients, since they are commonly infected with resistant organisms. Ultimately, optimizing antimicrobial therapy for the high-risk patient will be of importance not only in providing better treatment of the individual patient, but also in decreasing the ongoing development of emerging microbial resistance in hospitalized patients.

References

1. Weinstein WM, Onderdonk AB, Bartlett JG, Louie TJ, Gorbach SL (1975) Antimicrobial therapy of experimental intraabdominal sepsis. J Infect Dis 132:282–286
2. Rotstein OD, Pruett TL, Simmons RL (1985) Mechanisms of microbial synergy in polymicrobial surgical infections. Rev Infect Dis 7:151–170

3. Bohnen JMA, Solomkin JS, Dellinger EP, Bjornson HS, Page CP (1992) Guidelines for clinical care: anti-infective agents for intra-abdominal infection. A Surgical Infection Society policy statement. Arch Surg 127:83–89

4. Pasquale, MD (1998) Practice management guidelines for trauma. In: Trauma Practice Guidelines, www.east.org

5. Wolfe BM, Mathiesen KA (1997) Clinical practice guidelines in nutrition support: can they be based on randomized clinical trials? JPEN J Parenter Enteral Nutr 21:1–6

6. Oreskovich MR, Dellinger EP, Lennard ES, Wertz M, Carrico CJ, Minshew BH (1982) Duration of preventive antibiotic administration for penetrating abdominal trauma. Arch Surg 117:200–205

7. Dellinger EP, Wertz MJ, Lennard ES, Oreskovich MR (1986) Efficacy of short-course antibiotic prophylaxis after penetrating intestinal injury. A prospective randomized trial. Arch Surg 121:23–30

8. Fabian TC, Croce MA, Payne LW, Minard G, Pritchard FE, Kudsk KA (1992) Duration of antibiotic therapy for penetrating abdominal trauma: a prospective trial. Surgery 112:788–795

9. Bozorgzadeh A, Pizzi WF, Barie PS, Khaneja C, LaMaute HR, Mandava N, Richards N, Noorollah H (1999) The duration of antibiotic administration in penetrating abdominal trauma. Am J Surg 177:125–131

10. Kirton OC, O'Neill PA, Kestner M, Tortella BJ (2000) Perioperative antibiotic use in high-risk penetrating hollow viscus injury: a prospective randomized, double-blind, placebo-control trial of 24 hours versus 5 days. J Trauma Inj Infect Crit Care 49:822–832

11. Wittmann DH, Schein M (1996) Let us shorten antibiotic prophylaxis and therapy in surgery. Am J Surg 172:26S–32S.

12. Andaker L, Hojer H, Kihlstrom E, Lindhagen J (1987) Stratified duration of prophylactic antimicrobial treatment in emergency abdominal surgery. Metronidazole-fosfomycin vs. metronidazole-gentamicin in 381 patients. Acta Chir Scand 153:185–192

13. Smith JA, Bell GA, Murphy J, Forward AD, Forget JP (1985) Evaluation of the use of a protocol in the antimicrobial treatment of intra-abdominal sepsis. J Hosp Infect 6:60–64

14. Schein M, Assalia A, Bachus H (1994) Minimal antibiotic therapy after emergency abdominal surgery: a prospective study. Br J Surg 81:989–991

15. Taylor E, Dev V, Shah D, Festekjian J, Gaw F (2000) Complicated appendicitis: is there a minimum intravenous antibiotic requirement? A prospective randomized trial. Am Surg 66:887–890

16. Lennard ES, Minshew BH, Dellinger EP, Wertz M (1980) Leukocytosis at termination of antibiotic therapy: its importance for intra-abdominal sepsis. Arch Surg 115:918–921

17. Lennard ES, Dellinger EP, Wertz MJ, Minshew BH (1982) Implications of leukocytosis and fever at conclusion of antibiotic therapy for intra-abdominal sepsis. Ann Surg 195:19–24

18. Visser MR, Bosscha K, Olsman J, Vos A, Hulstaert PF, van Vroonhoven TJMV, van der Werken C (1998) Predictors of recurrence of fulminant bacterial peritonitis after discontinuation of antibiotics in open management of the abdomen. Eur J Surg 164:825–829

19. Solomkin JS, Reinhart HH, Dellinger EP, Bohnen JM, Rotstein OD, Vogel SB, Simms HH, Hill CS, Bjornson HS, Haverstock DC, Coulter HO, Echols RM (1996) Results of a randomized trial comparing sequential intravenous/oral treatment with ciprofloxacin plus metronidazole to imipenem/cilastatin for intra-abdominal infections. The intra-abdominal infection study. Ann Surg 223:303–315

20. Solomkin JS, Dellinger EP, Christou NV, Busuttil RW (1990) Results of a multicenter trial comparing imipenem/cilastatin to tobramycin/clindamycin for intra-abdominal infections. Ann Surg 212:581–591

21. Hatala R, Dinh T, Cook DJ (1996) Once-daily aminoglycoside dosing in immunocompetent adults: a meta-analysis. Ann Intern Med 124:717–725

22. Dougherty SH (1997) Antimicrobial culture and susceptibility testing has little value for routine management of secondary bacterial peritonitis. Clin Infect Dis 25:S258–S261

23. Bilik R, Burnweit C, Shanding B (1998) Is abdominal cavity culture of any value in appendicitis? Am J Surg 175:267–270

24. Mosdell DM, Morris DM, Voltura A, Pitcher DE, Twiest MW, Milne RL, Miscall BG, Fry DE (1991) Antibiotic treatment for surgical peritonitis. Ann Surg 214:543–549

25. Dellinger EP, Wertz MJ, Meakins JL, Solomkin JS, Allo MD, Howard RJ, Simmons RL (1985) Surgical infection stratification system for intra-abdominal infection. Arch Surg 120:21–29

26. Christou NV, Barie PS, Dellinger EP, Waymack JP, Stone HH (1993) Surgical Infection Society intra-abdominal infection study. Prospective evaluation of management techniques and outcome. Arch Surg 128:193–198

27. Bohnen JM, Mustard RA, Schouten BD (1994) Steroids, APACHE II score, and the outcome of abdominal infection. Arch Surg 129:33–37

28. Schoeffel U, Jacobs E, Ruf G, Mierswa F, von Specht BU, Farthmann EH (1995) Intraperitoneal micro-organisms and the severity of peritonitis. Eur J Surg 161:501–508

29. Ohmann C, Hau T (1997) Prognostic indices in peritonitis. Hepatogastroenterology 44:937–946

30. Wacha H, Hau T, Dittmer R, Ohmann C (1999) Risk factors associated with intraabdominal infections: a prospective multicenter study. Langenbeck's Arch Surg 384:24–32

31. Barie PS, Vogel SB, Dellinger EP, Rotstein OD, Solomkin JS, Yang JY, Baumgartner TF (1997) A randomized, double-blind clinical trial comparing cefepime plus metronidazole with imipenem-cilastatin in the treatment of complicated intra-abdominal infections. Cefepime Intra-abdominal Infection Study Group. Arch Surg 132:1294–1302

32. Hopkins JA, Lee JCH, Wilson SE (1993) Susceptibility of intra-abdominal isolates at operation: a predictor of postoperative infection. Am Surg 59:791–796

33. Montravers P, Gauzit R, Muller C, Marmuse JP, Fichelle A, Desmonts JM (1996) Emergence of antibiotic resistant bacteria in cases of peritonitis after surgery affects the efficacy of empirical antimicrobial therapy. Clin Infect Dis 23:486–494

34. Dupont H, Carbon C, Carlet J (2000) Monotherapy with a broad-spectrum beta-lactam is as effective as its combination with an aminoglycoside in treatment of severe generalized peritonitis: A multicenter randomized controlled trial. The Severe Generalized Peritonitis Study Group. Antimicrob Agents Chemother 44:2028–2033

35. Commetta A, Baumgartner JD, Lew D, Zimmerli W, Pittet D, Chopart P, Schaad U, Herter C, Eggimann P, Huber O, Ricou B, Suter P, Auckenthaler R, Chiolero R, Bille J, Scheidegger C, Frei R, Glauser MP (1994) Prospective randomized comparison of imipenem monotherapy with imipenem plus netilmicin for treatment of severe infections in nonneutropenic patients. Antimicrob Agents Chemother 38:1309–1313

36. Hoogkamp-Korstanje JA (1995) Ciprofloxacin vs. cefotaxime regimens for the treatment of intra-abdominal infections. Infection 23:278–282

37. Burnett RJ, Haverstock DC, Dellinger EP, Reinhart HH, Bohnen JMA, Rotstein OD, Solomkin JS (1995) Definition of the role of enterococcus in intra-abdominal infection: results of a prospective randomized trial. Surgery 118:716–723

38. Eggiman P, Francioli P, Bille J, Schneider R, Wu M-M, Capuis G, Chiolero R, Pannatier A, Schilling J, Geroulanos S, Glauser MP, Calandra T (1999) Fluconazole prophylaxis prevents intra-abdominal candidiasis in high-risk surgical patients. Crit Care Med 27:1066–1072

39. Abele-Horne M, Kopp A, Sternberg U, Ohly A, Dauber A, Russwurm W, Buchinger W, Nagengast O, Emmerling P (1996) A randomized study comparing fluconazole with amphotericin B/5-flucytosine for the treatment of systemic candida infections in intensive care patients. Infection 24:426–432

40. Nathens AB, Rotstein OD, Marshall JC (1998) Tertiary peritonitis: clinical features of a complex nosocomial infection. World J Surg 22:158–163

41. Mazuski JE, Sawyer RG, Nathens AB, DiPiro JT, Schein S, Kudsk KA, Yowler C (2002) The Surgical Infection Society Guidelines on Antimicrobial Therapy for Intra-abdominal Infections. Surgical Infections (in press)

Appendix: The Surgical Infection Society Guidelines on Antimicrobial Therapy for Intra-abdominal Infections

Selection of Patients Who Require Therapeutic (> 24 h) Versus Prophylactic (< 24 h) Antimicrobials

1. Patients with peritoneal contamination due to traumatic or iatrogenic bowel injuries repaired within 12 h (level 1) and those having gastroduodenal perforations less than 24 h old (level 3) are not considered to have established intra-abdominal infections and should be treated with prophylactic antimicrobials for 24 h or less.
2. Patients with a fully removable focus of inflammation, such as those with acute or gangrenous, but nonperforated appendicitis or cholecystitis, and those with bowel necrosis or obstruction without perforation or peritonitis, should be treated with (prophylactic) antimicrobials for 24 h or less (level 2).
3. Patients with more extensive conditions than those noted above should be treated as having established infections and given therapeutic antimicrobials for longer than 24 h (level 3).

Duration of Antimicrobial Therapy for Established

Intra-abdominal Infection

1. Antimicrobial therapy of most established intra-abdominal infections should be limited to no more than 5 (level 2) to 7 days (level 3). The duration of antimicrobial therapy for intra-abdominal infections can be based on the intraoperative findings at the time of initial intervention (level 3). Antimicrobial therapy can be discontinued in patients when they have no clinical evidence of infection such as fever or leukocytosis (level 2).
2. Continued clinical evidence of infection at the end of the time period designated for antimicrobial therapy should prompt appropriate diagnostic investigations rather than prolongation of antimicrobial treatment (level 3).
3. If adequate source control cannot be achieved a longer duration of antimicrobial therapy may be warranted (level 3).

Antimicrobial Regimens for Intra-abdominal Infections

1. Antimicrobial regimens for intra-abdominal infections should cover common aerobic and anaerobic enteric flora. The following antimicrobials or combinations of antimicrobials are effective for the treatment of intra-abdominal infections. No regimen has been demonstrated to be superior to another (level 1).

   Single agents:
   – Cefoxitin
   – Cefotetan
   – Ampicillin/sulbactam
   – Ticarcillin/clavulanic acid

- Piperacillin/tazobactam
- Imipenem/cilastatin
- Meropenem
- Ertapenem

Combination regimens:
- Cefuroxime plus metronidazole
- Third-/fourth-generation cephalosporin (cefotaxime, ceftriaxone, ceftizoxime, ceftazidime, cefepime) plus an antianaerobe
- Aztreonam plus clindamycin
- Ciprofloxacin plus metronidazole
- Aminoglycoside (gentamicin, tobramycin, netilmicin, amikacin) plus an antianaerobe (clindamycin or metronidazole)

2. For less severely ill patients with community-acquired infections, antimicrobial agents having a narrower spectrum of activity such as antianaerobic cephalosporins, ampicillin-sulbactam, or ticarcillin-clavulanic acid are preferable to more costly agents having broader coverage of Gram-negative organisms and/or greater risk of toxicity (level 3).
3. Completion of an antimicrobial course with oral forms of ciprofloxacin plus metronidazole (level 2) or with oral amoxicillin/clavulanic acid (level 3) is acceptable in patients able to tolerate an oral diet.
4. Once daily administration of aminoglycosides is the preferred dosing regimen for patients receiving these agents for intra-abdominal infections (level 2). Careful attention should be paid to prompt attainment of therapeutic antibiotic concentrations if divided daily doses of aminoglycosides are used (level 3).
5. Regimens providing enterococcal coverage are not necessary for the treatment of most patients with community-acquired intra-abdominal infections (level 2).
6. The routine use of intraoperative cultures is controversial. There is no evidence that altering the antimicrobial regimen on the basis of intraoperative culture results improves outcome (level 3).

Antimicrobial Therapy for the Higher-Risk Patient

1. In patients with intra-abdominal infections, treatment failure and death is associated with patient-related risk factors such as advanced age, poor nutritional status, a low serum albumin, and preexisting medical conditions, especially significant cardiovascular disease. A higher APACHE II score is the most consistently recognized risk factor for both death and treatment failure (level 1).
2. Disease and treatment-related risk factors, including a nosocomial origin of infection, the presence of resistant pathogens, and the lack of adequate source control, are associated with treatment failure and death (level 2).
3. Patients at higher risk for failure (particularly from non-community-acquired organisms) should be treated with an antimicrobial regimen having a broader spectrum of coverage of Gram-negative aerobic/facultative anaerobic organisms (level 3):

Single agents:
- Piperacillin/tazobactam
- Imipenem/cilastatin
- Meropenem
- Combination regimens:
- Third-/fourth-generation cephalosporin plus an antianaerobe
- Aztreonam plus clindamycin
- Ciprofloxacin plus metronidazole
- Aminoglycoside plus an antianaerobe

4. Routine addition of an aminoglycoside to other agents having broad spectrum Gram-negative coverage such as imipenem/cilastatin, piperacillin/tazobactam, or third-/fourth-generation cephalosporins, provides no additional benefit (level 2).
5. Higher-risk patients likely to fail due to *Enterococcus* such as those of advanced age, higher APACHE II scores, a nonappendiceal source of infection, a postoperative infection, or a nosocomial origin of infection may benefit from the use of a regimen covering this organism (level 3).
6. Addition of empiric antifungal therapy with fluconazole is reasonable for patients with postoperative intra-abdominal infections at high risk for candidiasis (level 2). For patients with established *Candida* peritonitis, antifungal therapy with amphotericin B may be preferable to the use of fluconazole, but the choice of therapy must be influenced by the risk of toxicity in a given patient (level 3).
7. Patients with tertiary peritonitis are likely to harbor difficult-to-eradicate organisms such as coagulase-negative staphylococci, enterococci (including vancomycin-resistant enterococci), multiply resistant Gram-negative bacilli, and yeast (level 2). Empiric therapy should be directed at organisms likely to be present based on the patient's history of previous antimicrobial therapy and local patterns of infectious organisms and resistance, and modified according to definitive culture results (level 3).

44 Epilogue

Moshe Schein, John C. Marshall

> I always wanted to write a book
> that ended with the word "mayonnaise".
> (Richard Brautigan)

How to conclude a multi-author scientific book is an unsolved dilemma. We could end simply by declaring this the last chapter, but this lacks the finality and festivity that a book deserves. A book has a head, a body and a tail, but should the tail merely repeat what has already been said in the body? Should the sporadic reader who labored through all the chapters, to arrive at the end, be exposed to a dry summary of what was already said?

Dear reader, rather than boring you, we decided to highlight what we consider the key messages of our panel of authors, decorating it with relevant aphorisms and quotations.

1 Introduction

- *The truth is that surgical decision making is based on the marriage of evidence from clinical studies, inferences from biology, and the elusive element of surgical experience.* (J.M.)
- *Time and Mother Nature are the surgeon's two greatest allies, and many a seemingly impossible situation can be converted to one that is merely a challenge by careful patience* (J.M.).

2 The Biological Rationale (D.L. Dunn)

- Host defenses are occasionally incapable of combating the introduction of microbes and establishment of infection, particularly when a large number of microbes is present or host defenses are diminished, or when an ongoing source of microbial contamination exists.
- Inadequate source control increases morbidity and mortality as much as seven-fold.
- *In surgery physiology is the king, anatomy the queen; you can be the prince, but only provided you have the judgment* (M.S.).

3 Experimental Models of Source Control (P. Wang, I.H. Chaudry)

- The CLP model of sepsis is associated with cellular dysfunction (such as hepatocellular depression) and upregulation of proinflammatory cytokines

(such as TNF). Furthermore, the ligated and punctured cecum can be excised at various intervals to serve as a source control model of sepsis. Such a model can be used for testing pharmacological agents in the management of sepsis.
- *Every operation in surgery is an experiment in bacteriology* (Berkeley Moynihan, 1865-1936).

4 Drainage (G.I. Gang, J.F. Moulton, J.S. Solomkin)

- Percutaneous abscess drainage (PD) is the preferred option in most cases.
- Operative intervention is indicated for failure of PD or when there are absolute contraindications to PD.
- PD can temporize, permitting delayed definitive management of an infectious focus.
- *Drain pus through the shortest route* (Mark M. Ravitch, 1910-1989).
- *Why is it fun to drain abscesses? Because you can't infect pus* (M.S.).

5 Debridement and "Peritoneal Toilet" (J. Bohnen)

- The degree of peritoneal contamination correlates with the severity of infection and outcome.
- The host responds to peritoneal infection by absorbing pathogens into the bloodstream and by mounting a local peritoneal inflammatory reaction; both responses kill bacteria but affect the host adversely.
- The goal of peritoneal toilet is to remove mechanically as many contaminants as possible to reduce the severity of infection and limit adverse host responses.
- *People claim that lavage is the solution to pollution by dilution of the contaminants – but remember that macrophages do not swim well.*
- *The phagocyte is the best antiseptic* (Alexander Fleming, 1881-1955).

6 Device Removal (V. Lazaron, G.J. Beilman)

- Make sure diagnosis of infection is secure.
- Determine whether device removal would pose significant risk.
- Assess complicating factors (virulence of infection, debilitation or immunosuppression of the patient, etc.) and history (has an attempt at conservative therapy failed?)
- When in doubt, take it out.
- *Too many Swan-Ganzes. The late NY cardiologist Bernard Lown wrote: "The reason for this shift includes a romance with mindless technology, which is embraced largely to maximize income. Since it is unnecessary to spend much time with patients… it opens floodgates for endless procedures."*

7 Definitive Versus Temporizing Therapy (D.E. Fry)

- Surgical choices at the time of achieving source control may require that the procedure be *temporizing* with the knowledge that a subsequent procedure will be required, or the choice may be *definitive* with the procedure designed to both control the source and also manage the underlying disease.
- The judgment to select a temporizing versus a definitive procedure requires an integrated assessment of
  a) the surgeon's knowledge about the underlying disease,
  b) systemic host factors, and
  c) the severity of the local inflammatory response.
- *To open an abdomen and search for a lesion as lightly as one would open a bureau drawer to look for the laundry, may mean lack of mental overwork to the surgeon, but it means horror to the patient* (J. Chalmers Da Costa, 1863-1933).

8 Deciding on the Extent of Surgical Therapy (G. Papia, J.C. Marshall)

- The more extensive the initial intervention, the greater the challenge of subsequent reconstruction: the optimal intervention is that which accomplishes the source control objectives in the simplest manner.
- *The larger the operation, the greater the trauma. The greater the trauma, the stronger the SIRS. The stronger the SIRS is, the sicker the patient is. The sicker the patient is the higher his M & M is* (M.S.).

9 Consequences of Failed Source Control (P.S. Barie, S.R. Eachempati)

- Failure of source control is more important than antibiotic failure in defining the outcome of surgical infections in general, and in intra-abdominal infections in particular.
- Source control of an intra-abdominal infection may fail because of a poor choice of operation or the correct operation performed poorly or with poor timing.
- Systemic consequences of failed source control include nosocomial infections, nutritional and metabolic disorders, and multiple organ dysfunction syndrome.
- *Surgeons are judged by the way they manage their own complications.*
- *What is alleged to be a "piece of cake" may become a sponge cake saturated in blood* (M.S.).

10 Diffuse Peritonitis (B. Gloor, M. Worni, M.W. Büchler)

- Aggressive initial surgical source control, including extensive intraoperative lavage, is sufficient in the vast majority of cases (~90 %).
- Continuous lavage, laparostomy and/or planned reexploration only if source control is not possible at initial operation.

- *The time will assuredly arrive when peritonitis will not kill, because we will learn that the effusions in the peritoneal cavity may be as safely evacuated as those in the pleural cavity* (James Marion Sims, 1813-1883).

11 Gastric and Proximal Small Bowel (D. Danielson, M.A. West)

- Primary closure can usually be performed.
- *We have no responsibility to such patients but to save their lives. Any procedure, which aims to do more than this, can quite significantly be considered meddlesome surgery. We have no responsibility during the surgery to carry out any procedure to cure the patient of his original duodenal ulcer* (Roscoe. R Graham, 1890-1948).
- *If anyone should consider removing half of my good stomach to cure a small ulcer in my duodenum, I would run faster than he* (Charles H. Mayo, 1865-1939).
- *In the era of Helicobacter pylori doing a gastrectomy for peptic ulcer is like doing a lobectomy for pneumonia* (Asher Hirshberg).

12 The Colon (D.H. Wittmann)

- Colonic perforations can be classified as traumatic perforation, perforation following localized necrosis from disease, and transmural ischemic necrosis due to impaired vascular flow.
- The choice of therapy depends on the general condition of the patient, the inflammatory response of the peritoneum, the magnitude of increased intra-abdominal pressure, and the pathology itself.
- Treatment options include simple suture closure, resection with anastomosis, exteriorization of the colon segment that is perforated, resection without anastomosis and formation of a terminal colostomy with or without a mucous fistula, STAR (staged abdominal repair) to secure source control by daily inspection during abdominal reentries.
- *Think about acute diverticulitis as a left-sided acute appendicitis which is, however, usually treated without an operation* (M.S.).
- *He who farts lives* (Nicholas Senn, 1844-1908).

13 Infection and Trauma of the Rectum and Anus (P.O. Nystrom)

- Perianal abscess and infected fistulae: incision and curettage for drainage of abscess, lay open associated low fistula, insert seton in high fistula, no drains or packing of wounds, antibiotics are of uncertain value.
- Fournier's gangrene: emergency action, broad spectrum antibiotics, wide excision of necrotic tissue, leave wounds open, and plan for revision, diverting stoma usually not necessary
- Anal and perineal trauma: debridement of devitalized tissue, suture of external sphincter if possible, leave wounds open, diverting stoma usually not necessary.

- Rectal trauma: defunctioning sigmoidostomy, suture of rectal wounds, drainage of presacral space, rectal washout.
- *Faecal incontinence after fistula is the result of aggressive surgeons, not progressive disease* (John Alexander-Williams).

14 Acute Appendicitis (J.M. Watters)

- Early appendectomy, open or laparoscopic, is standard therapy for acute appendicitis.
- Appendiceal phlegmon commonly resolves with antibiotic therapy alone.
- Appendiceal abscess may also respond to antibiotic therapy but will require percutaneous (or surgical) drainage in many instances.
- Appendicitis occasionally manifests as a more severe, potentially life-threatening problem, which may include generalized peritonitis, bacteremia, pylephlebitis, and/or liver abscesses, and requires appropriate surgical, antibiotic, and supportive therapy.
- *The experienced surgeon knows the pitfalls and dangers, which surround even the "simplest" operation. Perhaps he has himself lived through the sad experience of having a ligature slip when tying the appendiceal stump too short. He knows the dreadful penalty, which must follow... if he ligates the appendiceal artery improperly* (Max Thorek, 1880-1960).
- *The appendix is generally attached to the cecum* (Mark M. Ravitch, 1910-1989).
- *There are two things in life that I will never understand: women and acute appendicitis* (M.S.).

15 Bariatric Surgery (R.E. Brolin)

- Gastrointestinal leaks after bariatric operations can kill.
- Suture repair of leaks at the gastrojejunostomy is rarely successful in the face of florid infection. Conversely, leaks in the gastric staple line usually can be suture closed. If the leak involves the distal bypassed stomach, a tube gastrostomy should be performed.
- *Failure to demonstrate a leak radiologically in a patient with sign of a systemic inflammatory response, especially if progressive, should be followed by exploratory laparotomy* (N.V. Christou).
- *Anastomotic leaks are the Achilles' heal of this procedure as far as mortality is concerned* (N.V. Christou).
- *Patients who are naturally very fat are apt to die earlier than those who are slender* (Hippocrates, 460?-377? B.C.).

16 The Gallbladder and Biliary Tree (P. Götzinger, R. Függer)

- Early cholecystectomy is the treatment of choice in acute cholecystitis.
- Endoscopic sphincterotomy is the treatment of choice in ascending cholangitis.

- *Gallstones are not so harmless as was formerly thought* (Augustus Charles Bernays, 1854-1907).
- *It is better to remove 95 % of the gallbladder (i.e., subtotal cholecystectomy) than 101 % (i.e., to together with a piece of the duct)* (Asher Hirshberg).
- *When the gallbladder is "difficult" go fundus down and stay near the wall* (M.S.).

17 Pancreatic Infection (P. Dellinger)

- Prompt debridement when infection is diagnosed.
- Late debridement, when possible, is easier and safer.
- Sterile necrosis infrequently needs debridement, and then late in the course of the disease.
- Remove necrotic infected tissue.
- Avoid acute morbidity associated with necrotic tissue debridement: bleeding, fistula, devascularization of viscera, splenic injury.
- *Acute pancreatitis is the most terrible of all the calamities that occur in connection with the abdominal viscera* (Berkeley Moynihan, 1865-1936).
- *The pancreas situated high up in the abdominal cavity, and hidden behind such important organs as [...] is the least accessible of all abdominal organs, and on this account its affections, wrapped in obscurity, have for the most part constituted subjects for empirical medications* (Nicholas Senn, 1844-1908).
- Acute necrotizing pancreatitis: During the early phases of the disease "*our patience will achieve more than our force*" (Edmund Burke); later on, when called to operate on necrotic and infected complications, remember that "*patience and diligence, like faith, remove mountains*" (William Penn).

18 Liver Abscesses (I. Sayek, D. Onat)

- Liver abscesses are either pyogenic or parasitic.
- Early diagnosis and prompt treatment of the underlying cause reduce morbidity and mortality.
- Source control consists of drainage using surgical or US- or CT-guided aspiration and antibiotic therapy.
- Hydatid cysts of the liver can be managed surgically as well as percutaneously.
- *The liver confounds the surgeon's dependence on anatomy* (J. Foster).

19 Acute Mesenteric Ischemia (D.P. Raymond, A.K. May)

- Maintain a high degree of suspicion, the primary goal is diagnosis prior to bowel infarction – a complication that carries a mortality of up to 90 %.
- Aggressive use of angiography to make the correct diagnosis and plan surgical intervention appropriately.
- Restoration of bowel perfusion requires not only surgical intervention but also aggressive use of invasive monitoring to assure adequate resuscitation.

- Following resection of devitalized bowel, make a plan for a second look procedure based on the appearance of the bowel.
- *It is almost impossible to further increase the current mortality associated with acute mesenteric ischemia* (M.S.).

20 The Esophagus (J. Escallon, M.F. Jimenez)

- Early diagnosis, within 24 h (no associated esophageal diseases), requires primary repair.
- Delayed diagnosis, debridement and drainage, reinforced primary repair or exclusion and diversion.
- Cancer, megaesophagus, caustic stenosis: one stage esophagectomy with immediate or delayed reconstruction.
- Always leave adequate drainage.
- *In fact, I really do not think that the time of perforation should enter into treatment decisions to any significant extent* (J.D. Richardson).
- *I believe that an attempt should be made to close every perforation* (J.D. Richardson).
- *In my opinion, esophageal diversion should be reserved only for those patients who are almost certainly going to die unless diversion is done* (J.D. Richardson).

21 Pleural Empyema (T. Hau, E. Förster)

- Primary management of para- or postpneumatic empyemas is with antibiotics. Source control is a secondary measure whose aims are the evacuation of pus and full expansion of the lung; approaches to source control must be adapted to the stage of the disease.
- The objective of source control in postresectional empyema is to close any bronchopleural fistula and reexpand the lung, or, after pneumectomy, to stabilize or obliterate the thoracic space.
- *The pleural cavity and the peritoneal cavity are biologically identical; the bronchi, however, are sterile, while the gut is not* (J.M.).

22 Soft Tissue Infections (S.K. Lee, J.K. Horn)

- Necrotizing soft tissue infections (NSTI) generally involve the subcutaneous tissue, fascia, or deeper tissues. Therefore, a NSTI may not be readily apparent on external inspection of the skin.
- Treatment consists of urgent surgical exploration with drainage and debridement of nonviable or infected tissue. Wounds require frequent inspection until one is assured that tissues remain viable and infection is no longer spreading.
- *As long as surgical infections exist, surgeons must make never-ending efforts to control them. It may be described as a time when science and art can absolutely*

prevent bacteria from gaining a foothold in the human body and can abruptly terminate their activity, if they have already become established (Frank L. Meleney, 1889–1963).

23 Diabetic Foot (D. Vega, K. West, J.M. Tellado)

- Definition: syndrome involving pain, deformation, inflammation, infection, ulceration, and tissue loss of the foot in diabetic patients.
- Pathophysiology: neuropathy, ischemia, and infection are the principal pathogenic factors.
- Clinical features: neuropathic and ischemic ulcers and the infected diabetic foot.
- Diagnosis: should identify and grade neuropathology, osteopathy, and vascular pathology.
- Treatment: should relieve weight from the ulcerated area, eradicate infection – surgically and with antibiotics – and restore arterial perfusion.
- *Do not mistake the line of discoloration in gangrene for the line of demarcation. The former spreads, the later rarely moves* (Augustus Charles Bernays, 1854-1907).
- *A fresh wound of failed a bypass graft procedure is not a prerequisite to amputation* (M.S.).

24 Hand Infections (R. Saadia)

- Determine nature and extent of infection.
- Institute appropriate antimicrobial treatment.
- Perform surgical debridement and drainage, if necessary.
- Institute early measures to preserve hand function.

25 Head and Neck Infections (M.F. Jimenez, J. Escallon)

- Head and neck infections are generally controlled without the need for surgical drainage. Progression to abscess indicates the need of intervention to achieve source control.
- The clinician must identify infection and define the topographic diagnosis of the disease and the need for prompt and aggressive treatment.
- The presence of a purulent collection or cellulitis in a fascial space of the head and neck indicates the need for drainage for source control of the infectious process.

26 Vascular Graft Infections (M.S. Dahn)

- CT scanning is currently the most useful test.
- Infections due to methicillin-resistant *Staphylococcus aureus* (MRSA) and *Pseudomonas aeruginosa* are more virulent. Total graft removal is more

frequently required for infections involving these organisms. Infections due to
S. epidermidis are more localized and can frequently be managed with partial
graft removal followed by extra-anatomic or in situ reconstruction.

- Repeated radical debridement of the tissues surrounding an infected graft as
  well as debridement of all infected arterial tissue is pivotal for the control of a
  graft infection.
- Graft preservation is becoming increasingly popular to avoid extensive extirpative procedures in association with complex extra-anatomic reconstructions in frail patients.
- Arterial stents represent an infrequent but potentially catastrophic source of
  sepsis.
- *Do not place your trust in the graft but also search carefully the host factors into
  which it is implanted. They may be decisive* (Henry Haimovici).

27 Bone and Joints (R.Jan, A. Goris)

- Remove all dead tissue and scar tissue.
- Provide optimal soft tissue conditions around the infected area.
- Stabilize infected fractures, mobilize infected joints.
- Antibiotics are only complementary treatment and do not replace sound sur-
  gical practice.
- *Doubt as to the condition of the wound should incline one to pessimism rather
  than to mistaken optimism* (William Heneage Ogilvie, 1887-1971).

28 Incisional Surgical Site Infections (J.T. Lee)

- Incisional infections develop because host defenses cannot eradicate contaminating pathogens. Intraoperative contamination of normally sterile tissues
  by pathogenic microbes is the most frequent antecedent of incisional infections.
- Detection of incisional infections relies on the fact that infection is one cause
  of wound healing failure. Infection must be ruled out when routine postoperative incision examination suggests that healing is not proceeding as expected.
- Therapy of incisional infections is based on a simple anatomical classification.
  Source control always includes an element of mechanically altering geometry
  and content of infected spaces.
- *Keep them as neat and clean as possible, and disturb them as little as you can;
  so far as may be practicable, exclude the air; favor healing under the scab;
  and ... feed him as you would a women recovering from her confinement* (Felix
  Wurtz, 1518-1574).
- *The likelihood of wound infections has been determined by the time the last
  stitch is inserted in the wound* (Mark. M. Ravitch, 1910-1989).

29 Timing of Intervention (U. Schöffel)

- As a general principle, every established source of infection should be controlled as soon as possible.
- The urgency of intervention is determined by the rapidity of the evolution of clinical symptoms.
- In complicated infections, any additional insult must be kept to a minimum. Thus, rapid, minimally invasive, temporizing or palliative measures may be superior to definitive but lengthy and more traumatizing procedures.
- If the clinical signs of infection improve, the need for intervention must be reconsidered. There will be ample time for a thorough diagnostic work-up and careful planning of the therapeutic strategy.
- The time course of an infection can never be reliably predicted in the clinical setting.
- *Never operate on a patient who is getting rapidly better or rapidly worse* (Francis D. Moore, 1913-2001).

30 Complications of Source Control (M.A. Malangoni)

- Complications of source control often result from technical errors or local factors that impair healing.
- Diagnosis and drainage of local infection and correction of fluid and electrolyte disorders are important for successful treatment.
- Control of fistulous drainage and provision of appropriate nutritional support are important secondary goals of management.
- *Somebody's leak is a curiosity – one's own leak is a calamity.*
- *Attempts to close-suture postoperative intestinal leaks is an exercise in futility which promotes death* (M.S.).

31 Reoperation After Source Control for Intra-abdominal Infection (O.D. Rotstein)

- Timing: in general, reoperation should be delayed for several months following resolution of all complications arising from the source control operation.
- Definition of the anatomy: in all reoperative cases, it is critically important for the operating surgeon to fully understand the nature of the prior surgeries.
- Entering the peritoneal cavity: it is preferable to enter the peritoneal cavity through a "virgin area" of the abdominal wall.
- Reoperative surgery requires comprehensive preoperative preparation of the patient plus skill and patience in the operating room.
- *As can be said for many issues in life, "timing is everything" in operative management of these patients* (T. Fabian).
- *God, indeed, rewards those who enter the operating room with a prepared mind* (T. Fabian).

- *At times it seems as though there is a brain in the suction tip that allows it to find the perfectly appropriate adhesion plane between bowel wall and parietal peritoneum* (T. Fabian).
- *Lysis of all small-bowel adhesions is not required because I believe that the bowel is "locked in the open position" by these chronic adhesions* (T. Fabian).
- *If a granulating abdominal wound is allowed to chronically granulate… this substantially increases the rate of enterocutaneous fistula development* (T. Fabian).

32 Trauma (L.S. Kao, A.B. Nathens)

- An early assessment of the extent of anatomic injury, the degree of physiologic derangement, and the ability of the patient to tolerate a prolonged operative procedure are critical in the decision-making process.
- Primary restoration of gastrointestinal continuity may be safely achieved for most injuries.
- Early source control is of secondary importance to hemorrhage control.
- *We must realize that there is no magic potion for source control following trauma. Antibiotics, drains, massive irrigation, and colostomy all play limited and secondary roles* (E. Frykberg).
- On fistula from an injured abdominal viscus: *This new symptom, although in general very disagreeable, will not be dangerous, for all the danger is over before it can appear'* (John Hunter, 1728-1793).
- *Shock from severe wounds and hemorrhage always must take precedence of everything else* (William W. Keen, 1837-1932).
- *Simple closure of a wound of the colon, however small, is not warranted* (William Heneage Ogilvie, 1887-1971).

33 The Burn Wound (A.L. Dunican, W.G. Cioffi)

- Important risk factors for the development of burn wound infection include patient age, comorbidities, and extent of the burn.
- Burn wound sepsis is prevented through use of topical antimicrobials, early excision of the burn eschar, and barrier isolation precautions.
- Differentiation between wound colonization and invasive infection can be made by biopsy of the burn wound.
- Treatment of burn wound infection entails use of subeschar clysis and excision of the burn wound.
- *Infection remains the most common cause of death in extensively burned patients even though invasive burn wound sepsis has been "controlled" by current techniques of burn wound care* (B.A. Pruitt, Jr).

34 Organ Transplant Patients (T. Pruett)

- Transplant recipients frequently have surgical infections, requiring prompt control of the graft-host interface. The decision to invoke an operative or interventional radiological or endoscopic approach is dependent upon patient factors. Control of the source of the infection is key to successful resolution.

- Superinfection or concomitant systemic viral or fungal infection is common.
- The patient's underlying comorbid diseases and nutrition are significant determinants of the successful management of surgical infection.
- Removal of the allograft and the cessation of immunosuppressive agents is rarely required, but an option which needs to be contemplated.
- *The human body is the only machine for which there are no spare parts* (Hermann M. Biggs).

35 Tertiary Peritonitis (R.G. Sawyer)

- The term "tertiary peritonitis" has been applied to describe recurrent infection of the peritoneal cavity after a prior episode of secondary peritonitis.
- As tertiary peritonitis progresses, the opportunity for aggressive open surgical intervention decreases, and minimally invasive procedures are favored.
- The organisms associated with tertiary peritonitis are nosocomial in origin, often difficult to treat, but sometimes of unclear pathological relevance.
- Tertiary peritonitis is rarely cured rapidly and frequently requires long rehabilitation and secondary procedures weeks to months after initial presentation.
- *I have frequently thought that apart from Tertiary Peritonitis, there was not very much more we needed to study about the management of intraperitoneal infection* (J.L. Meakins).
- *Correct application of initial therapy, proper application of algorithms such as that presented and optimal clinical care will make Tertiary Peritonitis a rare entity* (J.L. Meakins).

36 The Role of Laparoscopy (P. Gorecki)

- Laparoscopic evaluation of peritoneal cavity enables magnified visualization of peritoneum and intra-abdominal organs with less tissue trauma as compared to laparotomy.
- Laparoscopy detects the presence of pus, feces, bile or blood – facilitating the detection of the source of intra-abdominal pathology and estimates its severity.
- Whether the therapeutic procedure is laparoscopic or conventional depends on the findings, the patient's condition, and the complexity of the planned procedure.
- *Source control is most necessary for patients with the most severe assault on their peritoneal defense mechanisms and systemic sepsis. These however are the patients least likely to do well with a laparoscopic approach* (Z.H. Krukowski).
- *Attempting translaparoscopic management of complicated postoperative peritonitis is like making love to a fully dressed harem woman* (M.S.).

37 Pediatric Surgery (G. Pitcher)

- The systemic response to sepsis in early life is different.
- The main challenge in abdominal source control is necrotizing enterocolitis
- The peritoneal cavity of newborns can be effectively drained.
- Nonresective management of pan-necrotizing enterocolitis is a viable option.
- *The management of a child with a surgical infection does not differ from that in an adult. What makes the philosophy of source control in pediatric surgery considerably different is the approach to the newborn and specially to the premature one* (W.J. Górecki).

38 The AIDS Patient (S. Sajja, V. Parithivel)

- Abdominal complaints are extremely common in the HIV population and clinical evaluation is often difficult. Serial clinical evaluation and frequent use of CT scan are essential to prevent nontherapeutic interventions
- Early diagnosis and prompt intervention are essential for non-HIV-related surgical pathology such as acute appendicitis and cholecystitis. Surgical intervention is also essential for complications of opportunistic infections such as cytomegalovirus(CMV) perforation. The morbidity and mortality for surgical procedures depends on the stage of the HIV disease and the nature of pathology.
- Surgical interventions should not be denied to this population because of the risk of occupational transmission and the fear of high complication rates. Relief of symptoms and improvement in quality of life are the chief considerations.

39 Clinical and Radiographic Assessment (M.P. Fink)

- Unfortunately, there is no single test that can provide the clinician with a clear answer to the question: has adequate source control been achieved?
- If ongoing intra-abdominal infection is suspected on clinical grounds, then an imaging procedure (usually computed tomography) should be performed prior to undertaking operative intervention.
- *In today's world, likely the best tool for diagnosis in intra-abdominal sepsis is the 3rd-generation CT scanner. Not only can the scanner detect "leaks", it can also demonstrate rather subtle amounts of edema resulting from inflammation or infection* (R.A. Mustard Jr.).

40 Monitoring the Course of Inflammation (A. Bauhofer, W. Lorenz)

- Complications resulting from inadequate source control result in a systemic inflammatory response; this response can be detected through changes in circulating levels of a variety of inflammatory mediators, including cytokines such as procalcitonin (PCT) and interleukin-6 (IL-6).

- Systemic inflammation is also manifested in changes in cellular expression of surface molecules such as HLA-DR and the receptor for TNF, and in the ability to generate cytokines in free response to microbial stimulation.
- Immunological monitoring of the high-risk patient holds the promise of earlier detection of correctable complications and so may lead to improved clinical outcomes.

41 Empiric Reexploration – Is There a Role? (P.A. Lipsett)

- The *need* for relaparotomy significantly worsens outcome.
- Planned reexploration of all surgical patients with signs and symptoms of infection will result in a small number of lives saved but at the cost of significant harm to others. Clear indications for planned relaparotomy do not exist.
- Reexploration based on localized radiological or physical findings may be beneficial; directed percutaneous therapy may also be beneficial.
- Undirected relaparotomy for MODS alone without supporting clinical or radiological data results in a 50 % - 90 % rate of negative explorations, without clear evidence of benefit. Supportive clinical data include prolonged ileus and pain, wound infection, and positive peritoneal signs. A computed tomographic scan is the most important radiological tool in the decision-making process for relaparotomy.
- *The last man to see the necessity for reoperation is the man who performed the operation* (Mark M. Ravitch, 1910-1989).
- *Early reoperation is a double-edged sword; we still have to learn how to use only the edge facing the enemy – the uncontrolled source* (M.S.).

42 Planned Relaparotomies and Laparostomy (M. Schein, R. Paladugu)

- A planned relaparotomy may be life-saving when the source cannot be adequately controlled during the first-index operation.
- The first week after the index operation – before the infective process has become localized and detectable by CT – offers a window of opportunity for planned relaparotomies.
- When the source is controlled and infection localized, a "direct" on-demand approach is safer.
- Laparostomy is indicated and beneficial when the abdomen cannot be closed or cannot be closed without creating significant intra-abdominal hypertension.
- Excessive or unnecessary relaparotomies may be harmful.
- *A negative relaparotomy is better than a positive autopsy but is not, nevertheless, a benign procedure* (Roger Saadia).

43 Antibiotics as an Adjunct to Source Control: Revised Surgical Infection Society Guidelines for Antimicrobial Therapy of Intra-abdominal Infections
(J.E. Mazuski, R. Sawyer, A. Nathens, J. DiPiro, M. Schein, K.A. Kudsk, C. Yowler)

- Antimicrobial therapy is an adjunct to primary source control procedures in treating patients with intra-abdominal infections.
- Therapeutic antimicrobials (< 24 h) are required only for patients with established intra-abdominal infections. Patients with limited exposure to contamination from a perforated viscus and those who have a removable focus of inflammation should be treated with prophylactic antimicrobials only (> 24 h).
- Therapeutic antimicrobials for intra-abdominal infections should generally be limited to no more than 5-7 days. Ongoing clinical evidence of infection should prompt a search for a new or recurrent infection rather than arbitrary prolongation of antimicrobial therapy with new or different agents.
- Antimicrobial regimens for intra-abdominal infections should cover common aerobic and anaerobic enteric flora. A number of different regimens are available, but the choice of antimicrobials for most patients with community-acquired infections should be dictated primarily by considerations of cost, convenience, and potential toxicity.
- Patients at high risk for therapeutic failure include those with preexisting physiological compromise and those with difficult-to-treat organisms, which many times have been acquired nosocomially. Antimicrobial therapy may need to be intensified in some of these patients to cover resistant Gram-negative aerobic organisms, enterococci, and yeast.
- *Our arsenals for fighting off bacteria are so powerful...that we're in more danger from them than from the invaders* (Lewis Thomas).
- *The most novel antibiotics and the best supportive care are meaningless – if principles of source control are not adhered to with obsessiveness* (M.S.).
- *Antibiotics for the fool is a tool which appears cool. But somebody pays the price as a rule* (M.S.).
- *Sepsis is not an antibiotic deficiency syndrome* (J.M.).

Dear colleague, the book was long but the final message to take home is short and simple: be prompt, bold, and radical but know when not to be bold and radical and remember that what you could not finish today, you can and have to do tomorrow. We hope that at least part of the book was enjoyable and of some use to you. Please send us any comment or criticism – we will reply.

Moshe Schein, New York
(mschein1@mindspring.com)

John C. Marshall, Toronto
(john.marshall@uhn.on.ca)

Subject Index